# William Richard Gowers
# 1845–1915

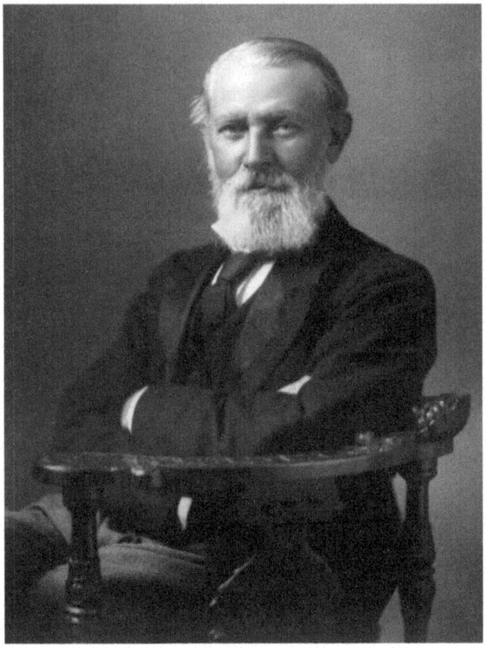

William Richard Gowers. (Queen Square Library, Archive and Museum.)

# William Richard Gowers 1845–1915

## Exploring the Victorian Brain: a biography

by

Ann Scott

Mervyn Eadie

Andrew Lees

OXFORD
UNIVERSITY PRESS

OXFORD
UNIVERSITY PRESS

Great Clarendon Street, Oxford, OX2 6DP,
United Kingdom

Oxford University Press is a department of the University of Oxford.
It furthers the University's objective of excellence in research, scholarship, and education by publishing worldwide. Oxford is a registered trade mark of Oxford University Press in the UK and in certain other countries



First Edition published in 2012



Published in the United States of America by Oxford University Press
198 Madison Avenue, New York, NY 10016, United States of America

British Library Cataloguing in Publication Data
Data available

Library of Congress Control Number: 2012944654

ISBN 978–0–19–969231–6

# Foreword

No name conjures up more vividly the period when clinical neurology 'came of age' than that of William Richard Gowers. Knighted by Queen Victoria in her diamond jubilee honours list of 1897, Gowers' name is inextricably linked to the early history of the National Hospital for Nervous Diseases, Queen Square, founded in 1860, where he worked as a member of the consultant staff from 1872 to 1910. Sir William Gowers was the quintessential clinical observer. He saw a great deal, remembered it in detail, and brought discipline and rigour to the basic methods of clinical neurology—history-taking, examination, localization, mechanistic interpretation, differential diagnosis, and, where possible, treatment. The documentary evidence lies in the thirty volumes of manuscript case-notes preserved at Queen Square relating to Gowers' clinical practice between 1878 and 1911. For many years, Gowers worked mainly in the outpatient department of the National Hospital, seeing referrals and demonstrating cases to students and trainees, but in 1892 he was granted leave to concentrate on inpatients and his private practice. The legend lives on: even now, the weekly postgraduate clinical conference at Queen Square, held for many years on Gowers Ward, is designated the 'Gowers teaching grand round'. Here, over the years, trainees have watched and listened but, in the Victorian tradition that Gowers represented, 'spoken only when spoken to' as generations of illustrious neurologists appointed to the consultant staff at Queen Square have delivered their weighty opinions.

*William Richard Gowers 1845–1915: Exploring the Victorian Brain* is doubly important. It brings to a wide readership the life and work of a great medical neurologist, offering additional insights into Victorian medicine more generally; and it makes available a rich store of archival material never previously published. The biographical appreciation of Sir William Gowers written by Macdonald Critchley in 1949 benefited from the contact Critchley had with neurologists who had known Gowers personally and observed his work at first hand, and from limited access to unpublished material. Now are considered all extant family papers rescued by Gowers' great-grandson in the 1960s, as well as the recent transcription by Ann Scott, the primary author and Gowers' great-granddaughter, of the 80,000-word diary written in shorthand that Gowers kept during his medical apprenticeship in the early 1860s—a skill that later allowed Gowers to moonlight as a medical reporter after he arrived in London in 1863—and material stored at Queen Square but not previously scrutinized.

We read of Gowers' embarrassment at fainting during his first surgical attendance in 1862 (aged 17 years); his valiant efforts to learn to smoke ('smoking is a blessing to a busy man and a curse to an idle one'), preferably with a few glasses of Mosel or gin-and-water; his adolescent eye for a pretty girl in church; distress over the suffering of a dog run over by a passing cart; relaxation through playing chess, reading Charlotte Bronte, and, later in life, playing billiards and table tennis with his children; the thrill of seeing his first publication in print; confusion over his widowed mother's male friendships; adventures as an amateur botanist; walking 23 miles during the course of his day as an apprentice to a doctor in general practice—which he was sorry to leave in 1863 although wondering whether his £150 apprentice fee had been value for money; mentorship from Sir William Jenner, to whom Gowers was introduced by the Reverend Philps before he became a student at University College London; and much else besides that shows the mentoring and intellectual development of the greatest English clinical neurologist of the nineteenth century.

Ann Scott, Mervyn Eadie, and Andrew Lees set out the early years of the National Hospital and the contributions of those with whom Gowers worked when he joined the hospital as its first medical registrar in 1870, his development as a clinician and researcher, and a more comprehensive analysis of his writings than has hitherto been available. Gowers had a lively and enquiring mind. He valued change, the opportunities afforded by technical advances, and the need to re-evaluate concepts and existing dogma: 'nothing pays except that which gives some new suggestion. The great thing is to create a feeling in the reader—I must not miss anything else this man [Gowers remained opposed to training women in medicine throughout his career] says'. Sir William Gowers' writings are the published versions of lectures, addresses, and clinical demonstrations, mostly delivered at the National Hospital or University College Hospital from 1879 to 1904; his two monographs on epilepsy (1881 and 1901) and the one on *Medical Ophthalmoscopy* (1879); and the three editions of *A Manual of Diseases of the Nervous System* (1886–8; 1892–3; and 1899 with Dr James Taylor, volume 1 only being published). What emerges is not only evidence for keen observation and vast clinical range but also the intellectual curiosity that led Gowers to the concept of abiotrophy as the basic mechanism of neurodegeneration and to appreciate the likely impact of genetics on the classification and understanding of neurological disease. He was ready and willing to interpret clinical problems in the context of the new neurology provided by the work of Camillo Golgi (1843–1926) and Santiago Ramon y Cajal (1853–1934) on the structure of the nervous system, and by Sir Charles Sherrington (1857–1952) on its function—studies that only came fully to fruition in the first decade of the twentieth century but with which Gowers, now nearing retirement, nonetheless kept abreast. We read of Gowers as austere and a 'gruff old bear', criticized by some of the more outspoken young men who gathered around him in the later years at Queen Square; but equally of the devoted family man with a few but strong personal friendships outside medicine, including with the somewhat younger Rudyard Kipling (1865–1936).

Although hagiography and the use of eponyms celebrating the work of individuals were not his style, readers will be indebted to Ann Scott, Mervyn Eadie, and Andrew Lees for making available such a rich store of material supporting the legend that makes the name of Sir William Gowers synonymous with the golden age of British clinical neurology.

Alastair Compston, Cambridge

# Preface

In 1949 Macdonald Critchley wrote *Sir William Gowers 1845–1915: a biographical appreciation.*[1] The immediate question, therefore, is why did we decide to embark on a second biography? There are two main answers to this. The first is that we felt it would be interesting to provide a twenty-first-century reassessment of the contributions Gowers made to the study of neurology. The second, driven by curiosity, was to take a closer look at those features of his life that were not devoted to neurology, drawing on resources that were unavailable to Critchley in 1949. Sir Arthur Hurst suggested to Critchley that a biography of Gowers should be written to do justice to his achievements when those of Hughlings Jackson were lauded so highly. Critchley asked Risien Russell, a colleague who had known Gowers, to undertake the biography. Russell said he would consult another colleague, James Taylor, who had known Gowers well. They told Critchley they felt that Gowers' *Manual* was a sufficient memorial. Fortunately, Critchley ignored this advice.

When the *British Medical Journal* noted in 1945 that 100 years had passed since Gowers' birth, readers were reminded that during his lifetime Gowers had earned an international reputation, that his name was still a household word among neurologists everywhere, and that 'historical justice therefore requires that we should now recall him as one of the founders of modern British medicine'.[2]

Critchley described Gowers' contribution to neurology in similarly glowing terms, claiming that 'to the study of nervous disorders, Gowers has probably contributed more than any other', and that he was probably 'the greatest clinical neurologist of all time'[3]:

> Neurology is inextricably bound up with his influence and the fruits of his endeavours, however lax we may be today in acknowledging our indebtedness to our elders. … Fourteen or fifteen years ago, the late Sir Arthur Hurst was deploring that no one had ever ventured a biography of Gowers. His brilliant achievements, he believed, had never quite received their full measure of recognition.[4]

Apart from Gowers' own writings, Critchley found that the details about his life were 'scant'. Even some of the sources that had existed in the 1930s had been lost by the time he wrote. In 1987, Henson commented on the somewhat negative portrait Critchley painted of Gowers' personality, and suggested that the full story of Gowers had not yet been told.[5]

What, therefore, can a new biography offer? The electronic research tools now available have opened up access to a far broader range of sources than were available to Critchley in 1949. Ann Scott's 'filial piety' towards her great-grandfather provided the impetus for re-examining some of the family sources available to Critchley, and she found that the Gowers family only provided him with excerpts taken from the limited transcriptions that had been made of the shorthand diary Gowers maintained as a medical apprentice. Either a complete transcription of its 80,000 words had never been made before or, if one had existed, it had disappeared. The family also held letters and memorabilia which had not been closely examined by Critchley because they were not relevant to the medical focus of his book. In addition, the archives at the National Hospital, Queen Square, were being catalogued at the same time as we were writing our book. We have drawn extensively on these archives, although the significance of two sets of Gowers' papers emerged late in the production process, so are dealt with in more detail elsewhere.[6]

The online archives and databases now available have allowed us to follow the kind of detective trail Gowers himself would have loved, allowing us to build up a more complete picture of his background and his life. It has been possible to compare the results of these searches with the family papers that survive, to obtain a broader view of Gowers, and to fill a number of the significant gaps in the story of his life. However, some gaps cannot be filled. In his prime, Gowers was one of the busiest consultants in London, but there are no records of the day-to-day management of the practice that he ran from his home in Queen Anne Street, nor of how he divided his time between the consultancy, his work at the National Hospital Queen Square, and his teaching commitments at University College Hospital. Gowers always sought evidence, and we have based our biography on the evidence available.

Not only have sixty years passed since Critchley wrote his assessment, but it is nearly 100 years since Gowers died. It is now possible to take a longer view of Gowers' contribution to neurological science.

The greatest challenge in writing the book was deciding on its structure. The first few chapters take the story of Gowers' life to 1870, the year he was first appointed to Queen Square. The bulk of these chapters is autobiographical, taken from the diaries Gowers kept when he was a medical apprentice, and occasionally when he was a medical student. But the diaries cease in the years between 1870 and 1890 which were, as he himself wrote, years in which he had time for little but his work. These were the 20 years in which he was most productive, and made his name as a neurologist. The middle chapters of the book focus on his approach to neurological inquiry: his clinical method, his research method, his findings, and the dissemination of his findings through publications and teaching. Here we have attempted to discern the developments in his understanding of disorders such as epilepsy, from the first of his publications on the topic to the last, spanning the 40 years of his working life from 1870 to 1910. These central sections of the book become more technical, although we have tried to make them interesting to the non-specialist reader. It is not until 1890, after his career had reached its peak, that the book returns to chronological biography, aided by the diary he kept for his children and by the letters that have survived. This chronology continues through to 1915, the year Gowers died. The book then finishes with an overview of the assessments made, both by his contemporaries and his successors, of Gowers as a colleague and a neurologist, and examines his place in the history of neurological science. Gowers searched for answers by gathering his own evidence. We have tried to follow his lead and, wherever possible, have used direct quotations from primary sources rather than indulge in paraphrase or speculation. Mervyn Eadie and Andrew Lees gave editorial control over the book to Ann Scott, so she has been responsible for these structural decisions.

# Acknowledgements

Without the foresight of Dr William Patrick Gowers, Ann Scott's brother, this book would never have been written. When William Richard Gowers' son Ernest died in 1966, Patrick rescued his library, papers, and other family memorabilia. This collection included many of the primary sources we have used, including Gowers' shorthand diary from 1862–3 which provided the raw material for two chapters; Gowers' 'children's diary' from the 1880s; miscellaneous correspondence; family documents; and Gowers' personal sketchbooks.

Emeritus Professor Roger Scott provided advice on imperial history, and made constructive criticisms as the book took shape. In addition, he never faltered in his support for the project, or in encouraging his wife to follow archival trails, however unlikely to bear fruit. Fortunately these were rewarded by some rich returns, not least a visit to Sydney made on the basis of a hunch, and a tentative hope that something of value might be found in the Morrison Collection housed in the Mitchell Library. Family archives often contain letters received, but it is rare to find the other side of an exchange of correspondence. Roger Scott was a patient, tolerant companion throughout the project.

Louise Shepherd, librarian at Queen Square, first became involved when Ann Scott was researching this book's 'prequel', her biography of Ernest Gowers, who had been chairman of the board at Queen Square for a number of years after World War II. The Scotts spent a memorable day with Louise exploring cupboards outside wards that contained a great miscellany of records and objects randomly stored after earlier library restructuring. In those cupboards we discovered an album containing the best of William Richard Gowers' holiday sketches. From then on, other Queen Square treasures gradually emerged, including many original drawings that Gowers made for his *Manual of Diseases of the Nervous System*, the manuscripts of two unpublished lectures, and Gowers' own hand corrections for the unpublished third edition of the second volume of his *Manual*, which had been referred to by Macdonald Critchley in 1949, but were thought to have been lost. Louise Shepherd located and arranged for the cataloguing and digitizing of these Queen Square papers. We are indebted to Louise for her help and support, as well as for that of archivist Martin Woodward, and all the Queen Square Library staff.

In 1862 and 1863 Gowers was a medical apprentice in the village of Coggeshall, in Essex. Shirley Ratcliffe, volunteer curator of the Coggeshall Museum and Heritage Centre, guided us to many of the illustrations used in the early sections of the book, and read drafts of the chapters on Coggeshall. We discovered the museum through the chance online discovery of George Beaumont's 1890 *History of Coggeshall*, republished by local historians Stanley Haines and Sidney MacKay in 2007. It was the 'index of places' and 'index of personal names' that proved crucial when Ann Scott transcribed Gowers' shorthand diaries.

Dr Kenneth Tyler, of the Department of Neurology, University of Colorado, has had a long-term project to transcribe the articles Gowers wrote in the shorthand journal the *Phonographic Record of Clinical Teaching and Medical Science*. He most generously provided transcripts of a number of articles he had already had transcribed. These included articles about the establishment of the Society of Medical Phonographers written by Gowers himself.

Dr Christopher Boes, of the Mayo Clinic in Minnesota, approached the Gowers family to see if there were any letters from William Osler in the Gowers archives. After learning that there were none, he most generously helped us to follow archival trails in the United States and Canada, as well as giving us access to a letter from Gowers from his own collection. He also kindly read an early draft of the book.

A number of other people have read and commented on drafts of the book. These include Professor Alastair Compston, Department of Clinical Neurosciences, University of Cambridge, and editor of *Brain*; Emeritus Professor Bob Milns, University of Queensland; Emeritus Professor Michael Swash, consultant neurologist and professor of neuropathology, the Royal London Hospital; and Mr John Topley, formerly registrar, Griffith University, Queensland.

We are especially grateful to Patrick and Caroline Gowers for allowing the nomadic Scotts to treat their home as a London pied-à-terre. Professor Sir William Timothy Gowers FRS, Department of Mathematics and Mathematical Statistics, Cambridge; writer Rebecca Gowers; and violinist Katherine Gowers made the project considerably more enjoyable by joining the Scotts in exploring Gowers' early haunts in Coggeshall, Oxford, and London.

The University of Queensland provided tangible support for the project, both through the School of History, Philosophy, Religion and Classics, and through providing access to the university's library with its extensive holdings and subscriptions to online databases.

Finally, our thanks go to the Delegates of the Press, Oxford University Press, for their act of faith in offering us a contract to write the book, and to all the people involved in its production, including Peter Stevenson, commissioning editor, Eloise Moir-Ford, senior assistant commissioning editor; Elizabeth Chadwick, assistant production manager Bridget Johnson, copy-editor; and Veena Deepak, project manager for Cenveo, Bangalore, for their support and advice throughout the project.

Libraries and archives that have provided many of the primary sources include:

Archive and Museum, UCL Institute of Neurology and the National Hospital for Neurology and Neurosurgery incorporating the Queen Square Library (formerly the Rockefeller Medical Library);

Coggeshall Museum and Heritage Centre, Coggeshall, Essex;

Library and Archives, Athenaeum Club, London;

Library and Archives, Royal Society, London;

Mitchell Library, Sydney, G. E. Morrison collection;

Online archives of the *British Medical Journal*; *The Lancet*; *The Times* (London), and the *Oxford Dictionary of National Biography*;

Osler Library of the History of Medicine, Montreal;

Special Collections, University College London Library;
Special Collections, University of Sussex Library;
The British Library, London;
The Heritage Centre, Royal College of Physicians, London;
University of Queensland Library, Brisbane.

# Contents

# List of illustrations

Chapter 1

# Family and schooling in Victorian England

## Gowers as a Victorian

William Richard Gowers was born in 1845, eight years after Queen Victoria came to the throne. His achievements as a neurologist were formally recognized by the Queen when he received a knighthood in the Diamond Jubilee honours in 1897. Gowers' career reflects many of the characteristics of the Victorian era identified by Asa Briggs:

> The key words of the times were 'thought', 'work' and 'progress'. Clear thinking was preferred to impulse or prejudice and the battle of ideas to the dictatorship of slogans; hard work was considered the foundation of all material advancement; and both clear thinking and hard work were deemed essential to continued national progress.[1]

Fundamental changes were taking place in science, medicine, religion, and political life throughout the nineteenth century. The impact that these interrelated changes had on Gowers' life and attitudes is sometimes clear from the evidence of primary sources. In other cases his views on contemporary events can only be inferred. The shorthand diaries he kept as a medical apprentice provide the starting point, and portray a devout Christian from a Congregationalist family, who was a hard-working but lonely young man. We lose the close insights into his beliefs when he becomes a medical student and is too busy to maintain a regular diary. As an adult, he only kept occasional diaries for his children, or once during a short convalescence. His biography therefore has to rely in part on other people's memories and draw inferences from the friendships he made and the colleagues he most admired during his later life.

The Congregational Church played a significant role in his life, not only because of the strength of his own faith, but for the support and guidance its ministers and mentors gave him. This support was evident from the moment when an aunt suggested to a Congregationalist doctor that he might accept the fatherless 16-year-old, who had shown no leaning towards a particular career, as his apprentice. It remains an intriguing mystery how Gowers' father, who grew up in Essex and established a business in Hackney, met his mother, who grew up in Yorkshire. However, it seems likely that the Congregational network played some part in it, because Yorkshire, Essex, and Hackney were all strong centres of Nonconformism in the early nineteenth century, and it is highly likely that Ann Venables visited Hackney connections and either met Gowers senior in Congregational Church circles or went to his shop to buy boots. The first railways opened in 1830, and 'railway mania' was firmly taking hold by 1837. One result was that railway travel from Yorkshire to London became possible. Hackney (Bishopsgate) station opened in 1840, and in 1846, the year after Gowers was born, the Great Northern Railway connected King's Cross in London with his mother's home town, Doncaster, 156 miles away, making a previously circuitous railway journey more direct.

Because of their exclusion from so many occupations, the Congregationalists were imbued with a strong bond of mutual support and self-help. In common with other Nonconformist 'Dissenters', such as the Quakers and Presbyterians, under the statutes jointly referred to as the 'Clarendon Code' at the turn of the century they were still prevented from participating in many areas of public life. The Acts that made up the Clarendon Code were passed in the 1660s to re-establish the supremacy of the Anglican Church after the years of religious strife that had engulfed England. The 1661 *Corporation Act* excluded Nonconformists from public office; the 1662 *Act of Uniformity* forced clergy who would not use the *Book of Common Prayer* in their services to resign their livings (leading to the 'Great Ejection' of nearly 2000 clergy). These Acts were followed by the 1664 *Coventicle Act*, forbidding a meeting of more than five people who were not members of the same household from worshipping together, which prevented Dissenting religious groups from meeting; and the 1665 *Five-Mile Act* which made it illegal for Nonconformist ministers to come within five miles of their former livings.

Nonconformists were not admitted into the teaching profession until 1779. Teachers and pupils at grammar schools were required to be Anglican. In the early nineteenth century Nonconformists were still excluded from the universities and the public schools. For a century and a half, strict religious tests excluded Dissenters (and Catholics) from holding public office and from being awarded university degrees. Under the *Test Act* of 1673 anyone wishing to hold public office had to renounce the doctrine of transubstantiation and take the sacrament in an Anglican Church. This *Test Act*, eventually repealed in 1828–9, required pupils in grammar schools and Oxford, Cambridge, and Durham universities to subscribe to the Church's Thirty-Nine Articles of Religion. It was not until 1871 that the *Universities Tests* Act was finally abolished and these ancient universities could award degrees to Nonconformists, Roman Catholics, and non-Christians. Scottish and Dutch universities admitted Nonconformists. Edinburgh established a medical school with teachers who had often qualified in Holland. The University of London was a secular institution established in 1826 specifically to cater for the groups excluded from the other English universities under the *Universities Tests* Act.

Throughout the nineteenth century debate continued within the Church of England about the damage caused by the exclusion of Dissenters. Proponents of the Broad Church, such as Thomas Arnold, argued that the Established Church was being weakened by their exclusion. The 'Tractarians' such as Pusey and Newman, favoured moving the Church closer to Roman Catholicism. Gowers' choices were affected by these debates, but one can only infer his shifting position over time from some of the decisions he took, and from brief glimpses of his home life.

Despite these disadvantages, Gowers was a man who had the intellectual ability to take advantage of the increased social mobility that the Victorian age offered. Born the son of a boot-maker, he studied for his matriculation by correspondence and then worked his way into the rapidly expanding professional classes. Later, his concern that his own sons should take advantage of the new careers opening up at the time affected the choices Gowers made for them, most significantly in sending them to Rugby, the school that Arnold had made famous. He also encouraged them to join the Civil Service, which had been gradually reformed in the second half of the nineteenth century after the 1853 Northcote Trevelyan Report recommended replacing the existing patronage system with a 'proper system of examination'.[2] The former selection system based on patronage was largely replaced by merit selection through a competitive entry examination.

Gowers was a medical student in London not long after men like Charles Darwin and T. H. Huxley had become the centre of religious and scientific controversy. Evolution was not only a challenge to scientific thought but also to religious thought. Men like Leslie Stephen lost their faith because of the challenge it presented, but Gowers never lost his. Gowers worked with and profoundly admired Hughlings Jackson, a man who, although married in a Congregational chapel in Yorkshire, was a 'convinced agnostic' who did not believe in any afterlife. Hughlings Jackson and Herbert Spencer (known for his theories on social evolution) were close friends, and Hughlings Jackson applied Spencer's doctrine of evolution to the nervous system. The closest one gets to Gowers' views on evolution is a section on 'hysteria' in his *Manual* in which he suggests that 'barbarous races' did not suffer from hysteria, and speculates about relative development of the cerebellum of 'civilized' and 'uncivilized' races. However, there is no hint he believes that they might be 'undeserving'. Spencer, like Hughlings Jackson was an agnostic. Leslie Stephen and Spencer were both members of the Athenaeum, the club to which Gowers was elected in the 1890s. Gowers clearly enjoyed the discussions that took place there, but his unqualified admiration for Ruskin seems to align him with the scientists who believed that applying their intellects to scientific inquiry would help them become closer to God.

A parallel Victorian preoccupation was imperialism, and Gowers became caught up in the prevailing interest in foreign lands and races. This was consistent with his admiration for Ruskin, and the view of the Congregationalists at the time. This fascination he had with explorers and with colonial politics only emerges clearly in the later stages of his life, through his correspondence and friendship with Rudyard Kipling, Leander Starr Jameson, and George Ernest Morrison.

## The Gowers family

Gowers had lost not only his father but all three of his siblings before he turned 12. It was only by chance that he was offered, and persuaded to accept, an apprenticeship to a country doctor five years later.

Gowers' father was born in 1810 in Great Coggeshall, Essex. Coggeshall is about 50 miles from London, lying on the ancient road which leads from Colchester to Braintree. The river Blackwater runs through the small town. Gowers was a descendant of the Dutch family named 'Goverts', Protestants who came to England in the sixteenth century as refugees from Spanish persecution. Weavers, they settled in the area where they first landed, East Anglia, which already had a thriving weaving industry.

However, Coggeshall's cloth trade started to decline in the eighteenth century, and was finally destroyed by the Napoleonic Wars, which cut it off from its European markets. Its place was taken by agriculture and also the production of medicinal crops such as coriander, hyssop, poppy, and caraway. Brewing and the cultivation of hops were also significant. Coggeshall became famous for its silk and 'tambour' lace. The town's economy was also supported by Swinborne's tannery which became a thriving isinglass (gelatine) factory, a gasworks, and several maltings, one of which was owned by the Gardner family in Church Street. There were many artisans such as tailors, boot-makers, blacksmiths, and wheelwrights. There were also several mills on the river Blackwater supporting the weaving trade through 'silk throwing' and treating woven material, or producing corn.[3]

The Gowers family attended the local Congregational chapel. Coggeshall, in common with much of the rest of East Anglia, was strongly Nonconformist. By 1810 the largest group of Nonconformist Dissenters were the Congregationalists, who had 'held the leading position' for well over a century.[4] After the 1662 *Act of Uniformity* a number of different dissenting groups gradually emerged, including the Quakers and the Congregationalists, both of which were strongly represented in East Anglia. Congregationalists believed that a local congregation should be completely autonomous under God and therefore should not submit to any outside human authorities, whether regional or national. Each 'congregation' was independent, with its own minister and chapel.

From 1815, after the Napoleonic Wars ceased, even agriculture collapsed in Coggeshall. Local unemployment was exacerbated by men returning from the fighting, and many young men left Coggeshall for London and elsewhere seeking work. William Richard Gowers' paternal grandparents lived in Coggeshall: his grandfather, John Gowers, was a 'gentleman's butler' who appears to have died relatively young. His wife, William Richard's grandmother Letitia, lived in Coggeshall most of her life. However, one of her sons, Gowers' father, after learning to be a boot-maker, probably at Pocock's, Coggeshall's main boot-making business, moved to Hackney, then a village outside London, where he established himself at 91 Church Street as a ladies' boot-maker. His younger brother John followed him, setting up nearby as a 'cabman' (the Victorian equivalent of a modern delivery-man).

The boot-maker married Ann Venables, from Cantley in Yorkshire, on 11 August 1835 in Headington, near Oxford. Most of the Venables family still lived in Yorkshire, but Ann's brother, John Venables, had moved to Oxford from Doncaster and established himself as a gun-maker in St Aldates. William Richard Gowers was born on 20 March 1845, in a room over his father's shoe shop in Hackney. He was the couple's fourth child. However, two of his siblings, a girl and a boy, had died in their infancy before he was born (Emily, born in 1836, died at the age of 3; William Venables Gowers, born in 1839, died at 2 years old). His other sister (another Letitia) died of scarlet fever in February 1852 at the age of 14, when on a visit to her grandmother in Great Coggeshall. There was one other family member in the household. William and Ann Gowers had provided a home for Ann's niece, Charlotte Venables, an orphan from Doncaster, who was three years older than young William.

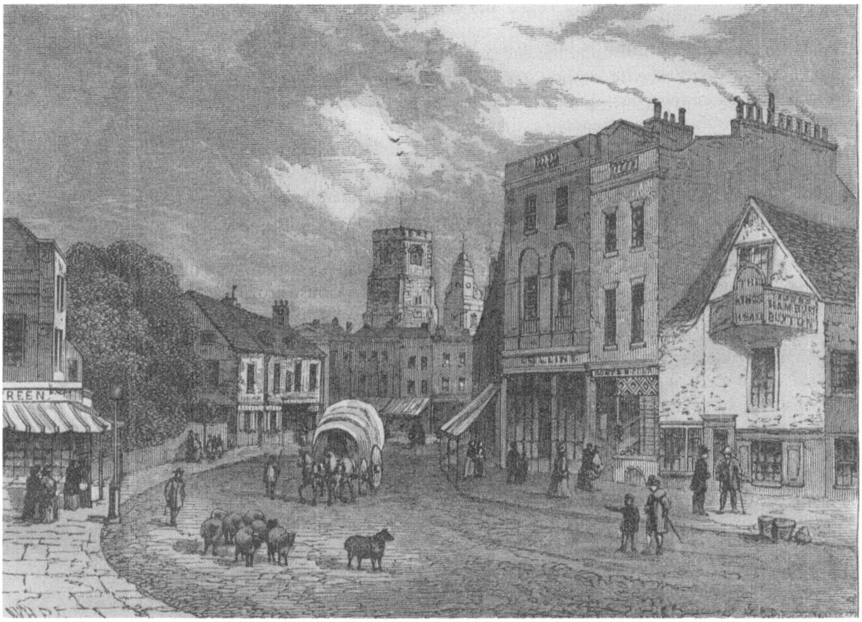

**Fig. 1.1** Church Street, Hackney, 1840.

The loss of all three of William's siblings was not an unusual statistic for the time. Waves of contagious disease were sweeping across Britain in the 1830s and 1840s. Between 1831 and 1833 there were two influenza epidemics, and cholera appeared for the first time; between 1836 and 1842 there were major epidemics of influenza, typhus, smallpox, and scarlet fever; between 1846 and 1849 there were waves of typhus, typhoid, and cholera. In 1840, scarlet fever was responsible for nearly 20,000 deaths.

Hackney, like Coggeshall, was home to a large number of Nonconformists. In 1802, the Hackney Academy had been established as a philanthropic non-denominational venture, particularly for the training of ministers. Bryan Dale, who became young William Richard Gowers' intellectual mentor in Coggeshall, trained there, as did the philanthropist Andrew Reed, into whose family Gowers eventually married.

The North London Railway opened its Hackney station in September 1850, located east of Church Street, and the street was renamed Mare Street after it was widened to make room for the railway. Many surrounding properties were demolished in the process. Perhaps for this reason, the boot-maker moved his family and business to Circus Road, St John's Wood, a rapidly developing area of London. A frequent visitor to the family was one of William's aunts from Great Coggeshall, Mary Gowers, who used to help her brother in the shop. She left the only description of William as a child, which was passed on through her daughter:

> Your father used to come into the shop as a little boy, and say Auntie Auntie let me. He wanted his Auntie to give him the yard measure with some slippers on each end, and he

would walk up and down the shop calling 'fat Rabbits, fat Rabbits' only he could not pronounce his words properly. His father would come in and see him sometimes, he would say 'that *naughty Auntie* I shall have to whip her for letting you do that'. 'No Daddy you must not whip my Auntie'.

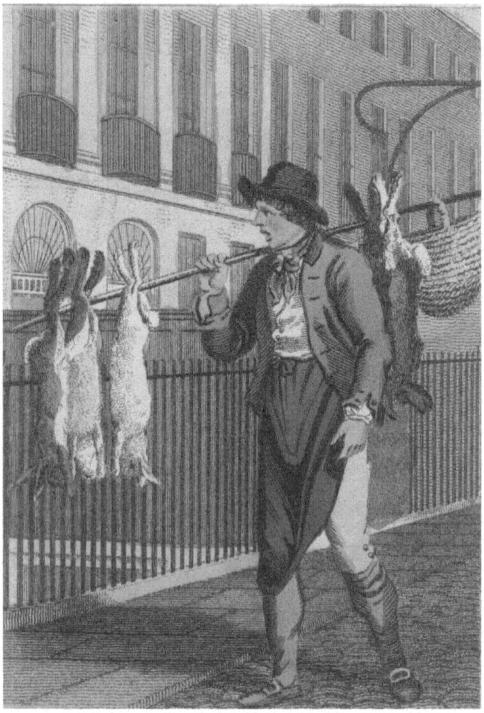

**Fig. 1.2** London street hawker selling rabbits, 1840.

There is no record of which London school, or schools, the boy attended. Tragedy struck the family yet again when the boot-maker's health failed and he died just before Christmas in 1856, aged 46. He bequeathed £10 to his mother Letitia, and stipulated that in the event of the death of his wife, £100 should be paid to his niece Charlotte Venables. The rest of his property, the house and 'all ways and means of trade', was left to his 'dear wife Ann Gowers'.

In later years his son, William Richard Gowers, was proud of his working-class ancestry, even though when an apprentice he was sensitive about his status in Coggeshall 'society'. His son Ernest recalled trying to interest him in George Meredith, then 'all the rage with young people who thought themselves clever':

> I remember the impatient disgust with which he threw aside *Evan Harrington*. 'Why on earth should the silly ass mind people knowing his father was a tailor?' he said, and that was the end of George Meredith for him.[5]

## Christ Church College School, Oxford

Ann Gowers sold the house and business in St John's Wood and took her son to stay with her brother's family in Oxford. Someone suggested that she try to get William accepted as a day scholar at Christ Church College School, just round the corner from the Venables' house in St Aldates. Her own father had left money in his will specifically for the education of his grandchildren. Ann could therefore afford the Oxford school's tuition fees.

She had lost her husband and her three other children and must have been desolate, uncertain about her own future, and wanting to do the best for her son. Her mother, Margaret Venables, was in her seventies and ailing, so Ann Gowers and her niece Charlotte returned to Doncaster to look after her, leaving William with her brother and his family in Oxford. The 11-year-old boy had a great deal to adjust to: without any of his immediate family, finding his feet in a new school, and in his out-of-school hours living at 99 St Aldates with six cousins, whose ages ranged from 7 to 27.

Unfortunately the Oxford school's records were destroyed in 1890, under the direction of over-zealous health authorities following an outbreak of ringworm. Critchley concluded that while a pupil there William 'gained an adequate acquaintance of French, German and Latin; a mastery of incisive English of peculiar beauty and clarity; and a most elegant penmanship'.[6] However, it is now clear from Gowers' diaries that some of these skills were acquired later, largely during his apprenticeship when he was studying by correspondence. He did not start to study German until 1863.

The school catered primarily for the cathedral's choristers, but it did also take day-boys who were not in the choir. William's son, Ernest, recalled that Gowers was not musical. Also, as a Congregationalist, Gowers may have felt uncomfortable in the ethos of the Established Church at Christ Church. He may well have found it difficult to fit in, either at school or in his uncle's family. William was clearly unhappy in Oxford. When an apprentice in 1862, he heard that his pet dog had died, prompting him to reminisce about the Oxford days in his diary:

> [The dog] was my sole companion during many a pleasant ramble about Oxford and Doncaster. Often we have raced together about the meadows near Iffley and along the side of the Isis, Bagley Wood, and old Hinksey. I have never had a brother or a near relation, or even a constant associate, and my little dog in a measure filled the place of one to me. I remember scores of places where we used to delight to roam together and where I used to be amused by watching him. How I and he used to jump the ditch by the side of the Abingdon Road at a little past Hinksey and he ran after the sheep and barked at them and after the horses, often escaping their hooves by almost a miracle. ... Everything in the old Oxford life looks pleasant now, but I know full well that it was not so when it was present.

## Choosing a career

William stayed in Oxford for three years, leaving school at the age of 15 to join his mother in Doncaster. Yorkshire was now his home. Most of his maternal relatives lived there, and it was where he had spent his recent school holidays. When her mother died in 1858, Ann and her niece Charlotte remained in Ann's house in St James Street.

However, although Ann was recorded in the 1861 census as an 'independent shareholder', she was far from well off.

After he left school, William had no idea what he might do for a living, and he was encouraged to try farming. It was a relative on his grandmother's side, local farmer Joseph Hurst, who offered William work on his farm to 'let him find out whether he would like to make farming his career'. Gowers spent less than a year working on Hurst's farm in Bentley. Ernest Gowers later recalled that his father spoke of his experience as an enjoyable one, but that he could imagine few occupations less suitable to his father as a career. Nonetheless, Joseph Hurst was a kindly man and Gowers grew to love him.

In October 1861 Ann Gowers took William to Coggeshall to visit her mother-in-law, Letitia Gowers, now in her seventies, who lived in West Street. Letitia's daughter Mary, who used to help in the Hackney shop, had by this time married Henry Foster, foreman of Swinborne's isinglass works further up the street. Letitia lived with them and their three young sons, doing the family laundry and helping with her grandchildren, moving into an adjoining cottage when the family expanded.

In 1926, a decade after Gowers had died, a younger cousin, Emily Foster, described what happened next in a letter to one of Gowers' daughters. It was Emily's mother, Mary Foster, who introduced Ann Gowers and her son William to the local doctor, Thomas Simpson. Dr Simpson asked Ann how her son was going to make his living. His aunt Mary Foster, 'as a joke', asked the doctor if he would take him on as a pupil. The boy, clearly unprepared for this exchange, said 'I would not like to be a doctor Auntie'.

Dr Simpson himself had been 'thrown entirely on his own resources' at an early age. He became a bank clerk but 'having set his heart on the medical profession, by dint of rigid economy and great perseverance he was enabled to go to college and afterwards enter as a student at Charing Cross Hospital'. After becoming an assistant-surgeon at nearby Halstead, he moved to Coggeshall to establish his practice. He was an office-bearing member of the Nonconformist chapel and was an 'ardent liberal in politics'.[7]

Simpson offered to take the boy on as an apprentice, and young William was persuaded to change his mind. Ann Gowers managed to raise the £150 premium, to be paid in instalments, covering his board and lodging as well as his tuition. On 15 October 1861, at the age of 16½, William Richard Gowers signed the indentures of a two-year medical apprenticeship.

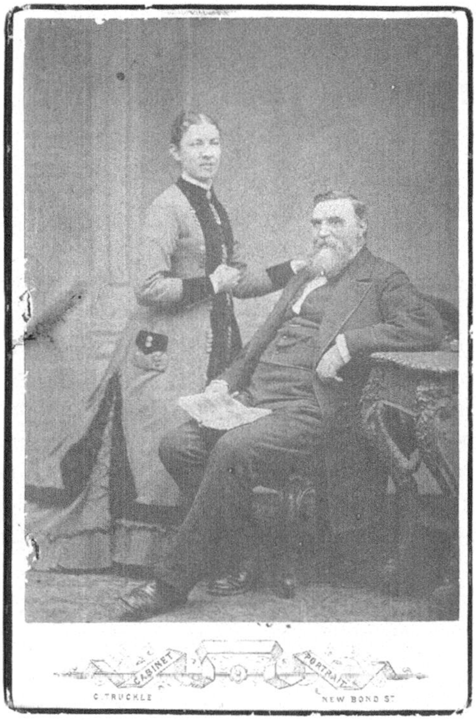


**Fig. 1.3** Dr Simpson with his second wife (*c.* 1880s). Sarah Ann Simpson, his first wife, died in April 1876 aged 49. Courtesy of Coggeshall Museum and Heritage Centre.

Chapter 2

# Apprentice years 1861–2

William began his apprenticeship in October 1861, three years after the belated enactment of the 1858 *Medical Act*. The new Act imposed some order on the previously chaotic structure of the medical profession. It established a General Council of Medical Education and Registration to control the training standards and licensing of members of the profession. Medical training had varied widely before 1858, ranging from university-based education to a 'broom-and-apron' apprenticeship in an apothecary's shop.[1] By the time William became an apprentice, the apprenticeship system was beginning to die out. He had set his sights on the University of London, so the first academic hurdle he faced was to qualify for a place by passing its matriculation examination.

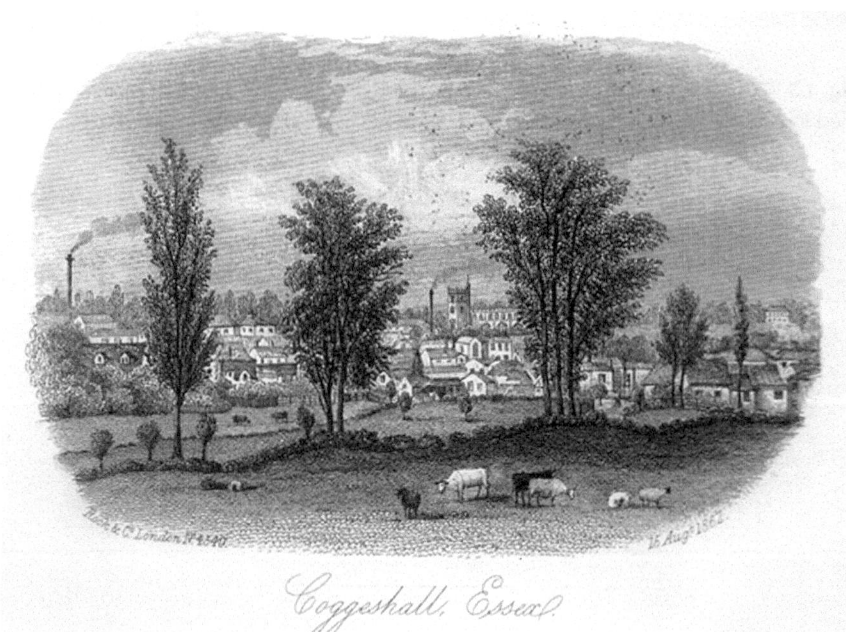


**Fig. 2.1** Coggeshall, 1862. (From Dale, B., *The Annals of Coggeshall, Otherwise Sunnedon, in the County of Essex* (London: A G Coventry, 1863). Courtesy of Coggeshall Museum and Heritage Centre.

Gowers became an 'inside' (resident) apprentice to Dr Simpson at 70 Church Street (later named Derwent House), the house that served both as the doctor's home and surgery, combining his duties as an apprentice with his academic studies.

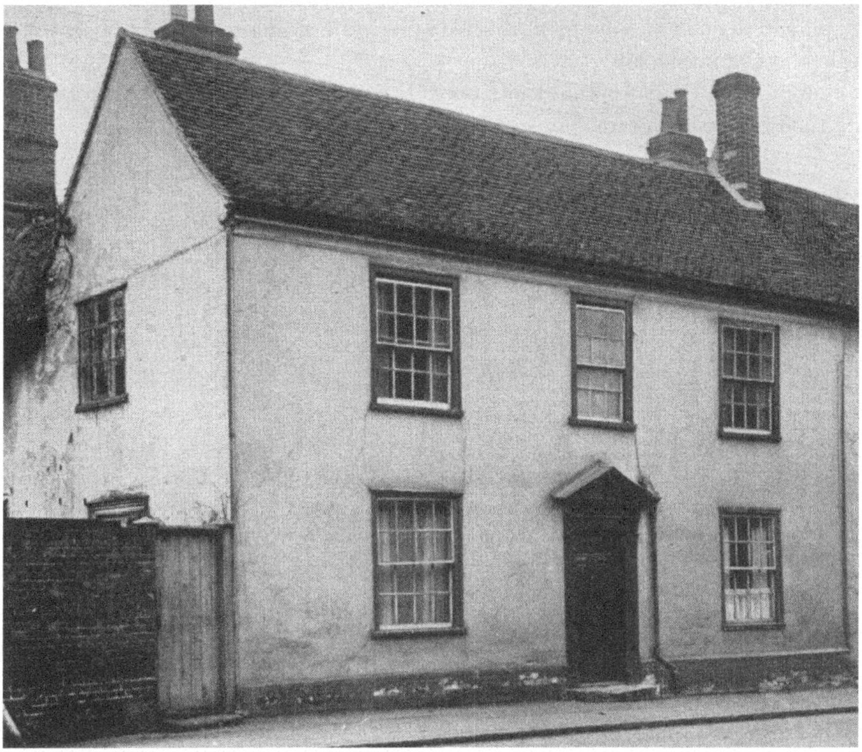

**Fig. 2.2** Dr Simpson's house, Church Street, Coggeshall (*c.* 1948). (From Critchley, 1949.)

## The shorthand diaries

There is no surviving record of the first months Gowers spent in Coggeshall. He started a diary, written in longhand, but this has since been lost. However, he decided to teach himself Pitman's shorthand, and soon began to practice his new skill by keeping a journal in shorthand. He also took down Sunday sermons in the Congregational chapel to increase his shorthand speed and 'became able to take down a sermon and think of the sermon or of something else all the time'.[2]

It was not unusual for educated men to write shorthand. In the seventeenth century Samuel Pepys wrote parts of his diary in Sheldon's shorthand. In the nineteenth century shorthand was used by journalists and court reporters. Charles Dickens taught himself Gurney's shorthand in 1830, at the age of 18, in order to become a court reporter. But Isaac Pitman's 'phonic system', first published in 1837, quickly eclipsed its predecessors. In December 1840, Pitman walked from Bath to London to promote his form of shorthand against its competitors. On one day alone, he trudged 40 miles through the snow from Stroud to Oxford, weighed down by shorthand primers. When he arrived in Oxford he left copies at most of the colleges.[3] In 1859 Gowers had 'acquired a slight knowledge of it, attracted by its intrinsic merits', probably just before he left his Oxford school.[4]

Gowers' diary bears a minute mock bookplate, drawn by hand, with the shorthand inscription 'constant occupation prevents temptation'.

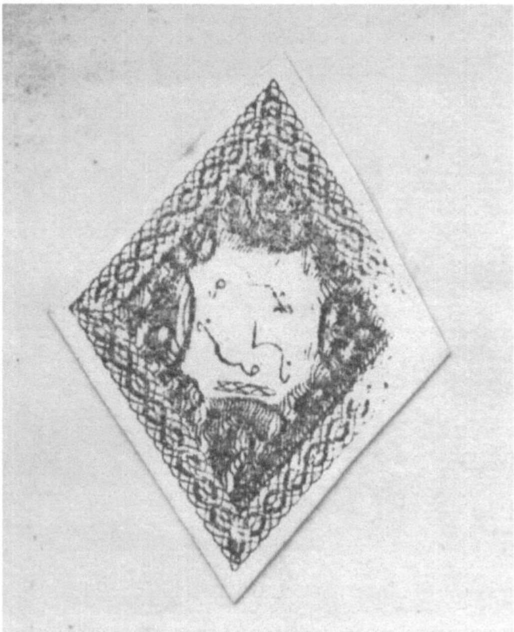

**Fig. 2.3** 'Constant occupation prevents temptation'; 'bookplate' drawn in the 1862 shorthand diary.

He recorded the first entry on 1 October 1862:

> I do not think that I need here give any remarks upon the origin and design of this journal, or at least none at any particular length. They are almost precisely similar to those with which I commenced the longhand one which I have continued to keep for the last three months . . . Longhand, however, I find is not calculated for journal keeping, at any rate not so much as phonography and so I intend in future to keep one regularly in shorthand. . . .
>
> I have now been with Mr Simpson rather more than a year although my indentures only date from the 15th of October. In a year's time today, if I am spared, I shall commence my three years' course of study at a London medical school and until then remain

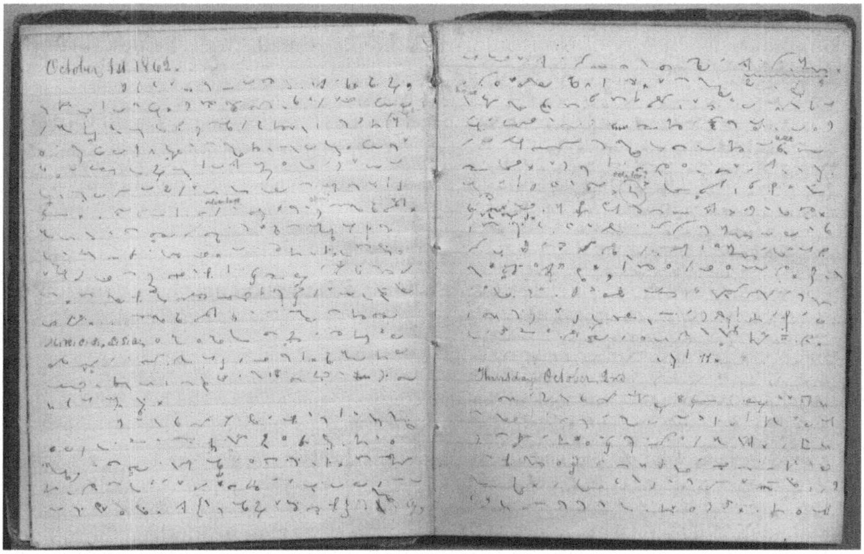

**Fig. 2.4** Opening page of the shorthand diary, 1 October 1862.

where I am. I am present studying for the Matriculation Examination at the University of London which I intend if possible passing next January.

The members of this household consist of my governor, Mr Thomas Simpson, MRCS, LSA, his wife [Sarah Ann], his wife's father, Mr Sharman, and myself, together with one servant, Myra, and a girl living in the town who comes every day.

I 'read' (by 'reading' in this journal I always mean studying) from breakfast to lunch. In the afternoon I read a little—made up some medicine and *wrote a letter to Isaac Pitman*. The latter is surprising and this is how it happened. I am practicing shorthand now chiefly in the hope that it will prove useful to me while I am at the hospital, but I met with one insuperable difficulty in the length and awkwardness of many of the medical terms and am very anxious to know whether there are any recognised grammalogues or abbreviations for the more common terms in use among medical phonographers. I was, however, at a great loss as to whom I should write to, to obtain the information, and at first thought of writing to the editor of the *Phonetic World*, but while sitting in the park this afternoon it suddenly flashed upon me—write to the author of *Phonography* himself. Which I have accordingly done. But I am afraid that the thought of receiving an actual letter from Isaac Pitman—one of those little neat concise and kind letters of which the writer of Isaac Pitman and Phonography in the last number of *Weldon's Registry* speaks, had almost as much influence as anything else.

Dr Simpson was not the only man guiding Gowers towards his future medical career. Mr Bryan Dale, the local Coggeshall Congregationalist minister acted as both his spiritual guide and his academic mentor during much of his apprenticeship. Educated at Western College, Plymouth, and University College London, it was Dale who guided Gowers through his otherwise isolated correspondence studies preparing for the matriculation exam. One of Dale's substantial achievements was the 300-page

*Annals of Coggeshall* published in 1863, shortly after he left Coggeshall, which included a comprehensive history of Nonconformism in Coggeshall.[5] In it, he described the ecclesiastical and educational institutions in Coggeshall:

> There are in the town, an Independent Chapel, Friends' Meeting-house, Baptist Chapel and Wesleyan Chapel, and three public schools—Sir Robert Hitcham's Charity School, the National and the Congregational. There is also a Mechanics' Institute and a Parochial Library.[6]

Gowers borrowed books from Dale and benefited from his encouragement, advice, and example. Observation of Dale's historical research method may have contributed to Gowers' later interest in the architecture and archaeology of East Anglia. Gowers visited Dale early in October, seeking advice:

> I went in to see Mr Dale and took his *London University Calendar* which I have borrowed. He talked about my studies, promised his assistance, lent me about ten books and gave me a good deal of sound practical advice. He thinks that by dint of hard work I can pass, but he says that I shall have to work very, very hard for the time is so short.[7]

The intensely self-critical Gowers adds the comment that time was indeed short 'but I have shortened it myself—work I must as I have never yet worked and am not working now'.

There were two rival adult education bodies in Coggeshall: the Coggeshall Mechanics' Institute, founded in 1847, and the Parochial Library and Reading Room, established by a group who resented the Nonconformists' control over the Mechanics' Institute. Both had libraries and regularly held 'penny readings'. The Mechanics Institute held about 600 books in its library. Its reading room also held daily newspapers, an unaffordable luxury for any but the well-to-do. Dr Simpson was an honorary secretary of the Mechanics' Institute, and his father-in-law, Samuel Sharman, was the librarian.

Gowers had also been introduced to a doctor from nearby Kelvedon, Edmund Marshall, who loaned him books. Marshall was offered a partnership in New Zealand with a surgery in a large practice where they 'were obliged to keep twelve saddled horses within the practice and need another doctor for they are the only medical practitioners within 200 miles around!'. Gowers recorded rather guiltily that his own distress at the man's leaving might partly be the loss of access to his books.

In a typical diary entry, Gowers wrote that his duties in Mr Simpson's surgery took up a great deal more time than he could afford, but says little about what these were, although it is clear that mixing medicines was a daily task. He mixed the potions with minimal supervision, although Mr Sharman sometimes helped him.

In October 1862 there was another scarlet fever outbreak. One Sunday he describes the deadly result of applying a treatment that had been advocated in the *Medical Times*:

> In the morning I went to Chapel and heard a very good sermon from Mr Dale on the text 'After that, he was seen of above five hundred brethren at once; of whom the greater part remain unto this present, but some are fallen asleep.' (Corinthians 1,6). A very good sermon. I have three pages of notes on it in my sermon book.
>
> On going home I learned from Mrs Simpson something which surprised me about as much as anything here surprises me now, namely that Mr Simpson, on going out this

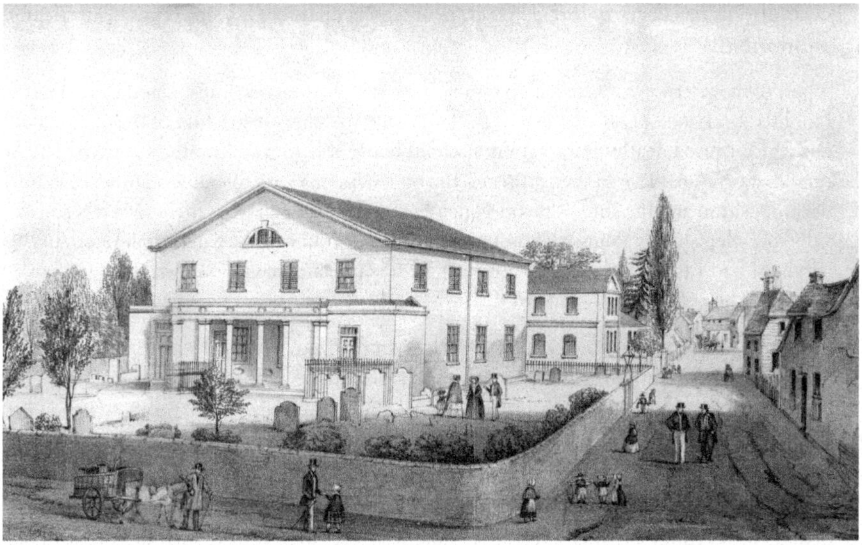

**Fig. 2.5** Congregational Church Hall, Coggeshall, 1860s. Courtesy of Coggeshall Museum and Heritage Centre.

> morning found two of his patients dead—both children and both died from scarlet fever, so that he now has three children lying dead from that disease. I believe, but I am not sure, that each case was incurable, but it is rather a curious fact that a new remedy has been used in each of these cases and in no others. It is that of carbonate of ammonia and is recommended in a recent number of the *Medical Times* as almost infallible for children in scarlet fever. Mr Simpson gave it to three children every one of whom now lies dead, not one having needed a second bottle.

The scarlet fever outbreak led to an increase in the surgery workload that threatened to interfere with his studies.

> The illness in Coggeshall appears to be on the increase instead of the decrease. It has never been at anything like half the height since I have been here—the entries for a day in our new broad day-book occupy no less than four pages and Mr Simpson walked actually about twenty miles. Unless this abates there will be but little prospect of my passing in January.

While lack of hygiene was not the cause of scarlet fever, people were becoming more aware of the relationship between public hygiene and people's health, and this was an issue of concern in Coggeshall. A Nuisance Removal Committee had been established in the town in the 1850s which appointed 'visitors' to report on conditions detrimental to health. Steps were taken to remove offensive smells caused by sewers, bad drainage, dirt lying about, and some appalling domestic sanitary arrangements. But it was not until 1864, just after Gowers had left, that a pump was erected to provide water for cleaning the sewer in Stoneham Street, one of the Coggeshall's main streets.

It was also many years before refrigeration was available. Gowers reports attending a post mortem:

> A part of the afternoon was taken up by a post mortem by Messrs Simpson and Christmas [another local doctor] on a patient of the latter who had died of stricture of the oesophagus which caused death by starvation, no food being able to pass into the stomach. The examination took place in the coffin and the body was in a very tolerable state as regards decomposition and the stink was consequently not very bad and what there was, was considerably alleviated by Poulton's smoking all the time. Poulton [the Coggeshall veterinary surgeon] had I think merely dropped in as he was passing, having known the deceased who was a horse dealer.

The London matriculation exam was held twice a year, with different set texts. For the exam Gowers planned to take in January 1863 the texts for classics were Homer's *Odyssey* (book ix); and Sallust's *Jugurthine War*; and for French, Racine's *Athelie* and Fenelon's *Dialogues des Morts* (xxxi–xl).[8] Gowers' diaries contain frequent references to his struggles with Sallust, Homer, and Racine (but little mention of Fenelon).

On the day he received Isaac Pitman's reply to his letter he was so delighted that he recorded in his diary both the letter he had written earlier, and Pitman's response. First, his own:

> Sir, I am a medical student preparing for the hospital and I have learned phonography principally in order to take notes of the lectures, remarks in the wards, etc. My chief difficulty arises from the length and awkwardness of most of the medical terms which so frequently recur. Phonography is I know extensively used by medical students etc. and I thought that there might be some recognised abbreviations or grammalogues for the more common medical terms and I am writing to you to ask you to be so kind as tell me if there are any and if so where or how I can procure them. I must beg to apologise for presuming to trouble you upon the subject but I know no-one personally to whom I can apply for the information. Phonography is I am sorry to say at a very low ebb in this little town there being only half a dozen and, of those, three write in accordance with the styles four or five editions back. Would you also be so kind as to tell me if I sign my name in the best way.

In his diary he wrote:

> I do not exactly know what were my reasons for writing but I believe that the chief moving cause was the wording of the account of his correspondence and phonographic letters in the article in *Weldon's Register*, and I suddenly found out that I wanted to know about medical grammalogues.

He then described Pitman's response:

> [It] was in nice little phonographic letters, written on both sides of half a sheet of phonography paper and devoted almost entirely to the explanation of his new 'improvements'.

Pitman described at length the changes he was making to his shorthand method, and gave Gowers advice on the various different ways 'Gowers' might be written:

> . . . I have no collection of medical terms abbreviated for the reporter. It will not be difficult for you to compile such a one for yourself. I see by your letter that you have a good knowledge of phonography.

Gowers' interest in developing medical 'grammalogues' (shortened forms, each unique to one particular medical term) was the beginning of a life-long crusade. It was over thirty years before Pitman's publishing house produced Gowers' *Phonographic Outlines of Medical Terms.*

Gowers was about to develop another interest: the history of buildings. His mentor and friend, Mr Dale, asked him to carry out a little research on his behalf:

> In the morning I went to Marks Hall with Alfred Gardner . . . I wanting to copy some inscriptions out of the church for Mr Dale. The church adjacent to Marks Hall is one of the smallest churches I ever was inside and the walls are covered with monuments to the memory of different members of the Honywood family whose seat the adjacent house is. One tablet records how one, Mary, the daughter of Robert Honywood Esquire had only one husband and had had 367 children lawfully descended from her. This is surmounted by a well-executed figure of a lady in the Elizabethan dress kneeling at prayer.

But the young man found himself too easily distracted by his fascination with shorthand:

> A tolerable day only, for I let myself be much too much taken up by shorthand. My five *Reporters* came down today and the list of the Phonetic Society. Gus got the *Phonic Journal* down also and when I went down to see him in the evening he lent it to me. I am very glad to see that Bunsen's lecture given on Macaulay is in my *Phonic Reporter.* Among the list of the Phonetic Society all those who can write 100 words per minute are marked with an asterisk, those who can write 150 words per minute with two asterisks and those who can write 200 words per minute (few and far between) with three asterisks. I think I shall join when I can write at the rate of 100 words per minute, that is to say if my views accord with those of the objects of the Society.

## Social life in an Essex village

The first anniversary of the day Gowers signed his indentures to become Simpson's apprentice was marked on 15 October 1862. He reflected on his momentous decision when describing a visit to his grandmother and the Fosters in West Street. Despite his initial reluctance to commit himself to medicine, there is no hesitation now:

> I must also not forget to record that I went down West Street today where all are pretty well. During dinner and afterwards I could not help thinking very much of another dinner party which took place here this day last year, namely that occasion on which my mother came to dine with Mr and Mrs Simpson and I had to put my name to a document which I have never for a moment regretted, and I do not think that I ever shall. Thus I have been apprenticed now just one year—I think I can say one happy year.
>
> It was October 15th—one year today has passed since I was bound to Mr Simpson—I remember it all as if it were yesterday, for the whole scene, including Mr Beaumont [the local solicitor], who came down with my indentures, are vividly impressed upon my memory, so vividly, in fact, that I do not think they will ever be completely effaced. And when I look back upon the twelve months that have passed since that day, I am anything but satisfied with my progress in any respect. I have obtained no very sensible increase of knowledge, at least nothing like so much as I ought to have done.

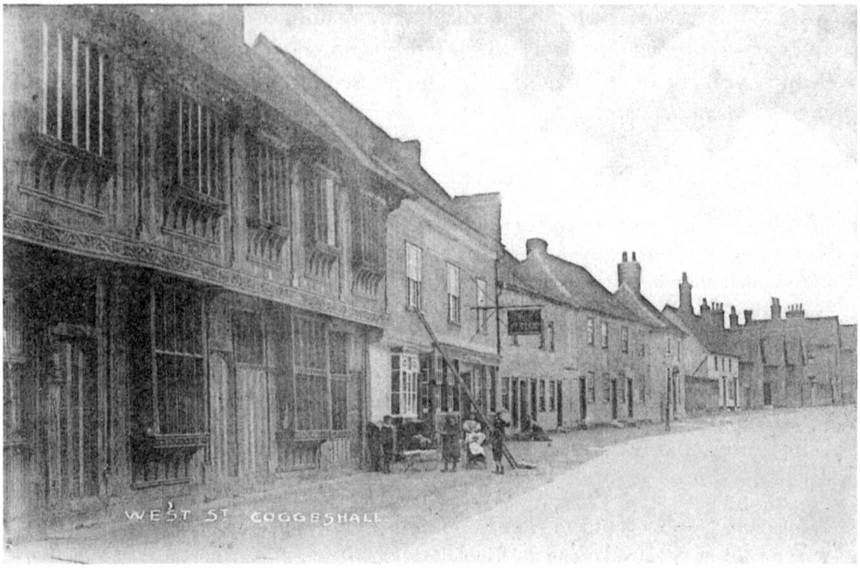


**Fig. 2.6** West Street, Coggeshall, 1910. Courtesy of Coggeshall Museum and Heritage Centre.

Gowers was ill-at-ease socially all his life, and at the age of 17 he certainly did not relish the prospect of an invitation to a dance in Coggeshall:

> Yesterday Mrs Simpson told me that she and Mr Simpson were going to an evening party at the Beaumonts tonight and I had been congratulating myself on having escaped, as it was to be a dance. But lo, when Mr Simpson came down this morning his first words were 'Beaumont's compliments to you and he will be glad to see you this evening'. And he seriously advised me to go.
>
> I had unfortunately no excuse that I could possibly plead, except that of not being able to dance, which Mrs Beaumont knew when she asked me. I felt the whole day as if there was some very heavy weight hanging over my head.

They went to the Beaumonts in the early evening:

> I enjoyed myself tolerably till the dancing began, and after that I cannot say that I enjoyed myself. The people who were there were Mr and Mrs Surridge and two of their nieces, very nice girls whose names were Miss Lully and their Mama was Mrs Lully. The party was given expressly for them. [He lists the guests]. I must not forget to mention Manthorp [Gowers never refers to his friend Manthorp's first name] who, with the exception of Arthur Gardner [father of Gowers' friend Alfred], was the only fellow in the room who had not on a dress coat. All, however, except Mr Beaumont and I, had knotted chokers on. I actually danced twice, which was much more than I expected to have done, but Marian Whitehead had compassion on me and told me that she would go through a polka with me if I liked, which of course I was only too glad to accede to. I got through two, or rather parts of two polkas with her, and she had promised to have the quadrille with me and told me all that I should have to do, but there was not the opportunity. I do not like to dwell upon that evening for I am only too conscious of having cut a very disreputable and ridiculous figure.

Gowers was anxious to conduct himself appropriately in Coggeshall. He was visiting his grandmother one day when the 81-year-old Sarah Unwin, from a well-to-do Congregationalist family of local farmers and brewers, also called in. He was uncomfortable to have been discovered in his grandmother's modest, worker's cottage, but wrote that Mrs Unwin had one day asked Letitia Gowers whether he ever came to see her, and when told that he came occasionally to read the Bible to her, Mrs Unwin had responded that she was glad that he knew his 'place and duty'.

Another example of his social sensitivities was when, on 23 October, he walked to Colchester, nine miles away. It was the year of the bicentenary of the 1662 *Act of Uniformity* which led to the 'Great Ejection of the Two Thousand'—the birth of Nonconformism. Gowers, propelled by a strong wind, walked to the town, partly to see a memorial stone being laid for the new Congregational church, but particularly wanting to hear a visiting preacher in the chapel nearby. On his way home he was offered a lift in her gig by Mrs Swinborne, wife of the Coggeshall tanner, who was accompanied by two attractive daughters. To his chagrin he was instructed to sit up beside the driver:

> But what a ride! I shall have to live to a considerable age I believe before I forget it. The wind which had been at my back to Colchester was full in our faces and although it was not quite so high, in its force was augmented by the motions of the carriage in the straightest opposite direction and I think I never felt a wind so much. I had no overcoat in having not expected that I should ride and the wind seemed to penetrate through my thin coat to the vary marrow of my bones to enter in between my overcoat and my trousers and get my loins with inconceivable severity and get in at my wrists and wind itself round and round my arms as it darted up them and sent itself like an icy knife into my blade-bones. And that was the way it was until I came to parts of the route which I knew, and although the ride was much better than walking I was not sorry when we came to the bottom of Starling Leeze where I got out, and thanked Mrs Swinborne for the ride, who was 'afraid that I was cold' and although I had just before resolved on what I would say in case I had the question put to me, namely that I should not be telling the truth if I said that I was not, what I actually said at the moment was 'Not at all', adding, however, that it was 'better than walking anyhow'. To which Mrs Swinborne said 'I should think so'. After cordial 'goodnight', I ran all the way from Starling Leeze to our house and warmed myself. After tea I went over at Mr Simpson's wish to chat with Alfred Gardner and had before I came away a glass of brandy and water and some apple pie! Went to bed, very tired, about 11pm.

## Gaining practical experience

By the end of October, Gowers was becoming increasingly anxious about the approaching matriculation examination:

> This has been a day of very hard working but not very much to show for it. Two pages and a half of Sallust occupied me till dinner and afterwards I did a little French, a little Latin—*Arnold's Practical Introduction to Latin Prose Composition*—a work which Mr Dale lent me, and which I am just going to do, a little geometry and a very little of Angus.

Angus was an examiner for University College London; this was probably his *Handbook of the English Tongue: For the Use of Student and Others.*[9]

At the beginning of November Gowers drew up a new work plan, distressed by his lack of application to his studies, and frustrated by Mr Simpson's casual attitude to his mentoring:

> The time is fast slipping away. I do not know that any amount of hard work can pull me through now but I must try hard—very hard. Mr Simpson never studies with me at all. I think he both might and ought to.

Early in November he was offered some practical medical experience by the local surgeon, Harold Giles, medical officer to Coggeshall district. Gowers was pleasantly surprised by a note he received from Giles:

> Dear Sir, I have got a case of a fractured femur in a child. Will you be so good as to come and help me put the splints on. Come to my house. Yours truly, Giles.

Gowers recorded the case of the fractured femur in considerable detail:

> I of course sent back word that I would be over in a few minutes, only too glad to get the chance. The case was that of a very little fellow, the child of a widow living down at the gas works. The right femur was fractured about the middle of the upper third. He was laid on a mattress on a table in the middle of the room and I had the task of making the extension while he [Giles] applied the bandages etc. His man was holding the child, and also the child's mother. The room was intensely hot but I got through it all well and think I was of considerable assistance to Mr Giles till after the bandages and splint were all on when I began to come over most awfully sick and just stepped out into the open cool air where I felt most awfully bad—I think worse than I have ever felt before. I thought I should have gone right off but, however, I did not. I walked about a step or two once or twice but at last I had to lean against the wall. I should think I was out about five minutes and then eventually I felt a little better. I opened the door and went inside again. But lo and behold! I could not see a glimmer! The whole room was perfectly dark. Mr Giles asked me to do something I did not know and I was obliged to say that I could not see. He told me to sit down for a minute or two and after a little time my sight began to return by degrees but by the time I recovered all, or almost all, was done and what little there was to do I could not assist in. However, I was able to take a quick look and criticise the leg before we left. When going out I apologised to Mr Giles for having gone off so and he said that it was most likely the heat of the room. It was considerate of him. He wanted me to go and have a cup of tea with him but I did not. I said that I should like to see the child again if he would have no objection to my looking in at him and he told me to call and go with him tomorrow morning, which I said I would. . . .
>
> I went to bed about 11pm feeling very much vexed with myself for my stupid fainting fit. Although the little boy cried out enough, I did not mind that one bit.

Dr Giles was married to a member of the Unwin family, and Gowers' descriptions of Mrs Giles, who was always aloof towards him, betray his insecurity about his social standing in the community. He records in detail whether she acknowledged his presence at all, and when she did, her distant manner. He went back to the Giles' house in East Street the following day:

> Just before we started Mr Giles took me into his study—a pleasant room with an excellent medical laboratory in it—and explained to me the chief bad complication of the case of the boy stating that the fracture was just before the place where the soleus muscle is

> inserted in the femur so that the tendency of that muscle was to contract and draw the small portion of the joint at the top in a different direction to the usual. We then went to see the boy who had passed a restless night but was tolerable this morning and the leg was in a pretty good position. On coming out Mr Giles asked me to call upon him at quarter past ten on the following morning and that we would call and see the child again.
>
> During the remaining few steps to his house we had a little conversation relative to the different medical schools in London at which I thought to study and recommended either Guys, Bartholomew's, St Thomas', or St George's. But I think I shall go to University College.

He visited Mr Giles several times over the next few days:

> The boy seems to be getting on nicely and had not disturbed the splint at all but Mr Giles asked me to come tomorrow morning at the same time and see him and if he complained of much pain in his leg it would be adjusted a little. . . .
>
> I went to keep an appointment with Mr Giles again this morning. I was first shown into the dining room and afterwards Mr Giles came and himself removed me into the room which I conjecture to be his study—a very comfortable little room—and had some chat with him on different things—scarlet fever, diphtheria, etc. He showed me the throat of a boy who came who had a kind of ulcerated sore throat and explained to me the difference between that construction of disease and the pure diphtheria.

In November he also learned that Sarah Unwin, his grandmother's kind visitor from Mount House, was critically ill:

> As we were coming from his house to the gasworks Mr Giles told me that Mrs Stephen Unwin was expected to die today—an obstruction of the bowels so that she brought up everything that she swallowed. It was a hernia he said. I am sorry for it for from what I have heard she is a woman universally beloved and liked by all and who has done a great deal of good.
>
> We went to see the boy who is doing well and some time in the afternoon was fixed for taking off the splint and exploring a little when he was going—what time—he said he would let me know but in the evening his man came up and sent his compliments and would I call for him in the morning at half past ten as he had not time to do it today.

His mother wrote in early November enclosing a Post Office order for £5, out of which he was to pay for his tuition up to December and to take off a sovereign for his grandmother. He had enough left over to buy a new pair of warm gloves and pay his tailor's bill.

He was becoming even more anxious about the London examination, now only two months away:

> I wonder if I shall ever pass. I do not see very clearly how I am to. Unless I alter very much I do not know whether the case is nearing past hoping for.
>
> Did some Greek this morning but that is all. The rest of my day was frittered away in the most, frivolous, trivial pastimes imaginable. A little time was occupied by reading up about piles for Mr Simpson advised me to do so for he said that he had seen Dr Giles who had told him that there would be most probably a slight operation when I came to his house tomorrow morning. Some reading connected with piles—for the removal of one I suppose—Mr Simpson thought I had better read up a little so that I do not appear entirely ignorant.

The following Sunday they attended the patient suffering from piles:

> Mr Giles came in and told me that he had to go to a labour and it was agreed that he should either call for me during the morning or I should call for him at half past two. However, the latter had not to be put to the test for I had not been at home long before Mr Giles came and we went, first to the boy who is getting on nicely and then to the man with the piles. It was a nasty place—dirty squalid children running about and a disagreeable looking woman kept on abusing the operation and Mr Giles.
>
> The piles were first examined as well as possible, the man kneeling on the chair, and after he was placed on a bed in the illumination possible and by means of a speculum one bleeding pile was touched with nitric acid.

Two days later he received troubling news from Doncaster. The Sunday had been busy, and that night he remembered that he had received, but not read, a letter from his mother. When he did, it upset him, and provoked an entry in the diary which he later tore out. But he kept the description of the contents of the letter:

> Just as I was going to bed I suddenly remembered a letter which I had on the day before (Saturday) received from mother. It was given to me at lunch and which I just broke the seal of it and put it in my pocket and—forgot all about!!! . . .
>
> To my astonishment and dismay I discovered that it was a letter consulting me about the purchase of a house in Spring Gardens which mother was thinking of buying and seeking what my probable expenses would be, especially the hospital fee, and *urgently and repeatedly demanding an answer by return of post as the final answer had to be given on Monday!* Here was a pretty fix. I put out the light, drew up the blind and got into bed and put on my considering cap. For some little time I began to get doubtful about certain pages in the letter and got out and sat up in bed and read it by the light of the lamp at the opposite side-road. I could not for some time arrive at any conclusion as to what I had better do but at last I decided that it would be best to get up early in the morning and write a letter and go over to Kelvedon and post it in time for the early post by which means mother would receive it the first thing on Tuesday morning which would I fear be too late. It was impossible that I could give her any opinion on the large purchase after she has told me so little respecting the house, not even how much it is or anything, but only that to buy it mother would have to appropriate one hundred pounds of the money set apart for my education (or which was once said to be set apart) as well as some money of Charlotte's.

He replied to his mother the next day, apologizing for the delay but also explaining why he was upset:

> I also said that I felt it a rather delicate matter to speak of the money which she was laying out on my education for the profession which she had selected for me, but if my dutiful, affectionate and upright conduct and my constant endeavours to do my best could prevent it, she should never regret the outlay. I must say that I have felt rather hurt at the manner in which she has got out of paying all she said, rather has imagined my being able to manage without laying out all the money she originally intended on me for when I first came here. She had £300 which she had saved up on purpose to expend on my education: £150 for Mr Simpson and £150 for my hospital money.

When Gowers and Mr Giles visited the boy from the gasworks with the broken leg again, they found him 'not so well', and in great pain:

> Mr Giles had no time now, but arranged to call at four and investigate the probable cause of the pain which he complained of in the foot which he did, but did not stop long only taking off as much starch bandage as we were able and arranged to put another starch bandage on in the morning.

Plaster of Paris, though invented in 1840, was not yet widely used. Its advantage over starch bandages was that it minimized the risk of subsequent displacement of parts of the bone: it hardened rapidly, taking about five minutes to set while being held in position by the surgeon, and allowed the limb to be inspected daily without removing all the apparatus. Starch bandages took several days to dry unless heat was applied to them.

The following day Gowers helped Dr Giles re-set the broken femur, an extremely painful and difficult process. But first he reported on one of his own cases that he was managing in the surgery:

> The boy who had the tip of his thumb cut off came this morning to have the bandages taken off and had it soaking for a long time in a tray but at the time appointed for me to be at Mr Giles it was not sufficiently saturated to come off and so I had to leave him. It was rather tiresome particularly as I had to wait for an hour at Mr Giles' before we started.
>
> When we got there [the gas works] Mr Giles wanted to take all the bandages off and put them on again without disturbing the splint if possible and tried to check for what remained of the old starch bandage but in cutting it off he scratched the boy's leg and made him cry and soon saw that it would be better to take it all off. When it was done the leg was in rather a mess, all the muscles being excited and the leg turned completely over, the ends of the fracture being, of course, completely out of place. Therefore it was gradually got into place and I put the 'containment-tailored' bandage on and we made a good job of it but I could not help thinking that it would have been much better to have put the new starch bandage on when the old one was taken off. Mr Giles decided on making the counter extension almost the entire fitting cloth sewn on to the left thigh, and strips taken from that to the top of the splint instead of the perineal band which was found cooling, so he got me to come and show the woman how it was to be done and afterwards to go and tie it on which I did, but which delayed me terribly and quite spoiled my day for it was just lunch time when I went home and an hour of the afternoon was occupied by seeing to it. That, together with some medicines that had to be made up and mending my gloves which I did with some surgeons' silk (!).

After dinner he made up some medicines, then recorded with relief:

> I am forgetting to mention that I received a letter from mother today. Fortunately my letter was not too late to be of some service for when she found that morning's post did not bring a letter from me she went to Mr Clarke, the agent for the house who is not the owner of the property which she was thinking of buying and asked for another day before she gave a final answer which was granted her and in the letter which I received today, as kind and loving and affectionate a letter as I have ever received from her (and that is every praise) she has gone into all the circumstances about the property but tells me that she,

after thinking a good deal about it, has come to the conclusion that it will be best not to do anything about it, for several reasons. I wronged my dearest mother, oh how much, when I spoke in the entry a day or two back about the probable causes of her thinking about the course—for she says that her sole reasons were to get a little more to her income.

And now I come to the great event of the day, the first 'penny reading' in conclusion of the year in this situation took place in the large room on Upper Stoneham Street. I dare say I have mentioned somewhere here that Mr Simpson is the Secretary to the Literary and Mechanics Institution here. There are two rival institutions here, the 'Church Parochial Library and Reading Room', the penny readings in connection with which have been commenced some weeks, and the old 'Mechanics' to which my Governor is secretary, and from which the others broke away, disenchanted in consequence of the books not being sufficiently anti-Nonconformist for them. Each has a set of penny readings conducted on essentially rival principles and held in the schoolrooms of the respective bodies: theirs in the 'National', ours in the 'British' schoolroom.

Ours very generally bears the palm as regards success in point of numbers for a larger room is generally better filled by far, partly in consequence most likely of the music being interspersed between the different readings which diversifies the proceedings and is a considerable attraction. I went with Mrs Simpson and although the time was only about a quarter to eight the room was well nigh full and nearly all the reserved seats already occupied. We got seating at the end of the room rather too near the pianoforte to hear the singing with great distinctness. The proceedings opened by Mr Dale reading some 'splendid pieces and splendidly read' but ill selected and consequently ill received. A glee followed, 'Forests sound the cheerful horn', or something of that sort, well sung by Prior, Coventry, Surridge and Collis. Abbott next read a selection from Burns, namely the 'Ode on Despondency' and 'Scots Wha Hae Wi' Wallace Bled'. The last was in my opinion the best read. Solos on the pianoforte followed by Miss Kate Prior. Mr Simpson then read 'Dissertation upon Roast Pig' by Charles Lamb—a very clever piece but which, in my opinion, might have been better read.

Mary Foster's baby, Emily, was seriously ill with scarlet fever and abscess. Gowers asked Mr Simpson how his infant cousin was getting on and was given 'a clear concise statement of the case in brief but decisive language'. The diagnosis was that she was very weak, but Simpson's prognosis was that 'still I think she will get over it'.

## Making his first diagnosis

Meanwhile, Mr Giles was exposing Gowers to more of his medical cases. Gowers was delighted when he made his first diagnosis, and annotated his diary later by marking the passage and writing 'first diagnosis'.

I was punctual at his house and he came and told me that he expected a man this morning with a hydrocele of the spermatic cord [a build-up of liquid in the scrotum] which he thought of tapping. The man arrived and Mr Giles, before tapping, endeavoured to get a view of its translucence by transmitting light, but in vain. He tried the sunlight, and then the room darkened and a candle held at the side of the scrotum, to no purpose. And then, not liking to operate without assurance for certain the character of the tumour told the man to come again at whatever o'clock in the evening when it would be dark. Soon after he went away.

> Burton the pile man came and had the pile repaired with nitric acid. We then went and saw the boy and I afterwards went back and placed a wedge under his pelvis. When I went home it was nearly 12 and in the little time that remained before lunch I was occupied by doing a little Sallust, and chiefly by reading up 'hydroceles'.
>
> Worked hard all afternoon trying to make up for lost time but in vain for after dinner I had some medicine to make up and then had quarter of an hour on Sallust before it was time to be off to Mr Giles. When I got there I went into the dining room. I have seldom seen a more comfortable looking room. It is such a good size and not too large with dark oak up to the ceiling on all sides, dark crimson window curtains closely drawn before the window and a nice cheerful fire in the grate.
>
> When Mr Giles came we adjourned into the breakfast room where we commenced by trying to discover some small degree of transparency at least, but it was in vain. However we had not been trying long before I had an idea in my mind and asked about its being affected by the man's coughing. That appeared to stir the idea in Mr Giles' mind and he inquired about how long it was going for, and on learning that it regularly went down at night, made the man lie down and succeeded in completely reducing it, showing at once that it was a case of inguinal hernia [abdominal contents protruding through a weak spot in the groin muscle, which causes a bulge in the groin or scrotum] and recommended the man to get a truss, and we returned to the dining room congratulating ourselves on the tapping not having been done which would have been a serious affair. I did not stop long, and when I came away Mr Giles said he was very much obliged to me for my suggestion. I had not, as perhaps I ought to have done, denied my claim to the merit of having suggested it but I received it without saying anything as I think I really did think of it first. What a lot of 'thinking'!

When visiting patients in their homes, doctors often had difficulty in finding enough light in which to examine them. Years later Gowers developed a 'triple-wick candle', to make it easier to use an ophthalmoscope on home visits in houses still lit by gaslight or paraffin lamps.

There was another case of fracture that November. This time it was one of Mr Simpson's patients who lived at nearby Bradwell Juxta Coggeshall.

> Miss Good's case was rather an interesting one so the next thing I did was to read up what Erichsen [*Science and Art of Surgery*[10]] says about fractures of the patella. These give readings about fractures of the patella and also the parts concerned in hernia and together with going once over a page of Sallust occupied me till lunch. After lunch I had a minute to spare for I had only just time to see to the people who came for medicine and packed a splint to take with me before it was more than time to start. The walk was a very pleasant one although a dreadful fog fell. However, I stepped out and did not mind it. I left the house here by 2.25 and got to Bradwell church at about two minutes from the appointed time. When I got to the house I found Mr Simpson already there. The patient is a very pleasant old lady who was feeding her chickens on Thursday morning and slipped on the slippery ground and fell, breaking her kneecap. The first business was to get her downstairs which was very well done considering the inconvenience of the stairs. She had been taken to the bedroom and was going to lie in a bed which been put in the parlour. I could not take many of the symptoms about the fracture for there was very little time.

They then had to place the splint and secure it with a bandage before finally bringing her downstairs to the parlour.

> After dinner whilst Mr Simpson and I were at work in the surgery a man, Blackwell from Pointell Lane came in for some medicine for his nephew who had his hand bandaged up and on inquiry he stated that he fell down in a field today and in extending his hand to save himself fell upon it and to use his own expression 'stucked his hand'. On examination the injury was found to be a fracture of one of the middle metacarpal bones, not quite so small a matter, seeing that it involved a cessation from work for at least six weeks. It was treated simply with a splint, with the bandage wound round the hand.

The following day he accompanied Mr Giles to check on the lad at the gas works. Fortunately they found that he was 'going on very well'.

## Stress of preparing for matriculation examination

Young Gowers was leading a lonely life in many ways and this, combined with worrying about his matriculation, seems to have been making him depressed, recording that 'I am not at all satisfied with my present way of going on for I am afraid I am getting into what a recent writer in the *Nonconformist* called the "corrosive habit of brooding"—in fact I am sure that I have and I should like to get out of it if I could—but how is the thing'. However, he was now concentrating better on his studies:

> Day of hard study has I am happy to say, brought me safely to the end of Latin subject for the examination of matriculation at the University of London. I am therefore exactly a month behind-hand in my studies for I was calculating upon getting the Geography which I have just finished, completed by the end of October, and at the same time the book of Homer which I am also reading up, that is to say going through both of them once. I have now just finished them the first time. I had hoped by this time to have been through both of them twice. My Homer I hope to finish tomorrow as I have only two pages remaining which by dint of hard work I hope to put behind me instead of before, as it is now. I did some Homer the first thing this morning instead of Sallust which I did not begin until twelve o'clock and I worked hard at it the whole day and had finished the whole translation and only three lines more to write out.

The last day of November was a Sunday:

> Went to chapel in the morning after breakfast and surgery work. I must not forget that although I did not get up <u>very</u> early I had been reading in bed a portion of a shorthand sermon from as soon as I could see. Mr Dale preached in the morning and a very fine sermon from the last two verses of the 84th psalm. Miscellaneous reading till dinner. What a nice dinner of duck and apple pie and I am happy to say that I succeeded in restraining myself and 'left off with an appetite' which is a pleasure—more than I can say for any of my three mails today. In the afternoon, in amongst several miscellaneous parcels, I wrote some short notes from memory of the morning's sermon and also read a little of Locke's 'Conduct of the Understanding'.

A month had passed since his last self-critical progress report on his studies:

> December is actually here! I have now a very serious doubt as to the possibility of my passing my examination in January or even being ready for it, however I don't mean to give it up without a very, very hard struggle. I was not up this morning in time to do any before breakfast, which I got over by nine after which I first got my washing ready as is my custom on Monday mornings and then sat down and did over the last two pages of Sallust

> which I finished on Friday. That and going to see some people who came occupied me till it was time to go to Mr Giles for it was the morning on which he had arranged to go and see the boy again. I had to wait some little time before he was ready and then we were occupied till past eleven and putting on the bandages afresh which had come off. When I came back I got down to reading as soon as I could but in spite of my hard work and I really have applied myself well as regards the amount of time today, but I cannot say the same about my mental application.

He received a newspaper from his mother, 'one edge of which, according to previous instructions I held to the fire when some light brown writing appeared telling me that all were well and that she should not write again until the sale was over which was advertised in the paper. Mother's name appears in the advertisement as the occupier of one of the houses adjoining the one which is to be sold'. Gowers did not explain why she used 'secret ink'.

Gowers' 'corrosive brooding' was exacerbated by his becoming overtired, and he records nearly making a lethal mistake:

> I have made an immense number of the most stupid blunders today that ever were counted. To begin with I made a stupid mistake with a name—a woman came and asked Mr Simpson to come and see what I understood to be Mrs Bryant's baby as soon as possible. I went and told Mr Simpson he was wanted to go up Tilkey to see Mrs Bryant's baby as soon as possible I suppose I added the name unintentionally for Mr Simpson went up there to see three Bryants and in the event none who had sent for him and came back and was very cross with me for not having taken the direction more explicitly as well he might. It afterwards turned out to be Mrs Bond who had sent for him, who did not live up Tilkey at all, and so I suppose I imagined that part of the message. Another blunder was that I forgot all about a bottle of liniment that I was to have sent to Eliza Swinborne. A third was a mistake about some powders in the evening—asking Mr Simpson about them and he told me to pulve gritty gum opiate so instead I went away with the idea that it was pulve antimony and calomel. The merchant did not have them, but it was not my fault that the child did not get killed. To crown all, I was to have gone to Mr Giles this morning to keep an appointment to go and see the boy with the broken leg but I forgot all about that too! . . .
>
> How fearfully the month rolls onward. Literally fearful for me because the time I have left grows shorter and shorter and I am filled with apprehension for the result. I went to Mr Giles this morning and he actually did not know that it was not this morning that he had appointed for me so I came off well in that quarter—no thanks to me though! I worked hard all day but I did not get a great deal of work done.

It is fortunate he did not attempt to make up a pulve of antimony (which is highly toxic) and calomel (mercury chloride), both of which were used as purgatives in Victorian medicine. On the Sunday he said goodbye to his friend Edmund Marshall, a farewell that sparked more introspection:

> After chapel, when I got home, I found Edmund Marshall here—and what is more he and Mr Simpson were smoking in the drawing room—over to say goodbye. He joins his ship the day after tomorrow and after a very few days sails for New Zealand. I fear it seems his parting words to me I shall not forget in a hurry and the tone in which he said them. They were 'Goodbye, I wish you success at university'. Nothing more. And with another goodbye he drove off waving his cap as he did so. And so I lost sight of him. He talks of coming

home in nine years. Where and what shall I be then? If I am not an MD then I fear I shall never be.

Where shall we all be? Marshall I suppose being four or five months on the passage not expecting to reach New Zealand till April. The practice to a partnership to which he is going is a very large one, being about 30 miles in diameter with different patients at a distance of thirty or forty miles from the place to which he is going—Christchurch. The opening is a splendid one for him and I should think that there is no chance but that he should get on.

By this time Dr Simpson was trying to expand his practice. In early December a deputation came to ask him to become surgeon to a Friendly Society at Feering, one mile from Coggeshall. Simpson agreed to attend a meeting when the voting was to take place. The deputation told him, erroneously as it turned out, that there was 'no chance but that he will get in'. One of the great attractions for Simpson's apprentice was that Simpson, if he was elected, would 'have to keep a conveyance at once and he thinks of getting the Beaumonts' which they are thinking of selling'. When the day of the Feering meeting arrived Mr Simpson's hopes were dashed when a colleague, Dr Christmas, just beat him.

## Sitting the matriculation examination in London

Gowers read *The Athenaeum,* a weekly literary review founded in 1822, with contributors including Robert Browning, Thomas Carlyle, and Charles Lamb. On 8 December Gowers received 'a very unwelcome notification by today's *Athenaeum* that the examination for matriculation at the University of London will take place on the 12th January, that is, on the second fortnight in the month instead of on the third as I was assured had been the case'. The following day, perhaps seeking reassurance, he went to dinner with Mr Dale:

> . . . and had a very pleasant afternoon and evening till nearly eight. We dined off a most beautiful turkey, tender as I have ever tasted one, and afterwards after some little conversation I got him to read. He got on the reading cue then could not be stopped, not that I wanted him to for he was reading well indeed. He read Wolsey's soliloquy from *Henry VIII*, Othello's speech before the court, and a great part of *The Taming of the Shrew*, which he advised me to read as it might soon prove useful (!). The last half hour was spent in going over some things in connection with my studies and he was so kind as to lend me his Smith's *Classical Dictionary* and also his large *Dictionary of Greek and Roman Antiquities.*[11]

From mid-December Gowers' studies took precedence over his diary. But on Christmas Eve he managed to find time to record the gist of correspondence he had had with the University of London:

> I sent my certificate of age to the Registrar of the University of London on Monday, accompanied by a notification of my intention to present myself as a candidate for matriculation and this morning I received a printed letter signed by the autograph of the Registrar, Dr Carpenter, stating that my certificate was perfectly satisfactory. The last two

days of the week preceding the examination is the time fixed for paying the fees and so I shall have to go up on the Friday.

I am not so forward in my studies as I expected a fortnight ago but I must do the best I can and in that confidence *wish* to pass and not feel unhappy if I do not. Such is my dear Mother's advice and I shall consider it worth following. I am studying very hard and I think I deserve to pass. I am sorry to say that my mother, according to a letter I received from her on Thursday, is very poorly indeed.

I have fortunately not been asked out to parties and hope that I shall not be for I really cannot afford the time. I shall have to go as a matter of necessity to Mr Pattison's next door tomorrow.

Gowers berated himself each month for not keeping to his own study plans. The final entry for 1862 was written two weeks before he was to sit the matriculation exam:

Wednesday December 31st—New Year's Eve—11.45pm:

From the necessity which there has been of the whole of my time being given to study if I would have anything like a chance of passing my examination I have thought it better not to keep this journal but I cannot allow this day to pass without putting a few lines upon it. The old year, 1862, is fast drawing to a close.

The last year indeed is nearly sped. But fifteen minutes more and 1862, with all its faults, with all its shortcomings, with all its wasted and misspent time, will have gone forever. Let me write it—1862—while I may—as it is fast going and will never, never, never come back.

Last year I was here. The year before—1860–61—I was in daily expectation of going for some months to Bentley to try farming. 1859–60 was my last New Year in Oxford—my old Alma Mater as far as school is concerned.

Six years ago the New Year opened in trouble and fear—my dear Father was lying in a fresh grave but a few days old and my mother put on for the first time her widow's weeds. Ah! many, many changes have taken place since then.

On 12 January 1863 he sat his matriculation examination. A few days earlier he went up to London. He started the day by walking to Kelvedon station to catch the London train:

I came third class but had a cab from the railway to Westminster. After a good dinner I went to Burlington House to pay the fee for my approaching examination. I had to wait some little time before I was ushered into the presence of Dr Carpenter. He is a younger looking man than I expected—tall, thin, with a long face, no hair on the top of his head but some brown locks at the side. In his behaviour he is exceedingly courteous. He asked me my name and then found my certificate and told me to sign my name in a large register with my present address and place of education. On the last item I asked him if I were to put my place of education or where I had been reading up for this examination for I said that I had been studying for it under a surgeon whom I was with. He asked me where I had received most of my education and I told him Christ Church College School, Oxford, and he immediately told me to put that. In the last column I put my place of birth—London—and then paid my fee; I was just going when he called me back: 'Mr Gowers—You have not got your certificate'. I did not know that I was to take it away.

## Awaiting matriculation results

Four days after he sat the exam he was about to travel to Doncaster to see his mother. He was convinced he had failed:

> A week has passed since my last entry. My examination is over but, if I am not mistaken, I shall be plucked. My English History and Algebra papers were so bad that I do not at all see how the examiners can pass me. But, however, I have not time to go into details now as I intend starting for Doncaster by the early train in the morning and if I do not go to bed I shall not wake.

He wrote another entry once he had arrived in Doncaster, on Saturday 23 January:

> I am sorry to say that I have not had time to write up my diary until now. I arrived safely in Doncaster on Saturday last after a very pleasant journey in which I was fortunate enough to meet with the most agreeable travelling companions I ever came across. In the carriage into which I got there were three other fellows who had all been up for the matriculation at the University of London. We went over every paper. One of the three, the oldest of them, was a teacher in a school at Bradford, in Yorkshire,—Gledhill by name—and seems a very clever fellow. Another of them is called Blackall. I asked them their names in order to be able to look and see if they have passed [Blackall and Gledhill both passed in the First Division].[12] At the station my mother and Miss Cunningham were waiting for me and I need not say that I was welcomed home.
>
> I wrote to Mr Simpson giving a detailed account of my examination and asking his opinion about it and received his answer yesterday saying that in his opinion I had passed. The weather since my arrival has been anything but pleasant consisting principally of high winds and storms and hail and rain.

Gowers received welcome news a few days before the results were published in *The Times* on 30 January:

> Although I heard the result of the examination on Tuesday last I have not yet had time to put it down. Let me give it a separate line, for it deserves it.
>
> I have passed—and First Division.
>
> It is useless to take time to express my feelings when I received Mr Holbrook's kind note.
>
> 'My dear Sir, I am very pleased to find your name in the first list of those who have passed. That this may be the prelude to the highest honours believe me. Yours very truly.'
>
> I thought upon more consideration that I might have passed Second Division but the First was far beyond me, although not beyond the occasional sigh. I am well rewarded for all my great anxiety and hard work and what different feelings can I now anticipate meeting my efforts from those with which I should have looked forward to had I been plucked!
>
> I need not say how very, very pleased my dear mother is of my efforts. The lists were published in yesterday's papers and I have got a copy of *The Times* for myself as well as one to send to New Zealand to send to Edmund Marshall when I know his address.

Many years later he wrote that he used his shorthand 'with great advantage in the various work, especially in classics, etc, for the matriculation examination for the University of London. I remember how strange it seemed to me that anyone should have lessons in shorthand. My chief help was the shorthand magazine called "*The Phonographic Reporter*", which was issued by Thomas Alan Reed'.[13]

He spent his Yorkshire holiday catching up with friends in Doncaster, Arksey, and Bentley, particularly spending time with farmer Joseph Hurst. It was the last time he would see Hurst. He enjoyed the holiday, returning south ready to study for the Preliminary Scientific Examination, the new introductory course for medical students at University College London. The course included botany, and although he again faced the problems of learning by correspondence, Coggeshall provided ideal surroundings in which to 'botanize'. The study of botany developed into one of his enduring interests.

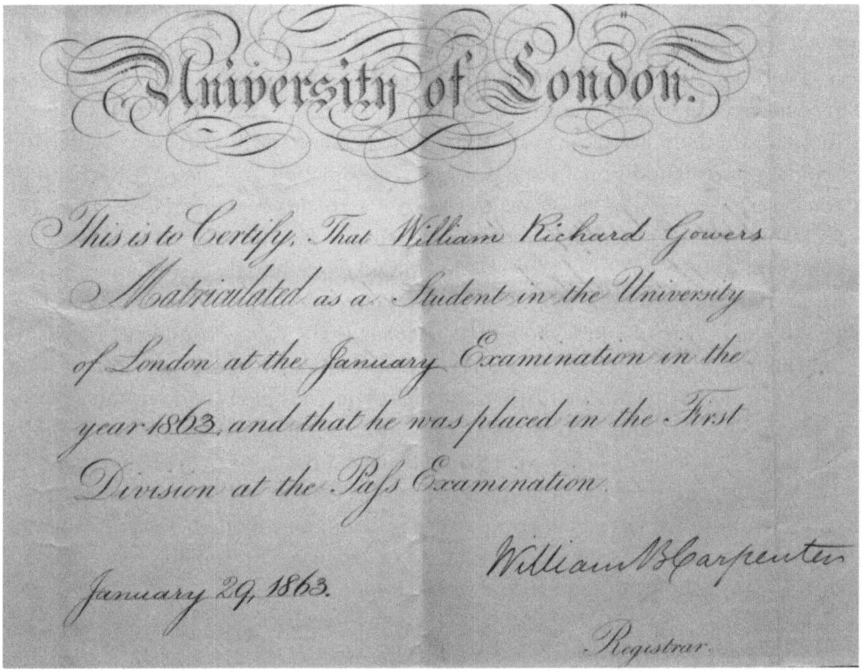


**Fig. 2.7** Gowers' matriculation certificate, 1863. Courtesy of Dr Patrick Gowers.

Chapter 3

# Apprentice year 1863

## Introduction of the Preliminary Scientific Examination

The enactment of the *Medical Act 1858* was followed by a new curriculum for medical students. This revived general science, 'inspired by the belief that the dramatic results of science could be applied to medicine, and that doctors ought to be taught to that end'.[1] The apprenticeship system was phased out, but Gowers never regretted having served with Dr Simpson. Nonetheless, the medical examinations he was to sit were part of the new regime, announced in 1862.

In 1860, the University of London had introduced the Preliminary Scientific Examination as an additional stage between matriculation and the First Bachelor of Medicine examination. In 1863 a major change was made when the Master of Surgery was created and the practical examination in surgery was transferred to it from the Second MB. At the same time surgery was omitted from the MD examination.

The Preliminary Scientific Examination was held each July, and was open to candidates who had turned 17 and who had matriculated. The course comprised mechanical and natural philosophy (statics; dynamics; hydrostatics, hydraulics, and pneumatics; optics; heat; electricity; magnetism); inorganic chemistry; botany and vegetable physiology; zoology and comparative anatomy. Candidates had the option of taking the exam in the same year that they were taking their first Bachelor of Medicine exam.

The subjects set out for the Preliminary Scientific, Gowers' second academic hurdle, do not mention further tests of competence in languages. Nonetheless, throughout 1863 Gowers taught himself French and German, languages presumably seen as essential in order to read European medical research reports.

## Return to London

At the beginning of February 1863, Gowers returned to London. While there he consulted his cousin Tom, seeking advice on preparing for the Preliminary Scientific as he now had to focus on languages and science.

> Left Doncaster this morning by the 9 o'clock parliamentary train and after a tolerably pleasant journey reached King's Cross terminus at a little before 4pm. I took a cab from the railway station to Tothill Street [Westminster] where I arrived in time to write a letter to mother before tea.
>
> I remembered, when I had got no further than Rossington, the first station after Doncaster, that I have left all my examination papers behind me. I therefore in my letter to mother asked her to send them to me by return of post. After tea I strolled to Regent Street in the hope of seeing cousin Tom. I found him not very well and also that the only

evening he would have at liberty was this one so I arranged to come at about 8pm for him. I employed the afternoon hour by taking a stroll down Oxford Street. At 8pm we started off and walked home to his house where his mother, my aunt, was pretty well.

I wanted to see Tom especially to get his advice about the best book from which to begin the study of German. He was so good as to lend me two books of Ollendorff's in the French [H. G. Ollendorff wrote both French and German language manuals], along which kind he learned from. He half recommended me not to begin German until I had perfected myself in French but the reasons which I had for commencing it now he allowed to have great weight: namely that I shall never have so much time for getting up the rudiments of the German language as I shall have during the next six months and the joy it would be to me to know enough to be able to profit by any evening class. Besides the two rather expensive books of Ollendorff's he also lent me three French books to read. He recommended me to get Flügel *German Dictionary* which he was going to get for me as he could get it for trade price. I had a capital supper with him and left at 11.

He also visited his old home in St John's Wood and then went on to Hackney:

... indulging myself, as I generally do, upon the underground railway, by paying 3d extra and travelling first class. I found all middling at Hackney but I had the greatest difficulty possible in preserving my gravity at the sight of Mr Coventry. The whole of the lower part of his face is one mass of hair!

He may have found this entertaining then, but Gowers eventually succumbed to the new fashion, sporting a luxuriant beard for most of his adult life.

## Coggeshall 'penny readings'; Tennyson, Arnold, and Coleridge

Gowers then returned to Coggeshall. The diary entries change in 1863, with few references to Mr Giles but recording his interest in botany, part of the new scientific curriculum. Gowers became preoccupied during his solitary walks with collecting plant specimens, or 'botanizing', which he took up with great enthusiasm. As he matured, and his confidence grew, he also became less solitary, taking long walks, playing chess, and indulging in social drinking with his friends Alfred Gardner and Manthorp.

I brought back with me from London a severe cold which confined me to the house on both Sunday and Monday. On Tuesday I ventured as far as Mr Dale's and went for a short walk, and on Wednesday I was so much better as to be able to go for a good long one as far as Bradwell to take the measure of Miss Gooday's knee.

I had a very pleasant companion in Mr Oliver Coventry with whom I had not before taken a walk. The weather since my return has been very pleasant; I think the most beautiful I have ever witnessed at this time of the year. I enjoyed the walk exceedingly going by West Mill where I had to see how a child was and returning by Water Lane and Stock Street where I called to see Maryanne Fenn whom I found very down in appearance from what she was when I saw her last. Her arms now seem to have literally nothing upon them but skin and bone.

I have now got regularly at work in my studies and I am happy to say that I should have every prospect of my getting very comfortably through them long before the examination in July. I have also got nicely to work at German and hope to get through the first of

> Ollendorff's books by July. I have had a great desire to read Coleridge's *Aids to Reflection in the Formation of a Manly Character* [1829] having been very strongly advised to do so by my sceptical friend of the railway train and I tried to obtain a second-hand copy at all the bookstores I could meet with in London but in vain. Fortunately, however, in Mr Dale's study the other day I found a copy and borrowed it. I am going to set to work and read it.

William Temple and Thomas Arnold, reinterpreting Coleridge's writings, were the founders of the Broad Church movement in the Established Church, and in the early 1860s there was considerable debate about their proposal to liberalize the church. Gowers remained a devout Christian throughout his life, but it is possible to trace a gradual shift in his views as he, like many contemporaries, adjusted to Dissenters being accepted within the Broad Church movement.

Early in the year Mr Simpson received the first half of a £50 bank note from Gowers' mother, the last of the three instalments for the £150 she had to pay for her son's apprenticeship. A few days later he received the second half (presumably splitting the note was a security measure).

Gowers started to come to grips with the new works he had to study, as well as the additional subjects he decided to learn. He mentions Arnold's *Greek Accidence* and the first book of Horace's *Odes*. He read Charlotte Bronte's *Shirley* for relaxation, but had great trouble understanding the Coleridge and decided he must not be clever enough.

On a walk with Alfred Gardner after chapel one Sunday he discussed Tennyson's *In Memoriam*, a best-seller at the time. Gardner particularly admired the verse:

> I sometimes feel it half a sin
> To put in words the grief I feel;
> For words, like Nature, half reveal
> And half conceal the Soul within.

Gowers replied that he could not exactly understand the way in which Tennyson 'half concealed and half revealed'.

> Alfred, however, said that he should think that it was the divine Soul that was appearing in Nature that was meant there. I could at once see it then for a true principle can never be obtained from the study of the Nature alone without the aid of revelation although the lesson which may be learned from Nature comes nearest to reality. It adds double beauty to the passage.
>
> When I came in I took up *In Memoriam* to read a little but I was not in a condition either to enjoy or appreciate it—I do not know why. Alfred, when I said goodnight to him, said to me 'Oh Gowers, I have but low chance of education—you have a splendid opportunity!'
>
> I have, and I must take care to make the best use of it that lies in my power. I am afraid that I am not at present. When I came in and thought over what he had just said a text came across my mind with startling force: 'To whom much has been given much shall be required.' [Luke: 12:48]

His diary entries reflect his growing appreciation of the beauty of the nature surrounding him on his walks. On 23 February he wrote:

> Along the side of a field through which the path from Tilkey to Marks Hall right of way runs is a small hill covered over with youngish trees. On this way are some pit-like places which have been dug out at some time for the purpose I should think of obtaining gravel. I thought that it might be possibly the remains of an old Roman camp for at a distance the holes do not look unlike the remains of a moat and so trespassed on to it and went to obtain a closer view. Although disappointed in that respect I found a quantity of the most lovely primroses in full flower. I think there could not have been less than some thousands about for they made the earth quite grey.

He also starts taking walks at night in order to try to conquer what he sees as his irrational fear of the dark, and these are described in detail. After one of his walks, he attended a penny reading:

> I just got home [after a night walk] in time to be off to the penny reading which took place this evening. So far as the readings and the music were concerned it was by far the best that they had ever had but there was a good deal of disorder occasioned by the intense crowding of the room which was fuller than it had ever been before. The floor literally shook and trembled, and a good many were trembling for it and Mr Pattisson, in his sermon, requested people to abstain from signifying their approbation by stamping on the floor but to clap their hands. The floor vibrated to the music, I suppose with the unconscious keeping time by those who were so enchanted by it.
>
> The pianoforte solo was played: 'The Maiden's Prayer', which I have heard before at one and only one place and played by one and only one person; the place: Highfields; the person: Amy Burton. I looked away from the piano and my thoughts as the notes fell on my ears went wandering back over the hundred miles which separated me from Yorkshire and into that little parlour at Snug Farmhouse on that hillside in Yorkshire, where, however, I do not suppose *she* is for I expect she is much nearer to me than that—in London. Of course I did not like it so well as when she played it—that was not to be expected. I sat during the evening next to Eliza Swinborne, from whom I had a congratulation on my pass and also a very hearty one from Mr Pattisson.

## Dr Simpson's practice expands and he buys a gig; royal celebrations; Gowers learns to smoke

Some good news in the Simpson household that month would soon provide a significant and welcome change in Gowers' routine, as well as that of the rest of the household in Church Street:

> Nothing important occurred to remark on this day. Stop! What am I talking about, something very important has occurred. Soon after lunch as I was sitting in the surgery Mrs Simpson came in and after a little conversation informed me she hoped to have some very good news to tell me this evening, namely that Mr Simpson was going to have Mr Christmas' practice, that it had been under consideration for some time and now it was only a matter of some ten pounds or so. And she had no doubt Mr Simpson himself would tell me at dinner. Mr Simpson, however, did not, and Mrs Simpson afterwards told me that it was all settled but that Christmas did not want it to be known about the town until Monday before which time it was not to be mentioned.

Not only was this to increase the number of patients Simpson visited, and therefore the number of cases Gowers visited alone, but also the area they had to cover.

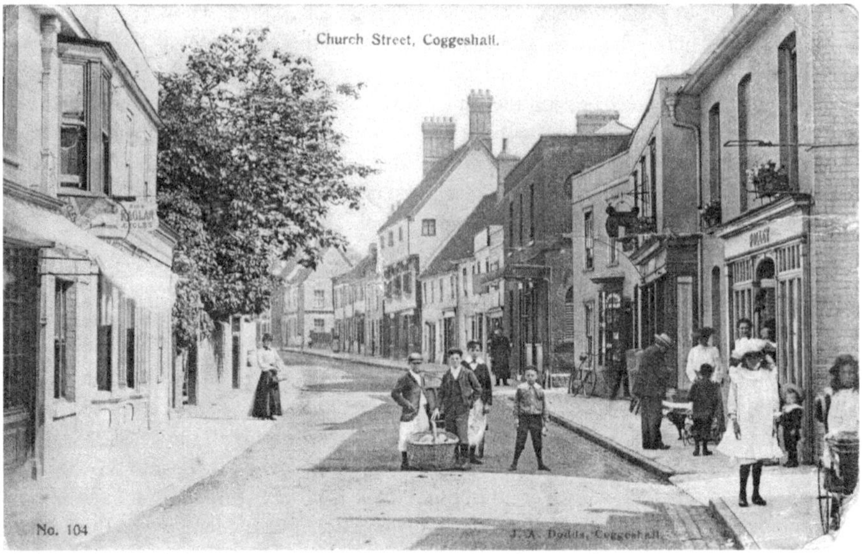


**Fig. 3.1** Church Street, Coggeshall (c. 1900). Courtesy of Coggeshall Museum and Heritage Centre.

The end of February came, and it was time for another, uncharacteristically brief, self-assessment.

> The last day of February has arrived. I have not accomplished nearly so much during this month as I should like to have done. Today, after lunch, I went down Stock Street to see the girl Fenn who was worse. I did during the evening German and French. I went to the Reading Room in the afternoon and there met Mr Dale who had returned. I borrowed from him Ollendorff's German dictionaries precisely the same work that I have borrowed from cousin Tom but in English instead of in French. I found it so extremely educational to get at the German idioms through the French idioms, so very, very much more out of them than from the English on account of the much greater similarity between the English and German languages than between French and German. In the evening I went out for half an hour's walk. The evening was exceedingly fine but I found the path I had chosen—down by the river—by Appleford and Barnard's Mills rather foggy and so returned sooner than I had at first intended. Mr Simpson has been very busy today seeing some of his new patients.

March began well. The Simpsons clearly needed a gig because the practice was now too large to manage on foot. Mrs Simpson took William to inspect one with her:

> I managed to get up soon after seven this morning but only looked over a little Latin prosody before breakfast. After breakfast I first ran over the whole of Chlorine, Bromine and Iodine and having some medicine to make up was not able to do anything else before eleven o'clock from when, till half past 12, I did botany, going over the epidermis and its appendages.

I walked in the afternoon down to the coach-builders with Mrs Simpson who went to look at a gig which Mr Simpson was thinking of buying. It is a small, low gig with, of course, two wheels. They settled to buy it.

A few days later Gowers was shocked when Simpson sent him off to see a dying patient without warning him of her condition:

After looking out Watson[2] on dropsy and heart disease, went up the Colchester Road to see an old woman who lives about a mile up there and who is ill. She is indeed dying of dropsy and heart disease. Her legs and the lower part of her body also, both of which she showed me without the slightest hesitation sitting in her chair, are swollen up to an enormous size. She seems almost dying; her lips have turned black within the last day or two. I have never seen her before for my governor only told me within the last few days. When speaking of the case to him after I came home that I wondered he had not told me about it before, he answered that he had not thought of it; I did not think that that was exactly right of him to forget so completely that he had a pupil.

At the beginning of March 1863 preparations were taking place across the country for celebrations to mark the impending royal wedding:

Arthur Gardner [the brewer's son] came in to tea, chiefly to talk about the rejoicings which are to take place here upon next Tuesday upon the occasion of the marriage of the Prince of Wales. There are to be scrambles for oranges, foot races, and climbing up the greasy pole and legs of mutton in the afternoon and in the evening a grand display of fireworks manufactured or purchased by Messrs William and James Surridge [auctioneers and estate agents from East Street].

I read Todd's *The Student's Guide*[3] for an hour or so and then did German for the rest of the afternoon. I am getting on with German nicely. The first book is divided into five months. Now by hard work I shall be able to get to the end of the first month on Saturday which will be just four weeks since I commenced the book. I did not do any French this evening. As for *Aids to Reflection* I have not been able to do anything much for some time but I must not leave off reading it.

There was also great excitement in the Simpson household when the gig arrived.

Mr Sharman and I had lunch alone together in the surgery. Mr and Mrs Simpson went out for a drive—this time in their own gig and harness but with Poulton's pony. They had a long drive—to Feering in one direction and to Pattiswick. Mr Sharman was dispatched immediately after lunch to Kelvedon by Mrs Simpson and I went out for a walk but before I got far I remembered that there was no-one at home except the servant and so I thought I had better go back.

After I returned I examined some specimens of leaves etc which I had brought home with me and then proceeded to do some German, for I had not done any last night and I am anxious to complete the first month's allotment by tomorrow evening.

Gowers was longing for an outing in the gig, and tried to be generous about not being offered one:

We have commenced lunching early in consequence of the gig being here every morning at twelve. Mr and Mrs Simpson had a long drive in it today running by the Teys, and Chappel and Colne as he had quite a few people to see. I wonder when I or Mr Sharman will get a drive, but it seems only fair that Mrs Simpson should wish to monopolise the

> possession of the second seat and that Mr Simpson should wish her to when one considers how fond they are of each other and how they must doubly enjoy the pleasures of the ride by each other's company. At times I feel rather grumbling at the monopoly but I always feel the utter unreasonableness of such dissatisfaction if it can be called so.

He and his friend Manthorp decided to walk to Braintree on Sunday afternoon to collect a dog for Manthorp. The entry is most notable because, during the course of the visit, Gowers received some surprising advice about preparing for a medical career.

> After dinner and dessert Manthorp and I started according to walk to Braintree. I had many, very many qualms of conscience about going and I felt plainly that it was an act of Sabbath breaking considering the object of the walk. However, having agreed to go I could not do otherwise and so we started. The day was tolerably fine though occasional dark clouds seemed to threaten.

They arrived in Braintree after being interrupted in their walk by a violent hailstorm which forced them to hide under umbrellas in the lee of a haystack:

> A rather equivocal day which was borne out by the actual experience of our walk. We first of all went to Reynolds, the man who it was that had the dog which was the object of our walk. He was not at home but the servant who opened the door informed us that Mr Christmas of Coggeshall was upstairs, and on going into a very fine large room we espied a man sitting smoking near the fireside.
>
> Now there are two brothers by the name of Christmas, one of whom has been in practice in Coggeshall, from whom Mr Simpson bought the practice a short time ago. The other, his brother, has been in Coggeshall for the last two months although I had never seen him and consequently did not know him by sight.
>
> When I went into the room I thought in my head of the elder R D Christmas, whom I know, and was rather astonished to see that he, as I thought, had shaved off all his whiskers except his lower lip just below his mouth and had his hair parted in the centre which he certainly did not have when I knew him. Nevertheless I concluded that it was the same and went unhesitatingly up to him and shook hands with him and presently remarked to him that it was a 'long time since I had seen him'. 'How long?' said he in a very queer kind of tone and looking rather hard at me. 'Oh, not since before I went up for my examination.' I said. He did not say anything particular, but by the conversation between him and Manthorp I soon discovered that it was not the Christmas I knew at all but his brother! . . . With him we stopped until nine, drinking and the two of them smoking, myself only having a glass of whiskey and water and all of us talking, especially Christmas and I on professional subjects. What an occupation for a Sunday evening!
>
> He is a jolly kind of fellow and recommended me to begin smoking for I should want it at the hospital and gave me a little advice as to the commencement.

London was a polluted, smelly city at that time, and London hospitals were only gradually learning about sanitation. Smoking must have protected doctors against the hospital smells, particularly post-mortems as Gowers had discovered in Coggeshall.

Gowers tried to contain his impatience while still waiting to be offered a ride in the gig:

> I felt rather stiff after the 12-mile walk as a thing which of late I have not been much used to. I was occupied during the whole morning by surgery work. I had the hope to have been

taken out with Mr Simpson today in the gig and took care to be dressed and with my boots on in case, but no: Mr Sharman went. It is the fifth day on which the governor has gone out and on the first three Mrs Simpson occupied the other seat and on the last two Mr Sharman has done so. I was greatly disappointed although I tried not to be and tried, and at times succeeded, in raising my spirits. My spirits are very, very easily disturbed and I do not know why it is but nowadays I seem to be continually put out. I think it is through spending so much of my time alone for I get into a brooding state which if I am not careful is very bad for me.

It is revealing that a book of essays by A. H. K. Boyd with the rather unprepossessing title *Leisure Hours in Town* made a great impression on him:

There is much in those essays which peculiarly affects me. Being brought into such intimate contact with the mind and soul of a good hard worker, of a genial soul which has no sympathy with idleness except so far as it cannot but have some sympathy with everything, such a soul, in a word, as is poured out in these essays, seems to have a peculiar action upon my own mind in making me thoroughly ashamed of my inactivity and backwardness, and of the little which I am doing to remedy that backwardness. The metaphor is a peculiar one, but the reading of a page or two of that Essayist's writings has the effect on me similar to the action of ergot of rye on women in labour, sharpening and restoring the pains which had well-nigh or entirely vanished.

Chapter headings in *Leisure Hours in Town*[4] give some idea of the essays that moved him: 'Concerning solitary days'; 'Concerning future years'; 'Concerning things slowly learnt'; 'Concerning veal: a discourse on immaturity'; 'Gone'; 'Concerning people of whom more might have been made'; 'Concerning people who carried weight in life: with some thoughts on those who never had a chance'. Boyd wrote of the weight of depression of spirits, of coping with loss, and of the need to resist giving up or going through life in a state of increasing bitterness. The essays are not all homilies, however. The final chapter, 'College life in Glasgow', is a colourful account of student life at Glasgow University.

Gowers may have been denied the experience of riding in the gig, but he was not going to delay taking the second Dr Christmas' advice about taking up smoking, summoning up considerable willpower to do so. In an entry clearly written under the influence of brandy, he wrote:

Immediately after lunch I went off to Kelvedon where I had announced my intention of going at breakfast and it might have been that which caused me not going with Mr Simpson as I cannot but think that it was in justice my turn and knowing how fond of riding with him, for I have often said so, Mr Simpson might have taken me. I felt that when Mr Simpson had taken everybody else and got tired of them he would take me!

I wanted to have my hair cut but I could not find a place which I thought would suit me. I entered a shop and bought an ounce of Warne's tobacco at a cost of 3½d and a small briarwood pipe for 8d together with a box of fuses. I had resolved to commence smoking operations in real earnest and accordingly came home through Felix Park and had several bits of smoke, about an eighth of a pipe apiece, and whenever I began to feel queasy leaving off and taking a little drop of strong brandy and water from a vial which I had in case of these consequences. In my last, however, I smoked at least a part of the whole pipe of which I congratulated myself. I think I shall get on; I like the pipe better than cigars. I was almost knocked up and so went to bed at about 11.

Gowers' sons remembered one of his favourite sayings in later life to be 'Smoking is a blessing to a busy man and a curse to an idle one'.

Study, the preoccupations with the gig, and smoking were all forgotten on the 10 March 1863, the day Coggeshall celebrated the marriage of the Prince of Wales to the Danish princess, Alexandra. Gowers enjoyed honing his descriptive powers for this diary entry:

> A day of days! A day of such rejoicing, such universal outburst of joy from every heart in England as has seldom been witnessed. Such a day as there has not been in England for the last quarter of a century; no day save that of the coronation of our Queen will bear comparison with it and even that half pales before the lustre on which the hope and heir of England took for his wife the fairest of all fair royal maidens in the world. The day has not been unworthy of the occasion. From every church tower and steeple have clanged out the notes of gladness all day long, in every village and town and city of the realm banqueted high and festively and from every place there burst forth the peculiar way in which the English like to testify to their joy. At least about here that has been the case and I believe over the kingdom. Hundreds and thousands of pounds of food have been consumed and hundreds of thousands of cubic feet of gas have been placed to illuminate, and hundreds and thousands of hungry poor have blessed the generosity of the loyal subjects of England from whom provisions had come. . . .
>
> The day was a general holiday here. All the shops etc. being closed. The afternoon was given up to sports of various kinds of races—both foot and donkey, climbing the greasy pole for legs of mutton etc, etc. Including, I am sorry to say, an intention which does not reflect very highly upon the members of the committee for arranging the games: races of women for dresses—however, fortunately for the credit of Coggeshall, none could be found willing to run. The evening was given up to fireworks and bonfires on Market Hill, a little open space in the middle of the town, where there was a good display prepared chiefly by William and James Surridge. I went down several times to see the games and fireworks. In the evening squibs, crackers and serpents were flying too in all directions among the crowd and all day long half a dozen young fellows were continually firing off pistols close to one's ears. I too kept the holiday for I did not do any study at all.

Three days later, he had another cause for rejoicing when he had his first ride in the gig:

> At last my long-expected turn came. Mr Simpson favoured me by taking me out with him today! It was a pleasant drive round by the Tey Road, Feering and Kelvedon and also West Street Coggeshall, being out, in all, three hours.
>
> I was occupied for almost the whole of the evening by writing to Charlotte whose birthday next Sunday is. She will be 21. I had several fractions of pipes today but taking care not to have too much.

For the remainder of his time in Coggeshall Gowers was amply rewarded for his enthusiasm for the gig. He was trusted to drive it, having learned to drive when working on the farm in Yorkshire, and from then on was frequently called upon not only to accompany Mr Simpson, but also to take Mrs Simpson out when she wished to go for a ride. He enjoyed displaying his skills in the driver's seat:

> I had a treat today. Mr Simpson was out and so I drove Mrs Simpson out for a couple of hours and we had a very pleasant round—going through Colne and thence round by

Chappel to Great Tey and so home. I have not studied well today I am sorry to record. The weather has been most splendid; today was a most magnificent day, weather of the height of summer—hot and cloudless as an August afternoon. I found I had not forgotten the art of driving, and coming home received a compliment from Mrs Simpson that I was a 'capital driver'.

He was growing up. His last entry as a 17-year-old describes being distracted in chapel by the presence of a beautiful young woman:

There is now staying at the Matthew Gardners' one of the most lovely girls I have ever seen: the elder of two cousins of Alfred's from Hackney. They were both at chapel this evening and I had great difficulty in restraining my eye from watching them more than was consistent with politeness. I have not spoken to them since they came a week ago, but soon after I first came down here they spent an evening here.

A new section of the diary starts on 23 March 1863, three days after his eighteenth birthday. In later life he had a fascination for inventing gadgets and medical instruments. At the age of 18 he was experimenting with hookah construction, perhaps as an alternative to smoking his briar pipe. Hookahs were fashionable in Victorian England. There is no suggestion that he used it for anything but tobacco, although later on he was an advocate of the use of cannabis for certain neurological disorders.

I have commenced my nineteenth year in circumstances anything but favourable to journal-keeping; for on the day before my birthday—I, experimenting in hookah-constructing when I ought to have been at my studies, managed to inflict an ugly cut on my thumb with a piece of glass tube, which utterly incapacitated me from holding a pen and writing at all legibly.

My birthday I spent much as other days. I went out for a drive with Mr Simpson, a longish one in point of time, although the distance over which we went was not great. On my return at four o'clock, coming into the surgery I was rather astonished to find no less than five letters upon my surgery table, one from Mother—a kind, good, motherly letter, another from my cousin Charlotte enclosing a very nice set of gold studs.

The Simpsons gave him a drink of sherry and they drank 'many happy returns', and then he visited his grandmother and aunt in West Street.

The end of March was unseasonably hot:

The weather for this time of year is certainly most surprising. Yesterday was a most intensely hot day. I took Mrs Simpson up to Mrs Marshall, but before I did that I had to wait for her in Kelvedon Street in the full glare of the sun which was not the most pleasant thing in the world.

A couple of days later he was able to report more positively on another outing with the doctor's wife, but visiting a patient on the way:

We went to Colne, and then a little way along the Halstead Road, and then returned by the high road to Coggeshall. We just called at the house and then went down Stock Street to see the girl Fane. I felt remarkably professional leaving the gig and going into the cottage to see my patient.

At the end of March he had another of his outings with his friend Manthorp:

At half past three I set off with my friend Manthorp for Colchester, our plan being to walk to Marks Tey and from thence take the train to Colchester. When we reached Marks Tey, however, we found that we still had three quarters of an hour wait, during which time we went into the Prince of Wales public house, and had a glass of porter. We didn't reach Colchester until nearly six, and it was quite six by the time we had climbed the hill and were fairly into High Street. We walked about a bit and then I, fancying that Manthorp wanted to go somewhere alone, told him not to scruple to leave me by myself if he wanted to go anywhere; so he did, having appointed a quarter past seven for tea at the Red Lion.

I then went and got my hair cut and then strolled about—down East Hill first, and on returning I saw a poor dog run over close to me—it was going along the road and didn't notice the horse and cart which was coming, when the horse, striking the dog with its shoe, knocked it over and just as it was getting up, the wheel passed over its loins. The poor thing ran howling away, but its cries soon ceased—terminated I should hope by death. It gave me a tremendous 'turn' for of all things I think I dislike to see dumb animals hurt in any way the most.

After a little further stroll down St Botolph's I returned to meet Manthorp and we went to the Red Lion to tea. I mustn't omit to mention that before getting my hair cut I went and got a pipe and a tobacco pouch. I could not get such a pipe as I wanted, and so contented myself with a nice looking briar pipe with a small amber tip, which cost me only a shilling. On being shown into the room at the Red Lion I was astonished at the set-out which was being prepared for us, for I had anticipated nothing but a bit of bread and butter and a cup of tea, and behold there was, besides tea and bread and butter, an untouched piece of cold roast beef and an untouched tongue, into which we pitched with a vehemency the effects of which soon became visible upon the eatables. Manthorp paid for the supper, which I must say had given me considerable apprehensions as to the price, but they only charged 3/6 for the two of us.

At eight we started to go home, having a companion for the first two miles, a very pleasant fellow, an exciseman who had been at Coggeshall about a fortnight. We had a tolerably pleasant walk, although I felt wretchedly tired; but when we got back to Marks Tey we stopped there and refreshed ourselves with some porter, managing to dispose of a pint apiece. We had intended to stop there only a quarter of an hour, but a very heavy shower nearly trebled the time. Manthorp and another man sang a song, and we were a jolly party in the room. I have no time to describe the company who were gathered there separately although I had intended it at first, but I don't think it would be worth the trouble. At half past ten we left there and had a nice walk to Coggeshall. This part of the walk Manthorp managed to enliven nicely by singing all the songs he knew, which were about a dozen. I was not sorry to tumble into bed soon after I reached home, where I found all retired, bar the servant who was sitting up for me.

Gowers was given practice in minor dentistry. In Coggeshall the major extractions were timed to coincide with the presence of the local brass band, who played loudly to drown the sound of the patients' protesting screams. Gowers' experiences were less dramatic. He was sent to borrow some 'tooth stopping instruments', before he and Simpson visited a girl who required her teeth stopping: Mr Simpson did one and Gowers the other. On another occasion the local innkeeper came in to the surgery to have a tooth extracted. Gowers examined the tooth, saw that it was already loose, and assured the man that he would have it out in half a minute, 'which I accurately did'.

Mr Simpson's expanded practice involved much more travelling for both of them. On one occasion Gowers recorded a round trip of 20 miles in one afternoon.

On Good Friday he had time to combine work, social life and an intellectual discussion:

> I was roused from my slumbers and reminded of the day it was by hearing at a little before eight the cry of 'One a penny, two a penny, hot cross buns', reiterated under my window, but the attractions and charms of bed were so strong that I did not rise until nearly half an hour after the time when I woke; but I came down before the bacon had been finished cooking.
>
> I studied for a little in the morning, and walked for about an hour from two to three in order to get an appetite for my dinner. At four we went, according to invitation, to dinner next door at the Pattissons. No-one else was there except Louisa Davids, daughter of the independent minister at Colchester, who is without exception the cleverest girl I have met, but unfortunately she is rather affected, which detracts considerably from her agreeableness.
>
> She is a splendid German scholar as well as very good at French, and knows something of Italian, Latin, and Greek. She has lately been chiefly employed in translating from German into English. I was fortunate enough to sit next to her during dinner and so had a good deal of talk with her. After dinner we played at croquet in the garden until it was quite dark and we could see no longer.
>
> Indoors afterwards I had some talk with Miss Davids about German. She does not speak at all highly about Ollendorff's work on which I am at work now, and I certainly think I shall not go on with it for several reasons. There is so very much repetition in it, and the exercises take me such an immense time to do that it will be September before I get through the first volume. The work seems to me calculated chiefly for working with under a master, and also for those who wish to learn the language with as little labour and real study as possible, and above all Miss Davids says that the German is not at all good. So that I think it will be much better for me to go on with Cassell's lessons in German[5] which Mrs Dale has lent me and by which I shall be able to get up the rudiments much more completely before I go up to London than if I kept on with Ollendorff.
>
> We had some music up in the drawing room and I had a game of chess with Miss Davids, and after a little supper we left at about half past ten.

## Gowers goes into print for the first time

One of Gowers' favourite relaxations in later life was chess, a skill he developed while in Coggeshall. He began to play regularly with his friend Alfred Gardner, son of the owner of the Little Coggeshall brewery, 'He and I anticipate having a good many games during this summer, and I sincerely wish we may'. However, he was about to lose one of his most reliable and valued Coggeshall mentors, Mr Dale. In March he had written:

> I am sorry to say there is a great probability of his leaving Coggeshall in a short time for he has been much wanted to take the pastorship of a church at Halifax in Yorkshire, and from the conversation I had with him yesterday, I think there is every probability that he will accept it. . . . I shall be very, very sorry for him to go, for he has been very kind to me, and I had been anticipating still greater things to be derived from himself and his library.

This prediction proved right. When Dale gave his farewell sermon in April the Congregational chapel was packed:

> The chapel was crowded, even up the whole of the pulpit stairs to the very door of the pulpit itself. The sermon was not so pathetic as I expected, but probably Mr Dale dared not trust himself to treat of that; indeed, as it was, he could barely get through the service.

Gowers had his first taste of writing for publication after he attended the public farewell for Dale:

> Last night was a great event to the congregational part of Coggeshall community, for a testimonial was presented to Mr Dale at a public meeting held at the Independent Chapel. Mr Davids of Colchester took the Chair, and the task of making the presentation speech devolved upon my governor, who got through it pretty well. Afterwards Mr Dale returned thanks. . . .
>
> I took some notes—tolerably copious—of the two first speeches, and today I wrote out a brief report and, for a spree chiefly, sent a copy of my short epitome of the chief speeches to Mr Bell, who is going to write the notice for a paper for which he is agent here: then I wrote out a complete, although brief, report, and sent it to Abbott, who said he would send it up to his paper—he also is agent and local correspondent for the *Essex Standard*, and then mirabile dictu—wrote out another copy of my little report and—sent it up to the editor of the *London Morning Star*!!!! I don't at all suppose he will put it all in, but I think it is just possible he may insert a notice of the meeting, and even put a full report in if he happens just then to be short of matter and with plenty of room.

The following day the Simpsons held a private farewell dinner for Dale, and the Surridges and the Beaumonts 'came down to have a last sight of Dale'. On 24 April Gowers called on the Dales to say goodbye. 'He said that I was quite welcome to keep the books of his which I have some time longer and he has asked me when I go to Yorkshire to go and see him at Halifax and I can then bring them with me.' Dale also gave him some books to keep.

Dale was succeeded by Alfred Downing Philps who, like Dale, had studied at Hackney College. Although he was not ordained pastor at Coggeshall until 1864 he took over from Dale immediately. Gowers referred later to the strong spiritual guidance he received from Philps. Philps was impressed by the young man, so much so that he took Gowers to London to meet William Jenner sometime that year (though this event is not recorded in the diaries).

The day after he said goodbye to Bryan Dale, Gowers recorded delight with his first publications:

> It is a queer sensation, that of seeing one's writing in print for the first time. I experienced that this morning, for I saw two newspapers in both of which my report appeared—the one I gave to Abbott slightly modified in one or two things by him, but in all other respects essentially my report. A word put in here and there, one sentence at the close of Mr David's speech, and a few 'hear hears' interspersed were all the difference from my own copy. In the *Morning Star* no notice has yet appeared, but its columns have been so occupied by other news lately that perhaps that may account for it.

## Death of the Yorkshire farmer

But Gowers had to suffer a more personal, permanent loss that April. He had heard in March that both Joseph Hurst and Charlotte Venables were ill:

> This morning's post brought me a letter from mother containing some very bad news, namely that my friend—I had almost said my brother—Joseph Hurst is very dangerously ill, and also that my cousin Charlotte has had the diphtheria but is now better. I am very sorry to hear such bad news.

A week later he heard that Joseph had died:

> By the midday post a letter came for me from my mother. I had been looking anxiously for one to tell me how my friend Joseph Hurst was. The letter told me he was dead. Mother broke the sad news as gently to me as she could in her letter, but it was sadly unexpected, as I had all along cherished hopes that today would bring me better news of him, but no—he died on Good Friday. . . .
>
> I hardly realise it, that Joseph is really gone, gone forever. I can hardly even now realise that he is dead. It is the first time that death has removed anyone dear to me since my father died. He was the oldest and dearest friend I have had, and, my father excepted, he was dearer and nearer to my heart than any other of my own sex. As a boy I worshipped him, my beau ideal of a farmer and a man, and as I grew up I learned to respect and love him, which was strengthened by the winter I passed learning farming under him previous to my coming to Coggeshall.

His mother had also formed a close attachment to Hurst and Gowers was concerned that she felt Joseph's death 'very very deeply I am afraid, but that is only what might have been expected from their close intimacy from so long'. Hurst was buried two days later in Arksey. Ann Gowers wrote to her son 'You will be sure I feel it deeply, for he had been much with us all and had looked upon me as a true friend and counsellor, which I trust I have been'. At the end of her letter, describing preparations for a great fair which was to be held on the Monday, and for which she had some little girls staying at her house, she wrote, to her son's obvious distress 'But I shall not be here, for I shall be at Bentley with my best lover'. 'The last word is a very singular one to be used by her' confided Gowers to his diary.

On the day of Hurst's burial Gowers confided his feelings to his diary once again:

> From what my mother has told me in her letter of his condition, I have no doubt that he is now with the spirits of the just men and perfect. I wonder if there are recognitions up in heaven? If so it is possible that my father and Joseph have met and talked together, and perhaps my father may have heard some news of me and may at this moment be talking of me. I wonder if the spirits of the happy dead are permitted to wander invisibly on the earth; if so, dear Joseph may be in this room at this moment, may be with me looking over my shoulder and watching into my most inmost thoughts. Oh death, what a mystery thou art! No spirit which has returned to this earth has ever been allowed to give the slightest information respecting the things that are 'beyond the veil' as Tennyson words it.

By May, Gowers was seriously weighing up whether it would be wiser to take the Preliminary Scientific Examination in the coming July or delay it by a year, as permitted under the rules:

> In a ride to Pattiswick I took advantage of the opportunity to speak to Mr Simpson respecting my July examination, and he quite agreed in the opinion I have formed respecting the practicability of going up now or in the following year; as, so far as I can find out it will make no difference whatever to the period at which I shall ultimately take my degree.
>
> It will be a very great deal better for me not to go up for this preliminary examination until the next year, when, after I have been at the hospital a year, and have been under the

practical and theoretical chemistry man. Williamson, who was one of the Examiners at the University of London, I have no doubt that I shall be able to get through very comfortably, and it will be much better for me not to risk it this July. In which case, according to a letter I received from Mother yesterday, I am not to go to Yorkshire this summer! It will be a disappointment for I had been calculating upon a trip to the North—Doncaster and Halifax—and shall be for many reasons very sorry not to be able to see the place again before I enter upon my London career, after which I shall not be able to for a long time.

May came, and by this time taking 'the governor' out in the gig had become a regular routine:

I didn't get up this morning in time to do any study before breakfast, and after the surgery people had been I didn't do as much as I ought to have done. I am very far from feeling satisfied with the manner in which I am going on now, for it seems to me that it is very far from what it should be. I did nothing of any importance from lunch—which was finished by twelve—to nearly two, and then went out for a walk—examined the plantation near Monk Downs, and then went to Ladywoods, which I didn't go into, however, as there were some workmen at work in it, and I didn't care to trespass before them for fear one of them should happen to be half a gamekeeper. After dinner and the surgery work Alfred Gardner came and asked me to come and join him in a game at quoits, to which of course I had but very little objection.

Soon after tea the governor was sent for to go to Pattiswick, and I went with him and drove him there. The case was a labour, but he was not engaged more than a quarter of an hour, as it was half over when he got there. The night was a very fine one, the moon being at the full, and I enjoyed half a pipe in the moonlight outside Pattiswick Church where I was waiting in the gig. After we returned we drove up to Poultons and then I stepped to Schofields and got a cigar for a treat for myself tomorrow, and as I was going back spoke to William Spurge who was standing at his door. He wanted me to come in and have a glass of wine with him, to which I saw after no objection and went in and stopped about half an hour and smoked a pipe and a half, to Amy [Mrs] Spurge's horror.

## Botanizing

Gowers' trips in the gig did not diminish his pleasure in walking, which was now enhanced by the excitement of botanizing, which he started to devote time to in May 1863. Botany was a popular pastime in Victorian England, and many medical men were interested in it. The eighteenth-century Swedish botanist Carl Linnaeus, the 'father of modern taxonomy' had introduced a new binominal naming system for plants. In the first half of the nineteenth century, when doctors first began to make physical examinations of their patients, the results were recorded using similar descriptive classification methods. Once qualified, Gowers applied these classification methods to his cases. The description of 'diseases' was advanced by correlating physical signs with post-mortem findings:

Medicine carried on the work of Linnaeus: just as he had described different kinds of plants and arranged them, by virtue of these descriptions into related groups, so the physical changes in organs discovered post-mortem were related to causal factors and clinical syndromes discovered during life and classified into a system of 'diseases'.[6]

Professor John Henslow had recently rejuvenated the study of botany in Cambridge, with Charles Darwin as one of his many followers. Darwin had studied medicine in Edinburgh, but he disliked the sight of blood and found his lecturers dull so left without a degree. His father sent him to Cambridge to study in the hope that he would take holy orders. However, Darwin gradually changed his focus to botany and other natural sciences. In 1831 Henslow founded the Botanical Gardens in Cambridge. A clergyman, in 1837 he moved to a living in Hitcham, Suffolk, where he founded the Hitcham Parish School in 1841 giving classes in botany and 'general scientific thinking'. He also was influential in the establishment of the nearby Ipswich Museum in 1847, based on 'natural history'. He published a *Catalogue of British Plants* in 1829 (with a second edition in 1835); *Principles of Descriptive and Physiological Botany* (1835); and *Flora of Suffolk* in 1866. So there was already a strong interest in botanical inquiry in East Anglia.

Botany was seen as a significant area of study for medical students in the second half of the nineteenth century. The surgeon and educator Sir James Paget was an enthusiastic amateur botanist as a boy, and at the age of 20 had published a botanical study of the Yarmouth area with his brother.[7] He remarked later that his botanical studies had no practical utility in his career, but although the knowledge was useless, the discipline of acquiring it was beyond all price.

> Plants are arranged by their external characters, among which there are innumerable affinities that cannot be seen and contemplated, without imparting acuteness to the faculties of observation, and establishing a habit of natural classification which is beneficial throughout life. In these respects, I know of no science that can be compared with botany.[8]

In 1864 a lecturer in botany from St George's Hospital responded to someone's criticism of how botany was taught, writing:

> It is not necessary to enter into detail as to the method pursued by botanical lecturers; suffice it to say that the course followed is one laid down for them by the authorities; and it is one which, in most if not in all the schools, involves a great deal of practical demonstration, while the pupils are encouraged to write descriptions of plants, or fill up 'schedules', which are corrected by the teacher. This practice of writing correct, terse descriptions is particularly valuable.

The writer bemoaned, as specialist teachers often do, that insufficient time was devoted to the subject in the medical schools, but suggested that really botany in medical school should be 'advanced botany':

> The pupil, with his elementary knowledge, would, when he entered upon the advanced class at the medical school, be far better enabled to estimate the bearings of the science on his medical studies than he now is; would be far more likely, should his tastes and means allow him to do so, to pursue it for its own sake.

He goes on to emphasize the benefits of practical experience pointing out that the Society of Apothecaries had reorganized the Physic Garden at Chelsea for the prosecution of botany.[9]

The time Gowers spent at Coggeshall in 'botanizing', taking advantage of the wild and diverse countryside around him, demonstrates one of the benefits of serving a country apprenticeship, and laid a solid foundation for his future work.

At about quarter past twelve I started off a good long walk to Greenstead Green, which is at least five miles off, to take a note from Mr Simpson to Mr Bentall to ask him what is the best work on British Botany. Mr Bentall is the celebrated manufacturer of botanical paper, for which he has some large works at Halstead, and he lives at a new house about three miles from the town. He was exceedingly kind and civil, bringing and showing me several books, but the two which he strongly recommended were Babington's *Manual of British Botany*[10] and Gibson's *Flora of Essex*[11], both of which, when I got home, Mr Simpson ordered.

He took me to a bog upon his land where he showed me several very rare plants, and we had a most interesting botanical conversation; and he is one of the very first botanists in the country. I hope I have profited by what he said. I stopped with him about an hour and walked home botanizing on my way, and being fortunate enough to find the white sorrel near Marks Hall deer park, a plant which is considered very rare in this neighbourhood. But the flower which we had brought to us a few days ago is of a plant which is only known to grow in one locality in Essex, so if we are right in our opinion as to what it is, and I do not doubt we are, we shall have the honour of having added another to its habits. After I came home, arranging and identifying my specimens took up a long time, until I could see no longer, and looking over botanical books occupied me for some little time after that.

He bought his botanical paper from Bentall's mill (which he found to his surprise was nothing to do with his friend Thomas Bentall, farmer and botanist). And there are other typical entries around this time:

Immediately after lunch I started off for Mr [Tom] Bentall's at Greenstead, which I reached in an hour from the time of starting, and had to walk pretty quickly for it. On approaching his house I noticed all his blinds down, and had made up my mind to an announcement of his absence from home, so it was an agreeable disappointment when on asking if he were home I learned that he was. He was exceedingly kind, for although he was rather pressed for time he gave up an hour to me and gave me three specimens of rare plants, as well as showing me his herbarium and press.

Not having had any walk at all yesterday, I resolved to have a good one today, so I started directly after lunch and went up by Curd Hall into Woodhouse Lane and down that, and then across Felix Hall part, and then nearly to Kelvedon, and then back again and about half a mile towards Rivenhall, and back home by the Kelvedon road, having had a most delightful walk of about eleven or twelve miles, and with a crammed tin case and a handful of specimens, having botanized on the way, with very good success. . . .

The greater part of the morning was occupied by me in seeing to specimens. At about half past twelve I set off and walked to Greenstead Green, but unfortunately Mr Bentall was not at home; but I took French leave and went and had a look over his bog, getting a nice little specimen of the alternate-leaved saxifrage, and also two of the myosotis, one of which, in consequence of some imperfection of the roots, has the flowers the same colour as the flowers generally are when the first burst forth. I had a very pleasant walk home through the woods, and found many flowers—four of them which I didn't know before I took them home and studied them and ascertained the names. After dinner I saw to the surgery, arranged my specimens, wrote a letter to my dear mother, whose birthday tomorrow is. . . .

> After breakfast I was busy in the surgery etc for some time, but afterwards managed to do a little bit of chemistry, and after lunch some botany. I was also occupied by clearing out a little in the surgery immediately after lunch, and then at about half past two I went out, first down to see grandmother, and then to Cooney for my umbrella, which was less money than I expected, and then walked as far as the plantation near Monks Down in which I found several plants, and amongst them one which when I got home I identified as the evergreen alkanet, a plant which is rather rare, only growing in about four localities in the country, of which the one I have found is not one, so I may consider that I have discovered it. It will be a little bit of news for Mr Bentall when I go over there. After my return at about four until dinner I was occupied by looking over and identifying the specimens I had brought in with me, and after dinner for some time I was busy changing the papers of nearly all the specimens I have dried.
>
> I did geometry, algebra, and some German, and also some German afterwards. After the surgery I studied chemistry etc until lunch, and afterwards I drew some diagrams of the pulley, and then did a very little botany, and [after going out] wrote out some notes on zoology and went and got a specimen of a plant growing in the small plantation near Monk Downs which I think . . . has not been found in Essex! If so, it will be the making of my reputation as a botanist, but I am afraid it is too good to be correct, and that I have made some mistake. However, I shall take it over to Mr Bentall tomorrow, and have his opinion about it.

One day that May there was a serious injury to a man in Coggeshall which, coming after a day of botanizing, resulted in a very long day's work:

> I was met by a man with the announcement that a man in Stock Street had been brought home with his thigh broken by a wagon having gone over it. I immediately set to work to find the governor; he was not at home, and as usual had not left any word as to his whereabouts, but by good fortune I found him at the first place I went to, where he was smoking a pipe and drinking gin and water. We came home and got splints and bandages ready and then set off on foot to Stock Street. We found the man lying on a bed on the floor of the cottage with his thigh fearfully crushed, the bone apparently shattered and a great loss of blood. I returned for an inclined plane and Mr Giles, both of which I brought back with me; and the leg was then moved into a little better position. We remained with him until past nine, and came home. If ever I was tired in my life it ought to be this evening, for I have walked at the least about 23 miles.

Another medical dilemma presented itself, within his own family. In 1853 vaccination for smallpox, the disease which had been a scourge in the eighteenth century, had been made compulsory. Many Dissenters refused vaccination on the grounds that deliberately implanting a disease into a healthy person risked breaching the Sixth Commandment, 'Thou shalt not kill'. Gowers did not agree, and was concerned about the welfare of his cousins in West Street, where his uncle Henry Foster had refused to have his children vaccinated:

> In the evening I was busy nearly the whole time in the surgery and also went down and had half an hour's conversation with Uncle on the subject of vaccination, trying to induce him to have his children vaccinated.

Despite vaccination being made compulsory, the century's severest epidemic of smallpox occurred in 1870.

The annual Coggeshall Fair was held on Whitsunday at the end of May. Gowers, who had been reading Charlotte Bronte's novels, and her biography, tries a new literary style:

> Coggeshall Fair Day! Certainly that sentence deserved to be written in longhand, if ever a sentence did. I walked through it in the afternoon—there were actually three cows standing there and a drove of sheep, a few beasts and calves and about half a dozen horses and several shows of various sorts upon the Market Hill—not omitting the omnipresent merry-go-round complete the category of this annual much-anticipated and I daresay much regretted event of the Coggeshall year. Anticipated by the servants of all kinds, to whom this day is the only holiday that the year brings, and regretted by many, very many I fear who make their first introduction to vice this day, and by many innkeepers whom deluding hopes induced to provide sumptuous repasts to remain uneaten on the table and who look in vain for custom where money there is none. What nonsense I am writing.

June started off with a trip to Feering 'to see a man who had been attacked with haemoptysis in the morning, or in common parlance had broken a blood vessel' (a rare Gowers inaccuracy, it means coughing up blood). The day ended with an eclipse of the moon, which Gowers stayed up late to watch.

In June he records being trusted to drive the Beaumonts' four-wheel pony trap.

> By means of going to bed at an early hour last night—namely ten o'clock—I fortunately woke at about five, and didn't lose much time in getting out of bed and my clothes on and myself in my surgery chair—distinguished from the others by means of a small square cushion and to work. On the whole, with the exception of the evening, I think I can consider this day a pretty good one. I did mathematics until nearly six-thirty, and then a little of an *Ode* of Horace until seven, and then German until breakfast. After breakfast my specimens, the surgery, and the arranging a glass tube in a cork for a castor-oil bottle in the surgery took up my time until eleven, when I did a little chemistry and botany for about an hour and a half.
>
> Mrs Simpson suddenly came in and asked me to drive her to Braintree in Mr Beaumont's pony and four-wheel, and I had no alternative but to comply, even had my inclination been opposed to it, which most decidedly it wasn't. We had a tolerably pleasant ride there and back hearing some thunder coming on whilst there, also some rain both going and returning, but we didn't reach home until nearly four, from which time until dinner I wrote out some notes on natural philosophy and botany.
>
> After a good dinner I felt but little inclined for any hard work, and so did first the surgery dispensing and then a scene and a half of a play of Scribe's [a French dramatist], and then copied out a little of the 'Ancient Mariner'. Then Alfred Gardner came and I had to go and have a game at chess with him, when to recompense me for going without my tea, he gave me some moselle; and having drunk about half a dozen glasses over a cigarette I admit I could not do anything when I came home, and finished by smoking a pipe and drinking gin-and-water with Manthorp here; which left me in a state not fit for writing my journal or for anything.

Evidently the Coggeshall Congregationalists were not teetotallers. Another day he describes a typical day's study, punctuated by his daily walk:

> I studied geometry and then a little Latin and then some German. From eleven to lunch I was busy at chemistry, also afterwards for about an hour. I then studied more natural

> philosophy and also some botany and some zoology. I went for a short walk before dinner. I happened to meet with Mr Giles and his son returned from Cambridge laden with honour, having taken off the first mathematical prize of his college. I walked along with them as far as they were going, namely about half a mile along the Colne road. The evening was swallowed up by the surgery, chess, a chat with Alfred Gardner about commencing French lessons, and a little of the exercises which Angus gives upon the syntax of the English language.

He agreed with Alfred Gardner that they would meet each morning to study French together. Gowers decided to reinforce his learning by keeping part of his diary in a special pocket book he started for French, so entries in his shorthand diary become less frequent. At the end of June he also made his first formal, social 'call':

> I got ready, and set forth on an expedition which I looked forward to with considerable mistrust, not to say dread, namely making my 'call' on Mrs Surridge after the party which I attended at their house on Friday last. Being about the first fashionable morning call I have ever paid, a certain amount of uneasiness respecting the way in which I should conduct myself was rather allowable, but the result, I am happy to say, proved that it was entirely unnecessary.
>
> On entering, after having first achieved a fair knock at the door, an operation I can seldom perform to my own satisfaction, I was shown into the drawing room, and upon the servant asking my name pulled out my card case and handed her a card—one of my own, and not that of a hairdresser nor of my friend Parker of Shamrock Lodge, which I had in there, and which I had seriously debated on my own account before going, as to whether I should remove them from a place where their presence might cause so terrible a catastrophe as the presentation of one of them. Presently Mrs Surridge came in and asked me to go with her into the office, where Mr Surridge was, and not to consider it a formal call. Accordingly I followed her and seated myself in an armchair there, and she brought another one and sat down, and we three chatted very pleasantly (although I am afraid rather stupidly on my part) for about twenty minutes, and then I left, at least not dissatisfied with my first call, but by no means sorry to have got it over.

## Meeting Cornelius Walford

Towards the end of June 1863 Gowers attended the local 'Hay Party', another event he had been dreading. However, he enjoyed himself far more than expected. He met the son of a well-known naturalist, Cornelius Walford, who lived at Park House Farm near Coggeshall. The son, also Cornelius, was interesting to Gowers for a number of reasons: he was an expert in life insurance (Gowers became an assurance assessor in later life); he was an experienced writer who had edited the *British Controversialist and Literary Magazine*, a journal 'devoted to the impartial and deliberate discussion of important questions in religion, philosophy, history, politics, social economy, and to the promotion of self-culture and general education'. He was also a member of the Statistical Society, which had been established in 1834 by a group including mathematician Charles Babbage. Finally, Walford was a strong advocate for using plain language when writing for publication, and the use of shorthand when drafting. Gowers described their meeting in detail:

> I am writing this morning, although I want it to be an entry of yesterday's events. The great, the dreadful, Hay Party is over. We went soon after two, and found ourselves among

> the first, the only ones who were there being Miss Denny and Mr Walford. This Mr Walford, being in his way rather a distinguished fellow, must have a few words of introduction. He is a nice-looking man of, I should think, about thirty-five years of age with a black moustache and a beard, thin face, tall figure. He is a very clever and rather notable fellow, being considered to know more about life insurance than anyone else in the country. He is also an important member of the Statistical Society, and is a frequent contributor to *The Times*. Before I went home I had a chat with Walford, which I enjoyed the most of all the afternoon's entertainments. I was standing by the door, and he and old Gardner [Alfred's father] were walking near, when I distinguished a word which fell upon my heart—'phonetic shorthand'. I went up to them and told Walford that the word struck a chord in my heart, and then we had about half an hour's chat, chiefly upon shorthand, literary composition etc, on both of which subjects he may be regarded as a tolerably competent authority, having been a phonographer for twenty years, and for six years having been editor of the *British Controversialist*. . . .
>
> One of the things he spoke of in reference to literary composition was the necessity of expressing one's thoughts in the briefest possible manner. He says that shorthand is perfectly available for literary composition. The way in which he does all his composition now is to dictate to phonetic secretaries, who transcribe it into longhand and—there it is! This is the way in which he has written two or three papers which he has read before the Statistical Society.

Walford became first president of the Shorthand Society when it was founded in 1881. Meeting him influenced Gowers in a number of ways, not least because it reinforced his conviction about the value of shorthand, and he later put into practice Walford's advice that day. Having had his interest in shorthand reinforced by such an authority, he decided to join the Phonetic Lines Society:

> Three or four days ago I made up my mind to join the 'Phonetic Lines', and accordingly sent a short note to the Secretary, Mr Henry Booth, to inform him of it, and to do the most important part—forward my subscription, which was not much, only sixpence entrance fee and one shilling annual subscription. Today I received an answer from him—a letter, a good long one too, in answer to some questions I asked relative to the present state of the 'Lines', and the probability of any important changes being made in the 10th edition, and by the same post I received a 'card of membership' neatly got up and having the objects of the Society printed upon it.

Gowers received packages of books through the Mechanics' Institute. The first Mechanics' Institute, dedicated to the education of working people, had been established in London in 1823 by George Birkbeck. By the time Gowers was an apprentice a network of Mechanics' Institutes had been developed, providing university education for people who could not afford to study full-time. Gowers' diaries record his studying German, Greek, Latin, chemistry, botany, zoology, mathematics, geometry, English language, and 'natural philosophy'. Typical entries read:

> I finished the *First Book of Euclid* in Lardner's Edition, and also the thirteenth exercise of Collins' *Algebra* and then did some German till breakfast, and afterwards, till the surgery people began to come, when I had to come up; and they bothered me for a longish time. Read chemistry, botany, natural philosophy, and zoology today, and altogether got on very well, not going for a walk in consequence of the rain, but doing some Latin just

before dinner. I finished 'Adrienne Lecouvreur', who dies—a very different sort of ending from what I expected, but I nevertheless liked it exceedingly, and have been much amused, as well as interested in its perusal. . . .

The postman has looked upon me with favourable eye today. By the early post I received two book parcels, one containing four French newspapers from Cousin Tom, and the other a lecture I had written up for, from Walton and Moberley on 'Self Training for the Medical Student'. . . .

Did no studying this morning except a little practical botany, a very little German and a little osteology, namely recapitulation of the scapularis, the humerus, the radius and the ulna. A great deal of time was occupied by dispensing. . . .

## Preparing to move to London; the search for lodgings; farewell to Coggeshall

By August 1863, Gowers' apprenticeship was nearly over. His mother had decided to leave Doncaster for good and provide a home for her son, and her niece Charlotte Venables, in London. She arranged to meet her son in London to start searching for somewhere to live. He went to greet her at King's Cross station:

> She had a heavy carpet bag and a basket nearly as heavy and I could not prevail upon her to take the subterranean railway, so we took an omnibus to the Tottenham Court Road, and thence by a yellow omnibus to Westminster. My dear mother is, I am happy to say, looking extremely well. Her poor gloves were far from immaculate, for they looked as if they had a good many times by actual experience the power of friction, and I made a mental vow when I could afford it, that is to say if she and I are spared until I am in receipt of five or six hundred pounds a year, to take her a new pair of gloves every time I took her out.

Gowers noted that the river 'seemed in a tolerable condition sanitarily considered, at least I noticed not the slightest disagreeable smell, although I am afraid that at low water there is a very appreciable one'. This was only four years after the infamous 1858–9 'Great Stink' when the Thames was so polluted with waste that people walked miles in order to avoid crossing one of its bridges. In 1862 *The Builder* had argued for changes in sanitation:

> On occasions of high tide the low-lying districts were flooded—not with water but with sewage . . . There are percolations of crammed churchyards, the rain washings of the streets . . . which carry away with them . . . filthy objects, horse and cattle dung, . . . refuse from hospitals . . . dead rats, dead dogs and cats, and, sad to say, dead babies.[12]

One of the early attempts to clean up London was the introduction of 200,000 water closets by 1857, but these emptied directly into the Thames via old sewers. A new network of sewers was constructed: the south side opened in 1865, and the north side, after the Thames Embankment was completed, in 1868.

Unfurnished lodgings were hard to find, and the week Gowers and his mother spent in London was unrewarding, although he did manage to visit the University of London. He returned to Coggeshall before the weekend, resuming the search alone at the end of the month. Planning was becoming a considerable distraction, even on Sunday, a fact which pricked his conscience:

> I received a reply this morning to a letter that I sent on Friday to the secretary at University College, and the perusal of that and consequent conversations with Mr Simpson were not of a character much in keeping with the day. I wonder if it was wrong to read the letter on the Sabbath.

In early September there was yet another outbreak of scarlet fever in Coggeshall, making him a little guilty about leaving.

> This morning I got up about 6.30 and at 8 had to go out with Mr Simpson to Skye Green where a man, Wood, is taken ill with scarlet fever. . . . There is a good deal of scarlet fever about now, and I am afraid it will be as bad this autumn as it was last and, if so, Mr Simpson will feel my loss the more. . . . There is a fearful amount of scarlet fever in the town; it has come on very suddenly and appears to be upon the increase.

He spent one of his last Saturdays in Coggeshall labelling all the bones which Mr Giles had lent him with the initials HG. The afternoon was spent in 'getting up' the femur and doing botany.

September, his last month in Coggeshall, prompts a final introspective entry:

> I heard from Mother by this morning's post, but not a very satisfactory one as regards the time of going to London. In one fortnight, if all is well, I leave Coggeshall as my permanent residence I expect, in all probability, for *ever*. I have lived here for two years and it is a very solemn thought, what good have I done here?—what good have I got here? I wish I could return a better answer to the first; to the second I can say, although not so good as I might have become, I have greatly improved in my mental powers, in my mental development, and, may I venture to pray, during the last few weeks in my spiritual development also?

He made his final round of farewells at the end of September:

> I went and wished my grandmother and my aunt and uncle goodbye. The rest of the evening was spent at home where Manthorp came in to have a farewell pipe with me. Thus I spent my last day at Coggeshall in multitudinous calling and in leaving cards. Mrs Simpson has been, of course, extremely pleasant and so was her husband whom I always have liked and loved, and always shall. With the exception of the negligence in giving me instructions, he has ever been a perfectly model master to me, and as the almost perfect gentleman he will ever remain in my mind. He gave me this evening a portrait of himself which he had taken for his wife a few weeks ago, and a most characteristic portrait it is. Although not one of his best expressions it is one which I have seen upon thousands of times when he has been giving me some information upon medical subjects.

The following day, 30 September 1863, Gowers left Coggeshall:

> I have left Coggeshall—left it as a place of residence for ever. And very sorry I am to do so, and I should be still more sorry were it not for the prospect which has opened up before me—the exciting and attractive prospect of a hospital career.
>
> I drove away from Coggeshall with rather painful feelings, for it was not very pleasant work taking my last looks at a place which has been my pleasant and comfortable home

> for the last two years, but leave it I have to, and I have great consolations in the pleasant field I am now entering upon, and in the prospect of occasional visits to Coggeshall.

Gowers' son Ernest later remembered that he had often heard his father say that his clinical experience at Coggeshall was of lasting value to him, regretting that the practice of apprenticeship to the medical profession had fallen into disuse. Ernest suggested that it was possible that, looking back, Gowers may have rated its value too highly, doubting whether Dr Simpson gave full value for his £150, 'but I have no doubt at all that he got full value out of his apprentice'.

Gowers did not forget his early Coggeshall training. There were four men, in particular, who provided him with help and guidance over the two years of his apprenticeship: Dr Giles, Dr Simpson, and the Congregationalist ministers, Dale and Philps. Dr Giles broadened Gowers' practical experience, serving as an additional medical mentor when he was studying for matriculation. Dr Simpson, who did not always live up to expectations as a teacher, remained a close friend, and it is interesting to speculate how influential his 'ardent liberalism' was on his apprentice. Thirty years later, in 1893, Gowers 'to his extreme satisfaction' went to Coggeshall to attend his old 'governor' when Simpson was dying. Simpson's funeral was conducted by the Reverend Philps, after which he was buried in the segregated Dissenters' section of the graveyard of St Peter ad Vincula on 20 May 1893, not far from several of Gowers' relatives. The Reverend Alfred Philps died four years later, after serving Coggeshall for 33 years. His memorial plaque in the chapel describes him as a man 'faithful in teaching, fervent in prayer, wise in counsel, and of stainless integrity'.

Bryan Dale had given Gowers the academic guidance that Dr Simpson failed to provide, and stimulated the boy's interest in history, architecture, and archaeology. The Reverend Philps, only ten years older than Gowers, provided strong spiritual guidance, mentioned on a number of occasions by Gowers in his diaries, and it was he who, impressed by Gowers' diligence, took the momentous step of taking the young man to London and introducing him to one of the crucial mentors in his university years, Sir William Jenner.

## Chapter 4

# Medical student 1863–70

## Reforms in medicine and medical education 1823–58

Gowers began his medical training at a time of great, and often controversial, changes in public health, medical science, and medical education. It was not until the mid-nineteenth century that it was discovered that bacteria might be the origin of infections. In 1854, Dr John Snow removed the handle of a water pump in Soho—thus demonstrating, having cut off that supply of water, that in the cholera epidemic then raging the 'impure water supply' of the Vauxhall Water Company had been responsible for far more fatalities than those in the population having the 'improved supply' of the Lambeth Company.[1] Snow was a generation older than Gowers. Born in Yorkshire in 1813, he served a long apprenticeship in the north before going to London. He graduated from London University in 1844, his training still conforming to the standards set by the 1815 *Apothecaries Act*. Despite his research, many people remained convinced that diseases such as cholera were spread through noxious air, or 'miasma'. Fortunately, the sewerage system was being modernized by the time Gowers and his mother made their permanent move to London.

In 1856, Florence Nightingale returned from the Crimea, where she had been nursing wounded soldiers, and started to press for a range of reforms. She initiated an inquiry into the 'scandalously high' incidence of syphilis amongst soldiers fighting in the Crimean War.[2] In her influential *Notes on Hospitals*, published in 1859, she described contemporary London hospital conditions: 'walls streaming with damp and often covered with fungus, dirty floors, dirty beds, overcrowded wards, insufficient food, and inadequate nursing'.[3] In the same year she published her *Notes on Nursing*, in which she asked readers to consider why it was:

> . . . that one in every seven infants in this civilized land of England perishes before it is one year old? That, in London, two in every five die before they are five years old? And, in the other great cities of England, nearly one out of two? The life duration of tender babies (as some . . . analytical chemist, says) 'is the most delicate test' of sanitary conditions.[4]

The reforms taking place both in the medical profession and in medical training had started with the passing of the *Apothecaries Act* in 1815, which first introduced a systemic curriculum for medical training. The Court of Examiners established regulations requiring competence in Latin; attendance at lectures on anatomy, physiology, medicine, chemistry, and 'materia medica' (the study of medicines and their sources, preparation, and use); six months' hospital attendance and five years of apprenticeship. Testing was to be introduced, rather than relying solely on interviews, in order to maintain a comparable standard.

The former three-tier system of physicians, surgeons, and apothecaries changed with the passing of the 1858 *Medical Act*. The new standards applied in the regulation of the professions led to a decline in the number of physicians and surgeons.[5] Medical training had been under scrutiny ever since the *Apothecaries Act* was being developed. But this Act was not the sole influence on changes to medical education, writes Newman: 'it was largely itself a part of the process of reform which involved the organisation of qualification, education, and much more besides'.[6] Increasing numbers of medical schools and the developing interest in anatomy had increased the demand for bodies to dissect, leading to various nefarious practices such as the practice of 'body-snatching' by 'resurrection men' stealing bodies from churchyards. The *Anatomy Act* of 1832 ended the practice by legalizing and controlling anatomical dissection. The principal source of bodies for dissection then became the parish workhouses and hospitals, a source of distress to relatives of the deceased.

Medical journals appeared, and became strong advocates for reform. Thomas Wakley, proprietor and editor of *The Lancet*, was largely responsible for exposing the medical profession's weaknesses. When *The Lancet* was established, there were only three other periodicals: the *Medico-Chirurgical Review*, the *Edinburgh Medical and Surgical Journal*, and the *Medical Repository*. Wakley founded *The Lancet* in October 1823 with three aims: first, to educate by publishing items such as case reports, lectures, and transactions of societies; second, to be a campaign broadsheet against the unreformed professional institutions; and, third, to be a vehicle for propounding his vigorous radicalism.[7]

Wakley campaigned aggressively against the three-tier medical system entrenched in licensing by the individual societies, and against the closed access to medical education and qualifications. Wakley, who had both medical training and competent shorthand, upset London lecturers, whose incomes were derived from charging attendance fees for their classes, by recording, transcribing, and then publishing their lectures. Sir Astley Cooper's nephew, Bransby, when accused in the journal of medical negligence, initiated a libel case against Wakley in 1828.

> The great excitement caused by the trial in the public mind, the publication of the proceedings in extenso in all the newspapers, and a separate issue in a pamphlet, could not fail to call the attention of the public to the position of the Medical Profession.[8]

Largely in response to Wakley's agitations, a parliamentary select committee was established to investigate medical education. At its hearings the committee revealed fundamental flaws in both the education and structure of the profession. The committee found that the existing Royal Colleges of Physicians and of Surgeons (and the Worshipful Society of Apothecaries) had 'failed to promote education or run fair and efficient examinations'. Reform, though inevitable, was extremely slow. It took 18 years from the presentation of the first Bill in 1840 to the passing of the seventeenth, enacted as the *Medical Act 1858*.

In 1840 a provincial medical association, established in 1832 in Worcester, started publishing its own journal. In 1856 the association had extended its membership to London doctors and changed its name to the British Medical Association; the following year it renamed its journal, the *Provincial Medical and Surgical Journal*, as the

*British Medical Journal* (*BMJ*). The association pressed for the nationwide registration of doctors at a time when all the professions were raising their standards of education:

> Professional reform was part of the movement elevating the status of all professions, ensuring that if the most interesting occupations were to be reserved for the most intelligent and rewarded by the highest remuneration, they should involve the obligation of an efficient and thorough education, rigid tests of admission, and adherence to a strict professional ethical code.[9]

Privilege gradually began to give way to academic merit in the selection of candidates for the medical profession. In his colourful autobiography, J. F. Clarke, a reporter for *The Lancet* for more than 40 years, described both hospital training and the role of the medical societies in the era before the reforms:

> If we turn to the Schools of Medicine and the Hospitals we find that the teaching was altogether unsatisfactory. Clinical teaching was all but unknown, and I recollect one of the earliest letters inserted in *The Lancet* was a complaint from a student of one of the larger Hospitals, that a Surgeon of eminence had gone through the wards without 'once opening his mouth'. In consequence of the difficulties in procuring subjects, anatomy was not completely taught, and the only Hospital Schools of Medicine at that time were attached to the larger institutions—the united Hospitals of Guy and St Thomas, St Bartholomew and the London Hospital [in Whitechapel].
>
> Turning to the Societies, we find them in an undeveloped state. The Medical and Chirurgical met in Lincoln's Inn Fields, the numbers present at the meetings being scarcely, on the average, a dozen, and this, too, when Sir Astley Cooper was the President. Discussion was not encouraged in any way—indeed, often discouraged; no reports of the proceedings were allowed to be published, on the ground that such publication might interfere with the sale of the *Transactions*. The Medical Society of London, then holding its meetings in Bolt Court, was somewhat under the influence of the 'cold shade of aristocracy.[10]

Apprenticeships continued to be common until the 1840s, but 'the isolated, one-to-one relationship of apprentice and master became only one part of the total experience of medical education, and progressively a less important one'.[11] This was of some concern to those who had formerly trained apprentices, as they lost a valuable source not only of practical help but also of income. Doctors depended for the bulk of their income on the fees of those patients who could afford to pay. Peterson cites two practices offered for sale in the *BMJ* in 1876: one offered an income of £500 a year, and the other, a 'prestigious practice calling for a purchaser with "high qualifications" who was accustomed to "good society"' offered an income of £1100 a year, though Peterson suggests that these incomes would be likely to have been inflated to increase the attraction of the advertised practice.[12] In the nineteenth century, friendly societies such as Foresters and Oddfellows offered working men insurance against sickness and old age. It is clear that Dr Simpson's Coggeshall practice was not only given a substantial boost when he was appointed doctor to a 'friendly society' in Feering; he also significantly increased his income when he took Gowers on as his apprentice.

The *1858 Medical Act* allowed the profession to control its own educational standards, examinations, and qualifications, making medicine a professional monopoly and enhancing its status and financial rewards.[13] Similar changes were taking place in the civil service at the time, the career Gowers eventually chose for his sons, with the introduction of the civil service examination which eventually changed a system that depended on patronage to one based on academic merit: changes prompted by the mismanagement of the Crimean War.

Fundamental changes were also taking place in the understanding of diagnosis and disease. Together with developments in anatomy and physiology, these had far-reaching effects on medical science and practice:

> They include the growth of knowledge about the relationships between symptoms, physical signs, and the findings of morbid anatomy, and the resultant shift away from mere 'history taking' in diagnosis to the 'invention of diagnosis by physical examination' of the patient. Less reliance was placed on the patient's description of his own symptoms and more importance placed on the medical man's evaluation of the physical signs of disease which he observed in the patient. In a subtle way, authority about the patient's physical condition shifted from patient to doctor as the doctor became less dependent upon the patient for knowledge of the patient's condition. As a result, training in anatomy and physiology and experience at the bedside became increasingly important aspects of a medical student's life.[14]

## The establishment of University College London

University College London (UCL) had been founded in 1826 and started offering medical classes in 1828. King's College, London, was established in 1829. Both colleges, therefore, pre-date the founding of the University of London, which was initially established in 1836 to act as an examining body for its colleges and other 'approved institutions'. The University acted solely in this capacity until 1858.

Referred to by its detractors as 'that Godless institution in Gower Street', UCL had come into existence as a result of strong pressure and financial support from Nonconformists. The intellectual 'father' of UCL was the utilitarian philosopher Jeremy Bentham, and its founders included Thomas Wilson (a Congregationalist benefactor of chapels and educational institutions); James Mill (father of John Stuart Mill); and Henry Brougham (the Whig politician who served as Lord Chancellor from 1830 to 1834). Brougham had been involved with Birkbeck in forming the Mechanics' Institutes. The Dissenters had planned a university of their own, but were persuaded of the merits of a more open institution. Its establishment was a direct challenge to Oxford and Cambridge as it was modelled on Edinburgh University, where Mill and Brougham had both studied. The aim of the new secular institution was not only to to provide a university for students excluded by Oxford and Cambridge, but also to offer a variety of subjects not previously recognized as part of the university curriculum.

Despite their exclusion from university degrees, there had been a tradition of medicine amongst Dissenters over the previous two centuries: 'steering "another course" around all obstacles ... Puritans and Dissenters had carved a permanent niche for themselves within the medical profession, a niche that would continue to produce outstanding doctors well into the nineteenth century'.[15] That this continued through the nineteenth century was amply demonstrated by the many Dissenters who, like

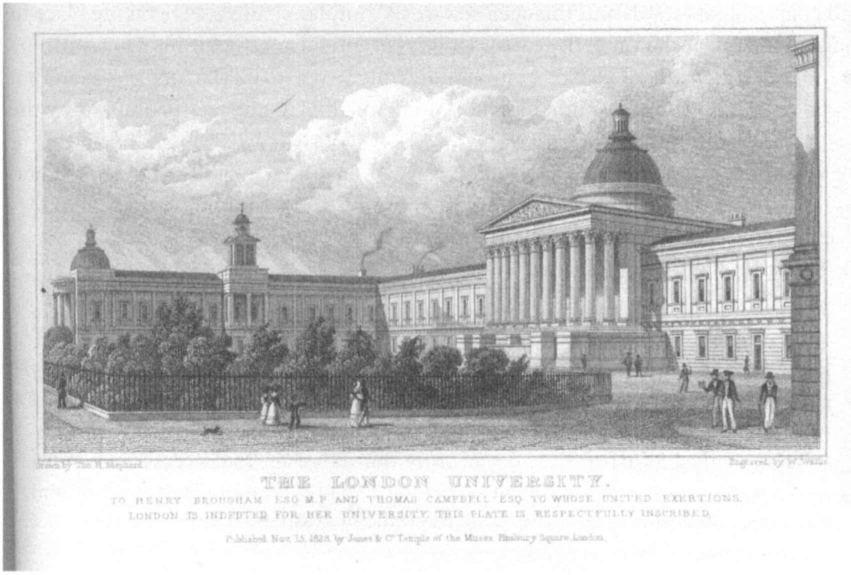


**Fig. 4.1** The London University, 1828: 'To Henry Brougham Esq MP and Thomas Campbell Esq to whose united efforts London is indebted for her university this plate is respectfully inscribed'. Published by James & Co, Temple of the Muses, Finsbury Square, London. Drawn by Tho H. Shepherd. Engraved by W. Wallis. Courtesy of Ash Rare Books, London.

Gowers, studied medicine at the University of London and went on to become leaders in the medical profession.

G. M. Young has described the impact the new university made on the English university system:

> It was strongly Radical in origin and affinity, it was entirely secular, and its curriculum was very much wider than the old Universities. The foundation of the University of London marks the conception of a University as training for a specific profession, for medicine, law, engineering, or teaching which was in England a novelty to which the examples of both Germany and Scotland both contributed. But as a seat of instruction University College rose at once to the first rank.[16]

Clarke recalled the state of medical education in England before UCL opened its doors to medical students in 1828:

> The system which then prevailed of election to medical offices in the large endowed hospitals was most vicious and detrimental to the interests of the Profession. The influence of money and family connections were paramount. This was especially the case in the great united hospitals of Guy's and St Thomas's, and in that of St Bartholomew's. The system was simple enough; the surgeons in particular took 'apprentices' with immense fees, with the understanding that at a convenient time they should be appointed to posts of honour, to the exclusion of all other candidates, whatever might be their claims to receive such distinctions. . . .

It was in the midst of these circumstances that the 'University of London' was established. The council of that institution had a wide field from which to select their lecturers on Medicine and the allied sciences. They made their selection from men 'who had been left out in the cold,' but these consisted of a formidable phalanx. . . . Such men . . . could not fail to attract large classes to the new institution.[17]

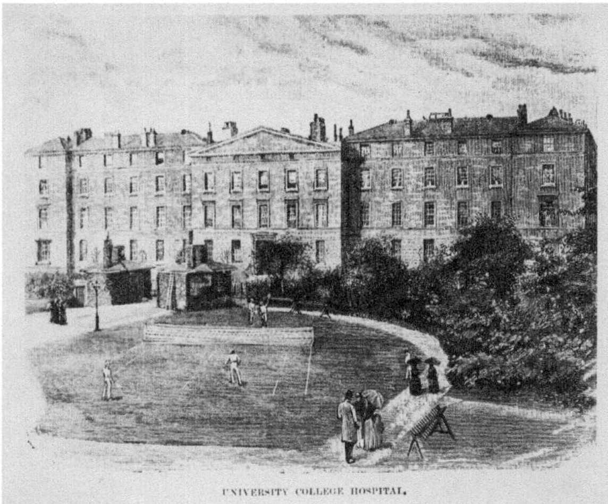

**Fig. 4.2** University College Hospital, 1835. University College London Library Special Collections.

## The medical school and University College Hospital

Gowers had set his sights on the medical school at UCL despite Dr Giles' advice that he should train at one of the long-established London medical schools that did not offer a degree. In 1863 London was still the only English university that awarded degrees to Nonconformists, but it was also founded as a non-residential institution, intended to serve the middle-classes and to be inexpensive compared with Oxford and Cambridge. It was another example of the more egalitarian approach to education that had led to the formation of the Mechanics' Institutes, one of which had served Gowers so well in Coggeshall.

The UCL medical school had a large field of potential students to choose from as a result of opening its degrees to Dissenters. Previously, Edinburgh had been the primary medical centre in Britain offering systematic scientific and clinical teaching.[18] The London medical school was unusual 'because it was here, rather than at any other metropolitan school, that a student would come in contact with the view that the basic sciences, particularly the experimental sciences and especially physiology, should be the foundation of all medical education, practice, and progress'.[19]

The new medical school immediately attracted outstanding staff, including the Quain brothers: Jones Quain became professor of general anatomy in 1831 and Richard, professor of descriptive anatomy in 1832. Richard Quain encouraged William

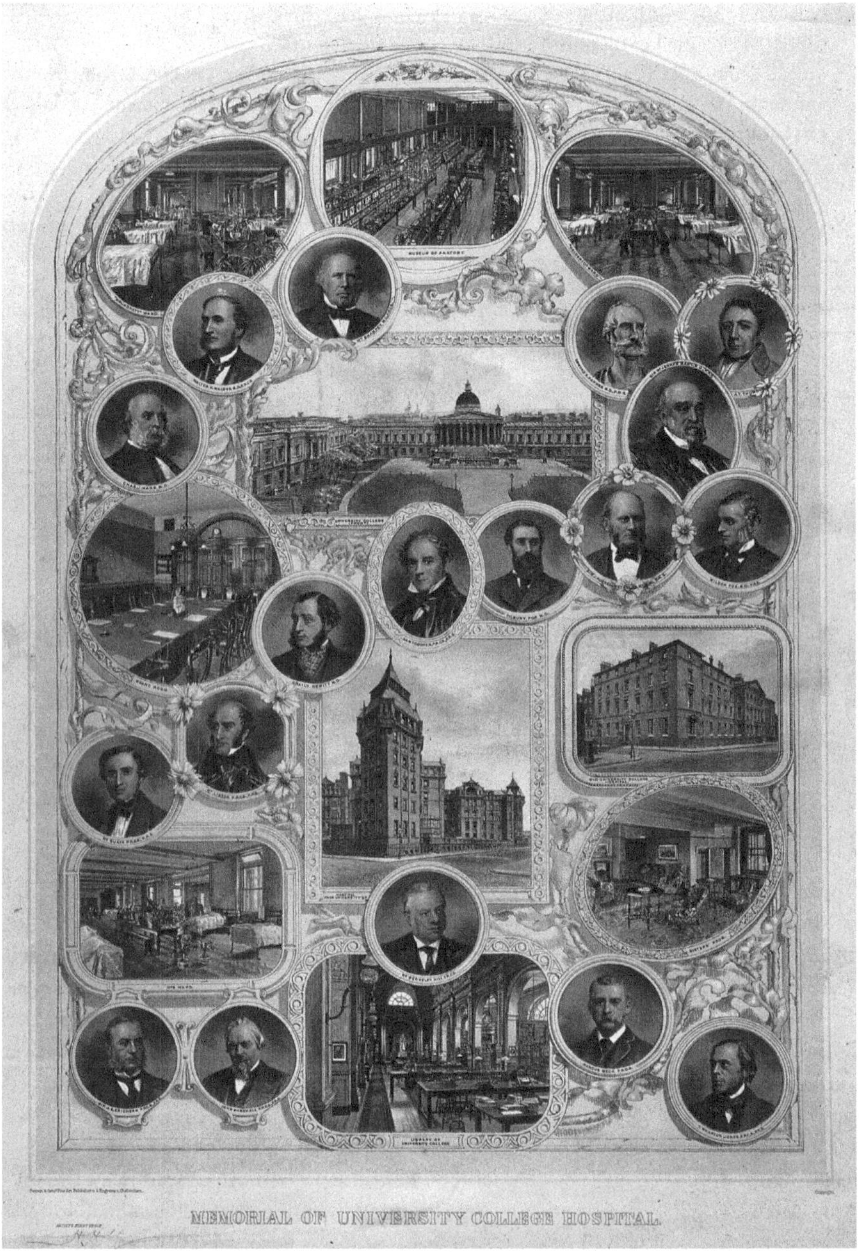


**Fig. 4.3** Buildings and famous early alumni of University College Hospital, London. Courtesy of Wellcome Library, London. Top to bottom: Sharpey, W. (1802–1880); Parkes, E. A (1819–1876); Walshe, W. H. (1812–1892); Thomson, A. T. (1778–1849); Hare, C. J. (1818–1898); Jenner, W. (1815–1898); Hewitt, G. (1828–1893); Cooper, S. (1780–1848); Fox, T. (1836–1879); Reynolds, J. R. (1828–1896); Fox, W. (1831–1887); Quain, R. (1800–1887); Liston, R. (1834–1892); Erichsen, J. E. (1818–1896); Marshall, J. (1818–1891); Beck, M. (1843–1893); Jones, T. W. (1808–1891).

Sharpey to apply for the new Chair of anatomy and physiology, a position he held from 1836 until he retired in 1874. Sharpey taught the first course in systematic physiology to be offered in England, a subject previously treated as an appendage to anatomy, and was still lecturing when Gowers was a student. William Jenner was appointed professor of pathological anatomy in 1849.

Both the University of London and the Mechanics' Institutes experienced a dip in popularity in the 1850s when Oxford and Cambridge adjusted their courses to meet changing demands. The medical school enrolments in the late 1830s started to fall from a peak of 497 in 1837–8, not beginning to recover until the 1860s. In 1863, Gowers was one of a cohort of 161 students who enrolled.

A lectureship in practical physiology was established in 1856 to provide instruction in using the microscope 'examining the textures and fluids of the body'. Revolutionary changes in physiology teaching began in 1867, towards the end of Gowers' studies, when Michael Foster was appointed Instructor in Practical Physiology and Histology, a man whose 'instinctive perception of ability and a power to inspire effort enabled him to gather round him a band of capable and devoted disciples'.[20]

Initially UCL had no hospital of its own, depending on the main London medical schools to provide practical experience for its students. London hospitals had provided hospital-based training from the beginning of the century, drawing students from Oxford and Cambridge and from apprenticeships in the provinces. The founders of UCL knew they needed a hospital, and in 1828, as an interim measure, opened a university dispensary, managed by a resident apothecary, which acted much like a casualty department. The trigger that led to the foundation of University College Hospital six years later was a decision by the Middlesex Hospital not to allow students from UCL to cross its threshold. As a result, the 130-bed North London Hospital central block was opened opposite UCL in 1834 to provide hospital-based training for the UCL medical classes. In 1837 it was renamed the University College Hospital (UCH).

UCH was one of several hospitals which became the centres of medical teaching in London. Established before UCH were St Bartholomew's (c. 1123), St Thomas' (c. 1207), Westminster Hospital (1719), Guy's (1721), St George's (1733); the London Hospital (1740), the Middlesex Hospital (1745), and the Charing Cross Hospital (1823).

When the UCH medical school opened in 1828 five consultants had been appointed to its staff. Six years later the hospital received some unfortunate notoriety after John Elliotson, who had been appointed in 1834, carried out popular, but dubious, public demonstrations of mesmerism. He was forced to resign in 1838. Robert Liston, who joined the staff in 1835, performed the first recorded major operation in Europe using an anaesthetic (ether), when he amputated a man's leg at the hospital in 1846. The most significant influences on Gowers as a student, William Jenner and John Russell Reynolds, were appointed consultants to the hospital in 1850 and 1860.

Judging from a contemporary newspaper clipping in the archives, the students gained some notoriety for their dress habits around the streets near the hospital. It is noticeable that Gowers was not the only student who learned to smoke before starting his medical studies.

## CURIOSITIES OF COSTUME.

A SORT of academical epidemic has broken out among the medical students at the northern end of the town; and the youths at the University in Gower Street have not only trenched upon the collegiate trenchers, but have assumed the gown, which ill assorts with the paletot of private life. This strange association of the garb of learning

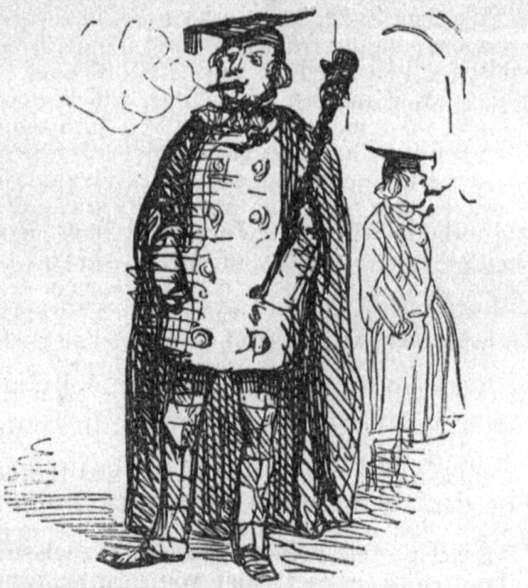

with the habits of the medical students as they live, produces a curious effect; and the neighbourhood of Gower Street has been accordingly startled by the appearance that the combination presents.

We have not heard by what authority the assumption of the toga has taken place among the youths of Gower Street; and indeed it requires no less a person than old GOWER himself to come forth and explain the mystery.

**Fig. 4.4** 'Curiosities of costume' (1846).

Joseph Lister, a Quaker 'Dissenter' and founder of antiseptic surgery, attended Liston's operation as a London University student in 1846. When he graduated in 1847 he wanted to broaden his experience by travelling abroad but was advised by Sharpey to go to Edinburgh. He moved from Edinburgh to Glasgow in 1860 where he read about Pasteur's germ theories and began trials using carbolic acid as an antiseptic treatment for wounds. He wanted to move back to London, but UCH failed to appoint him when he applied for a chair in 1866. This was a decade in which wound disease appeared to reach epidemic proportions in British hospitals.[21] But the medical establishment in London strongly resisted Lister's claims. In 1945 Herbert Brown recalled that Lister's work was accepted with enthusiasm on the continent of Europe, 'but in

London at the time my hospital training began (1880), antiseptic surgery existed in only two hospitals—University College and King's'.[22]

Lister's biographer, Rickman Godlee, gives an idea of the number of operations performed at UCH in the late 1860s, when there were about 80 surgical beds, served by three surgeons and two assistant surgeons:

> There was one small theatre and one principal operating day, on which the whole surgical staff assembled, except one of the seniors who preferred to have a date to himself. The number of operations performed in a year was about 200, of which more than 40 were amputations.[23]

The mortality rate from amputations at UCH in the 1870s was about 25 per cent. Buckston Browne described the conditions in 1872:

> Surgeons and dressers wore old coats, often stiff with dried blood, and we washed our hands in a small basin on the ward table. The wards were full of hospital gangrene and cases of septicaemia. Hospital gangrene was a shocking thing, almost invariably fatal.[24]

The reluctance of London surgeons to accept Lister's theories endured. In the 1880s Christopher Heath, then senior surgeon at the hospital 'had taken to Listerian surgery only under protest and still operated in an old frock-coat, turning green, which hung on a hook outside the theatre'.[25] Although the risk of infection made operations almost as risky to surgeons as patients, it was a long time before London surgeons were persuaded to wash and dress properly before operating. Gowers' colleague Victor Horsley, however, was one surgeon who was an enthusiastic convert to antisepsis.

Another of Florence Nightingale's reforms had an impact on Gowers' later research. She forcefully advocated collecting medical statistics and persuaded a number of hospitals, including UCH, to use her 'Model Forms'.[26] She argued that the high mortality rate in large hospitals was preventable. Sir James Paget commented that her *Report on Hospitals* appeared to be 'the most valuable contribution to sanitary science in application to medical institutions that I have ever read', and hospitals created 'almost as many diseases as they cured; there was hospital gangrene, hospital pyaemia, hospital erysipelas, hospital fever ...'.[27] The Statistical Society published comparative hospital statistics in 1862. However, as with many of the medical innovations at the time the medical establishment remained sceptical about the benefits of statistical collection. The Royal College of Surgeons referred the subject to a committee, which reported adversely on Nightingale's forms.

## Gowers as a medical student

Gowers and his mother had found lodgings in Roxburgh Grove (now Belmont Street), Camden Town, not far from UCL. They established their first London home here (still providing a home for cousin Charlotte Venables). When Gowers sat his Preliminary Scientific with the First MB in July 1864, he was awarded a University Exhibition in Biology, which provided him with £40 a year for two years.

The photograph of UCH medical students taken in 1865 (Fig. 4.5), does not identify the individual students, nor why they were photographed. However, a close comparison with a photograph of Gowers taken ten years later at the age of 29 (Fig. 5.8) suggests, both from his features and the clothes he is wearing, that Gowers is the young man on the extreme right of the picture. It may have been a photograph of a group of prizewinners. Gowers was awarded his first university prize when he passed the Preliminary Scientific Examination with flying colours in 1864. The young man stands apart from his more confident peers. It is likely that this is the insecure but intensely studious and devout young man who wrote the diaries in 1862 and 1863.

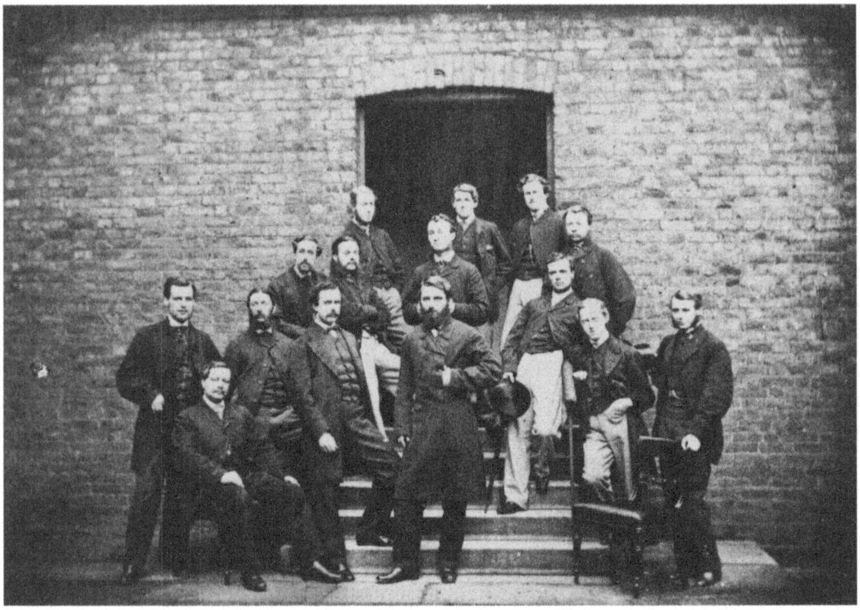

**Fig. 4.5** UCH medical students 1865. From Harte, N and North, J, The World of UCL: 1828–2004 (UCL Press, 2004).

Gowers took down his lectures in shorthand, later reminiscing that:

> In the case of all the chief subjects, Medicine, Pathology, Surgery, etc, I used no textbook. I found no textbook comparable to them. I trusted entirely to my notes (among others) of Russell Reynolds's lectures on Medicine and Bastian's on Pathology, Marshall's on Surgery, a course given by Michael Foster on Medical Jurisprudence, even for the University of London.[28]

Critchley notes that with Reynolds and Charlton Bastian on the staff there was 'already a bias towards neurology' at UCH.[29] Gowers stopped keeping a daily diary once he became a student in London. He had ample opportunity for practising his shorthand when recording his university lectures, the purpose for which he had acquired the skill. However, the absence of a regular diary means that we no longer have an intimate record of his day-to-day routines and impressions. Nonetheless, it is possible to picture the changes in his life as a medical student compared with his previous, often solitary, life in quiet Coggeshall. The University of London had been founded as a non-residential institution, on the assumption that students would live at home under the guidance and supervision of their parents, so his mother's decision to provide a London home for William was in keeping with this aim. There had also been considerable debate about whether a residential college would require some form of religious education, and this would contradict the principle of access to all, whatever their faith. One effect was that medical students did not mix with arts students.[30]

Gowers now lived in a family home with his mother and cousin Charlotte for the first time since his father died, and had a central role around which the small family unit revolved. The student atmosphere, on the other hand, would have been a considerable contrast to the strict proprieties of Congregationalist Coggeshall. London medical students at the time had a tradition of 'bawdy boisterousness, so much so, it was said, that in respectable company some were unwilling to admit to being medical students. Teachers of anatomy, in which a great many very dull facts had somehow to be committed to memory, relied heavily on indecent mnemonics'.[31]

He was also exposed to controversial developments in scientific thought, which may have posed challenges to his Nonconformism. It was an era in which English society's 'practical ideals were at odds with its religious professions, and its religious belief was at issue with its intelligence'.[32] But there is no record of his reactions to the new ideas on issues such as evolution, though he clearly remained a devout Congregationalist. But, given his innate intellectual curiosity, he would undoubtedly have given considerable thought to the controversies of the time. Buckston Browne recalled the impact of going to hear T. H. Huxley's lectures:

> These lectures made a life-long impression upon me. Huxley was the apostle of Charles Robert Darwin who, just ten years ago, had shaken the whole world, especially the theological world, by his publication of *Origin of the Species.* Controversy had run, and still ran, high. It was bitter, and often very bitter. Darwin was a figure of intense interest to me. I saw him only once in the flesh and this was at one of Huxley's afternoon Jermyn Street lectures. Darwin came in, sat amongst us and waited patiently for his interview with Huxley after the lecture, at 4pm. I shall never forget his tall figure and massive high-domed head. He wore a long black cloak and carried a large black sombrero hat. His general appearance was grave and impressive and could nowhere pass unnoticed.[33]

On 20 March 1865, Gowers turned 20. Despite the two-year gap in entries, he marked the event in the diary he had started in Coggeshall in October 1862. He was still self-critical, hard-working, and devout:

> Once more my birthday comes round to remind me that I am living, and to startle me from my too great apathy with the question 'How?'. For many months—ever since before I left Coggeshall, I have felt a yearning for something higher, nobler than the poor miserable worthless life I was then leading. Since I came to London the desire has been growing still more intense, and has been constantly attempting to realize itself to outward, and, to a certain extent, inward goodness. Virtuous but not religious attempts. During the last ten months, however, I trust a really religious spirit has been growing within me. And especially through the preaching and example of Mr Philps at Coggeshall and Mr White

in London, whose chapel I have attended for the last six months. Through all of my life, and especially through the last two years, I can see God's guiding hand, plain and definite.

I am writing this under difficulties, and must soon desist. Being far from well tonight through some indisposition—temporary, I hope, from eating too much pork or something of that kind—I am sitting with my feet in hot water in my pleasant snug little study at Roxburgh Grove. My mother and Charlotte have just gone to bed—the former with needless admonitions to take care of myself and not to stay up too late.

The first *Pure Food Act* had been passed in 1860. In 1863 a report to the Privy Council stated that one-fifth of meat sold came from diseased cattle.[34] Pork must have been even more dubious. This is the last time Gowers mentions his cousin Charlotte Venables. She married a man from Oxford, Edwin Knibbs, 'common room man' at Queen's College, at a ceremony in Camden in September 1868, at which Gowers was the witness. The last that is known of the couple is that they had two children and Mr Knibbs became a wine merchant in St Ebbes, Oxford; the family eventually settled in Gloucestershire, where Mr Knibbs had bought a hotel. The diary ends:

I am busy working for the examination in physiology and histology and devoting my whole time to it. I rose this morning at about half past six, and studied until 9.30 with an intermission for breakfast and received two kind presents—a handsome Russian leather purse from my mother, and a silver fruit knife from Charlotte.

I then went down to college and heard Doctor Sharpey's lecture 10–11. Worked in the library till 12.30, returned home to dinner—after which instead of going for a good walk as I had promised myself on this, a day as clear as I ever remember the 20th March to be, but with as high a wind and as much dust as to make the streets very unpleasant—instead of this walk I had to go down to college for an extra lecture from Dr Sharpey on muscular electricity. After tea attempted to study and a little microscopic work.

## Recuperation in Bournemouth and a glimpse of Tennyson

Gowers kept a new shorthand diary, briefly, when at the beginning of January 1866 he took a break from his studies. Ann Gowers took her son down to Bournemouth, leaving him there for two months. The seaside town had built up a reputation as a health resort for those suffering from pulmonary diseases, and a Royal National Sanatorium for Consumption and Diseases of the Chest had been built there in 1858. However, Gowers gives no explanation for his two-month break. He carried with him a letter of introduction from a London doctor to a 'Dr F':

Dr F looked in at eleven but was not able to stay. Later in the day, however, he examined my chest, which he found tolerably sound. At his recommendation I went up before dinner to the sanatorium, a sort of convalescent hospital which is erected here, in a sheltered situation, capable of accommodating about forty patients. I saw the house surgeon, a Bartholomew's man, who after weighing me (at nine stone eleven pounds) showed me over the place, a tolerably airy building built of stone, but the original space is not completely filled up. The ground floor is occupied by the men, the upper by the women. The sleeping places looked to me somewhat crowded but possibly not injuriously so as they only use them as such.

Gowers took solitary walks around Bournemouth, sometimes taking Tennyson's *In Memoriam* with him. G. M. Young describes the widespread crisis of faith at the time largely brought about by the debate over Darwin's theories of evolution:

> The natural sciences in all their branches—rocks, fossils, birds, beasts, fish, and flowers—were a national hobby; the *Vestiges of Creation*, issued with elaborate secrecy and attributed by a wild surmise to Prince Albert, was a national excitement; translated into golden verse by Tennyson, evolution almost became a national creed. *In Memoriam*, which is nine years older than the *Origin of Species*, gathered up all the doubts of Christianity, of providence, of immortality, which the advances of science had implanted in anxious minds, and answered them, or seemed to answer them, with the assurance of a pantheistic and yet personal faith in progress.
>
> *In Memoriam* is one of the cardinal documents of the mid-Victorian mind, its ardent curiosity, its exquisite sensitiveness to nature, and, not less, perhaps, its unwillingness to quit, and its incapacity to follow any chain of reasoning which seems likely to result in an unpleasant conclusion. In his highest mood, Tennyson sometimes speaks like an archangel assuring the universe that it will muddle through.[35]

Gowers was undoubtedly deeply influenced by Tennyson's work. It is touching that on his journey home from Bournemouth at the beginning of May he actually caught sight of the poet:

> Returned to London this morning from Bournemouth. The only thing worth recalling concerning the journey was an incident which occurred at Bishopstone. The train stopped there for some ten minutes. Walking up and down the platform I passed several times a tall man with a black moustache and beard. He stooped slightly and was clad in a very long black cloak reaching below his knees, below which showed the end of another black coat and a pair of black trousers. On his head was a 'chimney pot' [hat]. After passing him once or twice I looked at him quite well, and on noticing his face it struck me that I had seen that face before somewhere. I looked again, thought for a moment, and it flashed upon me. There could be no mistake about that face and its moustache and beard. It was Tennyson. I went up to Dr . . . who was standing upon the platform. 'Do you know Tennyson by sight? Is it possible that man in the long cloak is he?' He thought for a moment and then said 'Yes that is true enough'. I passed him half a dozen times at least and took a good look each time, and thought of *In Memoriam*. Strange to say no-one seemed to notice him, no-one looked at him, familiar as his features were through photographs which are so abundant. He was walking up and down talking to a boy who was with him, who appeared to be his son, a pleasant looking lad of some 12 or 14 years of age [Tennyson had two sons: Hallam, born in 1852 and Lionel in 1854]. Tennyson's features are crosser than I should have thought, though talking and laughing with the lad the easy expression of his face was pleasant and jocular, not sceptical. He walked off at Basingstoke with the lad, carrying over his shoulder a cricket bat and a fishing rod.

## Arnold, Darwin, William Jenner, John Russell Reynolds, and Ruskin

Gowers also read Strachey's *Life of Arnold* while in Bournemouth. The liberal Anglican 'Broad Church' movement had suggested that the authority of the Bible and the

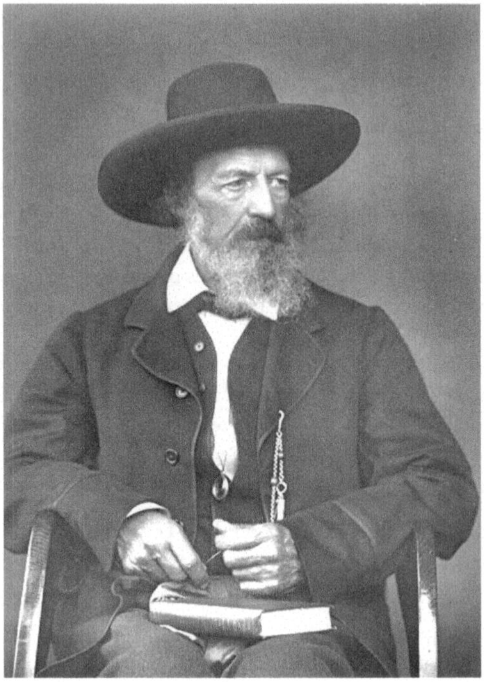

**Fig. 4.6** Alfred, Lord Tennyson.

Church might be subjected to historical and scientific criticism. Debate on the issue began to undermine the insistence by the Established Church on the 39 Articles, which had been a sticking point in the awarding of degrees to Nonconformists by Oxford and Cambridge.

Thomas Arnold, the reforming headmaster of Rugby school, had written his *Principles of Church Reform* in 1833, in which he argued that Church of England litany and government might be reformed to allow for the inclusion of Dissenters. He argued that a Church Establishment was essential to the well-being of the nation; that the existence of dissent had always impaired its usefulness 'and now, from peculiar circumstances' threatened its destruction. He suggested that trying to extinguish dissent by persecution would be both wicked and impossible, and that there therefore remained 'a hitherto untried way, to extinguish it by comprehension'.[36]

Religious controversy between Low Church evangelicals who viewed the Bible as 'inerrant', High Church 'Tractarians' moving towards Catholicism, and the 'Broad Church' movement founded by Arnold and Coleridge reached its peak in the early 1860s. While still an apprentice, Gowers had battled with Coleridge's *Aids to Reflection*, and in 1866 he was reading about Arnold. The Tractarians, or Oxford Movement, had been publishing their tracts in the 1830s and early 1840s. In 1860, seven authors, six of whom were clergymen, published *Essays and Reviews*, introducing German biblical criticism into England.[37] The Oxford classicist, Benjamin Jowett, in his essay on the interpretation of scripture, questioned whether all the new peoples and religions being discovered by the adventurous Victorians would be denied access to the Kingdom of Heaven if they had not been converted to Christianity, and also argued that a more critical approach to interpreting the Bible would lead to greater religious tolerance. The publication of *Essays and Reviews* unleashed a four-year controversy which represented 'a crisis of faith contemporary with that provoked by Darwin's *Origin of Species*, but more central to the religious mind'.[38] It was in 1860, the year the National Hospital for the Paralysed and Epileptic opened, that T. H. Huxley had earned the nickname 'Darwin's bulldog' when he argued for Darwin's evolution theory with Bishop Wilberforce at a meeting of the British Association in Oxford (Darwin was ill at the time). Darwinism became a new component in the debate already taking place within the Established Church between liberal and conservative theologians. It was a clash that significantly affected the general relationship between religion and science.[39] Gowers, like so many of his contemporaries, must have been wrestling with these new and highly contentious issues.

Gowers had initially aspired to a country practice after he graduated. However, as Petersen notes, even when a young man came to London 'with modest plans for a country practice', the experience of assisting one of the great medical men opened up a new medical world and new aspirations.[40] The 'great man' in Gowers' case was Sir William Jenner, thanks to an introduction by the Reverend Philps from Coggeshall. In 1951 Gordon Holmes, told the story of how this meeting came about:

> Nearly 50 years ago I spent a weekend with a friend whose father was vicar of Coggeshall, where Gowers had served his apprenticeship. The vicar, then an old man, asked me if I had met Willie Gowers, and told me he never knew a more intelligent, industrious, or conscientious boy. He became so interested in him that when his apprenticeship ended he brought him to London and introduced him to his friend, Sir William Jenner, then one of physicians to University College Hospital and President of the Royal College of Physicians, who promised his help and advice. Jenner appears in fact to have used him during his undergraduate career as a secretary and assistant, and by the meagre salary he paid him enabled him to live in moderate comfort. This association continued even after Gowers qualified in medicine.[41]

Gowers' mastery of shorthand played a critical role in determining his future, and was no longer limited to taking lecture notes. One of his obituaries later noted the importance of his shorthand in his gaining the position with Jenner:

> The influence of his shorthand had another great effect on his career—namely, that of determining the fact that he became a physician in London instead of a practitioner in the country. It brought him also the post of secretary to Sir William Jenner, who referred in the preface of one of his works to the fact that his lectures on abdominal tumours were reported by 'his able friend and former pupil, W R Gowers'.[42]

Bellot described Jenner, an innkeeper's son born in 1815, as 'unquestionably one of the greatest clinicians of the Victorian period, a teacher who had a most impressive personality, combined with an extraordinary shrewdness in estimating at their true value the signs of disease, and also a sound and wide knowledge of disease'.[43] In 1847 he had begun a study of the causes of continued fever and published papers describing

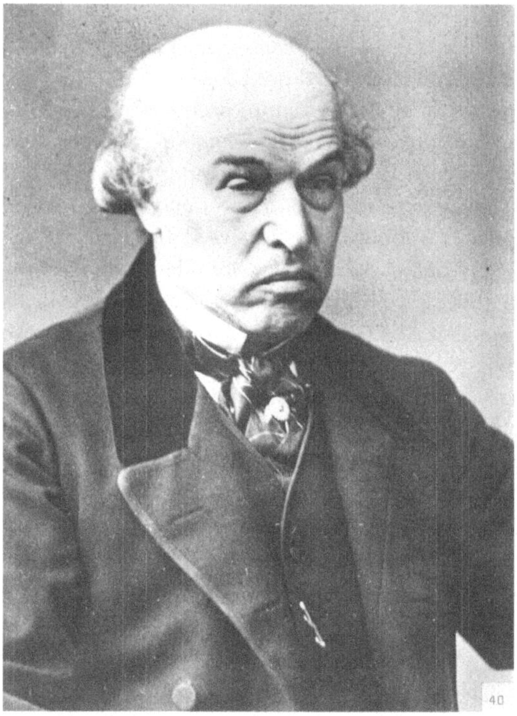

**Fig. 4.7** William Jenner. Image courtesy of the Museum and Archive, Great Ormond Street Hospital for Children.

the separate identity of 'two common and often confused fevers, typhoid and typhus'.[44] His papers included descriptions of cases and of post-mortem findings which were 'models of careful, accurate observation'.[45] Jenner was also a great clinical teacher, and had many eminent patients, including Queen Victoria and other members of the royal family. Philps had introduced Gowers to an ideal mentor, a leader in the profession, who was at the height of his illustrious career in the 1860s.

Gowers' shorthand skills also enabled him to earn money as a medical reporter and, as he himself put it, managed to bridge over the interval between 'the impecunious student and the impecunious physician'.[46] In the second half of their medical degrees students worked in the hospital, and at this point, in 1867, Gowers became Jenner's assistant house physician. Critchley comments that while it was important in bringing Gowers into close contact with the activities of such an able medical man at the height of his profession, it might have been 'ill-fated, for both were men of strong and rigid personalities'.[47] However, Gowers was in his twenties, thirty years younger than Jenner, and it is unlikely any of this 'rigidity' had manifested itself at that stage, but Jenner's directness of manner might have rubbed off on the younger man. Throughout his life Gowers held Jenner in the utmost respect, writing that acting as his house physician was the 'culminating privilege' of his student days. Gowers was in 'the closest relation with him as private secretary' and was sure that any powers of reasoning displayed in his own books, or in the method in which the subjects were discussed, was due to the influence of Jenner 'in a degree that no ordinary person would suspect'.[48]

Gowers and his mother moved to 32 Mornington Crescent, St Pancras, in 1865, within walking distance of UCH, though some distance from Jenner's rooms in Brook Street, Mayfair. Gowers appears to have earned a little extra money as a census recorder, because the 1871 census return for Mornington Crescent is written with particularly fine penmanship, and his recently acquired medical qualifications are recorded with great precision and obvious pride. They lived there until they moved to their permanent home in Queen Anne Street, Marylebone.

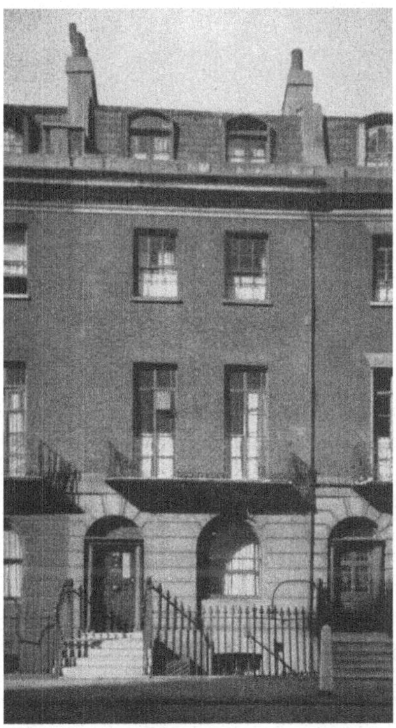

**Fig. 4.8** 32 Mornington Crescent in 1948. From Macdonald Critchley biography, 1949.

The experience of working for Jenner left Gowers with a 'lasting veneration for his old chief'.[49] When Jenner died, the *BMJ* invited Gowers to write an appreciation of him as a clinical teacher and physician. Gowers, who himself became renowned for the quality of his teaching, observed that it was hard to conceive that any equally effective clinical teacher as Jenner ever existed:

> Facts observed, certain relations definitely perceived, dominated him and his teaching. Pathological observation, scrupulously precise and thorough, was applied to the elucidation of symptoms, and the results were expressed in concise, terse, emphatic words, which fixed themselves in the memory of those who heard him. It was the same with the clinical facts of disease, and his keen observation and retentive memory made his observations in early life of service in later years.[50]

John Russell Reynolds was another influential mentor, and also became a friend. Reynolds was also a Nonconformist. He and his brother, the Reverend Henry Reynolds (Congregationalist minister in Leeds, and later principal of Cheshunt Theological College) had been educated by their father before going to UCL. Russell Reynolds entered his medical training in 1846, and had a brilliant career as a student. In 1859 he became assistant physician at UCH, remaining attached to the hospital for the rest of his life. He succeeded Jenner as professor of the principles and practice of medicine in 1865.

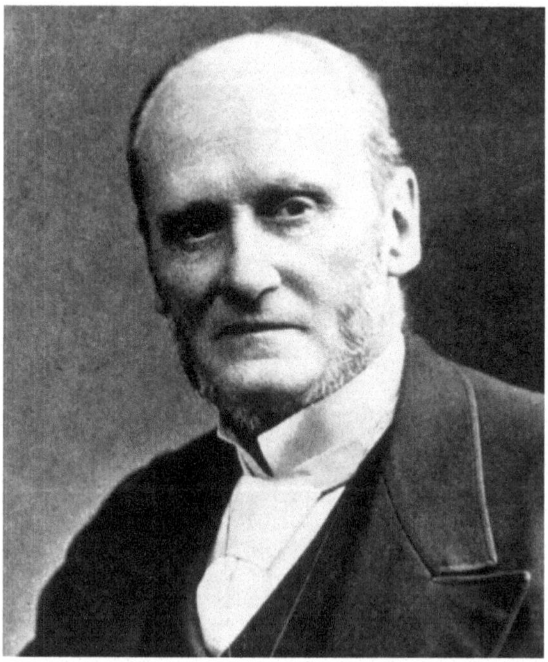

**Fig. 4.9** John Russell Reynolds. Image courtesy of the Queen Square Library, Archive and Museum.

In a book on epilepsy, published in 1861, Reynolds demonstrated the use of statistical method in medical research. The book, which included statistical tables to support each of his conclusions, made him an authority on diseases of the nervous system.[51]

He was also an excellent lecturer, noted 'for his love of precision, order, and classification, his reluctance to make general statements, his dry humour, and the ease of his delivery which concealed the care of his preparation'.[52]

After Reynolds had given a series of lectures on the clinical uses of electricity in 1870, the recently qualified Gowers asked him why they had not been published when the profession needed to learn about the subject, and told Reynolds that he had taken down a verbatim shorthand record. In 1871 the lectures were published, thanks to Gowers' intervention.[53] Between 1866 and 1879 Reynolds produced his five-volume *System of Medicine* with a large number of contributors. It is evidence of his regard for Gowers' abilities, that Reynolds asked him to contribute sections on the heart, covering atrophy, hypertrophy, dilation, fatty diseases, and fibroid diseases.

In its obituary for Reynolds, the *BMJ* cited Gowers' comments on his student shorthand notes as an example of the excellence of Reynolds' lectures:

> All those who attended them would be willing to bear testimony to their many excellences, but we may perhaps best quote a statement from a small shorthand pamphlet, the preface to which is signed by the initials 'WRG' which will be readily recognised as those of one of Sir Russell Reynolds' most distinguished pupils. After giving notes of a lecture as specimen of the kind of notes taken, the writer adds: 'Although the words given are only about a third of those uttered by the lecturer, such epitome will be felt to be adequate for all the needs of the student, and, as a matter of fact, as stated on a previous page, these notes constituted the only source of knowledge of systematic medicine which sufficed for the medal at the MB and MD Lond. examinations.[54]

Gowers qualified in 1867 when he passed his Second MB. He was awarded a Gold Medal in Anatomy, and in November 1867 was also admitted as a Member of the Royal College of Surgeons.[55] He continued his studies, however, sitting the Second MB in 1869. He was an outstanding student, achieving gold medals for botany, physiology, anatomy, and materia medica; and silver medals for pathological anatomy, and practical physiology and histology. He sat his MD in 1870, and was awarded the University Medal.

Between leaving Coggeshall and qualifying as a doctor, Gowers had also taught himself to draw. This was not an unusual skill for doctors at the time, and there were plenty of role models. John Marshall, who beat Joseph Lister to the chair in surgery in 1866, was a teacher of anatomy who had a long-term interest in 'artistic anatomy' (he was made professor of anatomy at the Royal Academy in 1873, his application supported by Dante Gabriel Rossetti who was one of his patients). Russell Reynolds was also an accomplished painter. Henry Thompson, a close friend of Reynolds, professor of clinical surgery at UCH from 1866, also had paintings hung at the Royal Academy.

In 1867 UCL introduced public lectures at which its own professors lectured but also guest speakers, such as Huxley and Ruskin. In 1869, Ruskin delivered the first part of a series of talks later published as *The Queen of the Air*[56], and in 1870 gave his lectures on art in Oxford. In the inaugural Oxford lecture he urged 'you, youths of England' to help found colonies in the expanding empire:

> Within the last few years we have had the laws of natural science opened to us with a rapidity which has been blinding by its brightness; and means of transit and communication

> given to us which have made but one kingdom of the habitable globe. One kingdom;—but who is to be king? . . .
>
> And this is what she [England] must either do, or perish: she must found colonies as fast and as far as she is able, formed of her most energetic and worthiest men;—seizing every piece of fruitful waste ground she can set her foot on, and there teaching these her colonists that their chief virtue is to be fidelity to their country, and that their first aim is to be to advance the power of England by land and sea.[57]

Ruskin reflected the mood of the day, exhorting his audience 'to have a fixed purpose of some kind for your country and yourselves'. This imperial evangelism, compatible with liberal Nonconformism, was one that Gowers responded to, as will be seen from the friendships he cultivated in later life.

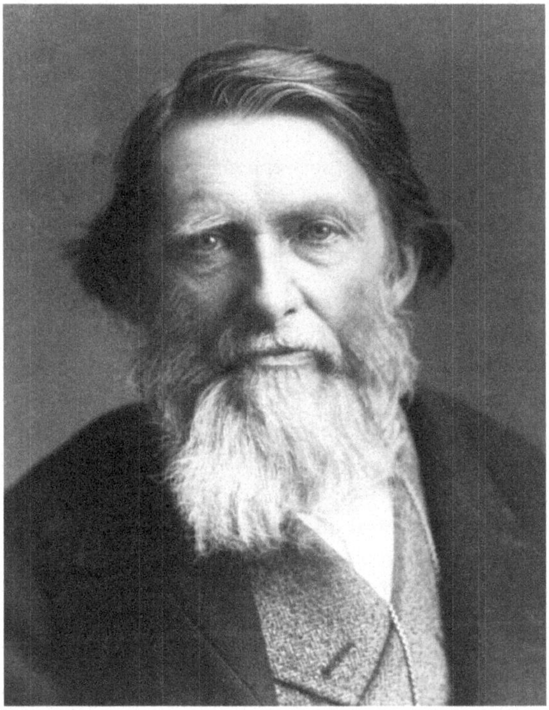

**Fig. 4.10** John Ruskin. (Courtesy of Mr Charles Seper.)

Ruskin lost favour in the twentieth century, but for almost fifty years 'to read Ruskin was accepted as proof of the possession of a soul'. He was admired 'as one of the unassailable masters of English prose', and to be 'one of the greatest social reformers of his time'.[58] But he also approached art through nature. 'For the first half of his life he believed that nature—by which he meant the mountains, rocks, trees, plants, skies and rivers of Western Europe—was a direct revelation of God's glory, designed for the edification of man; and that it should be interpreted as an expression of His Word'.[59]

It seems highly likely that Gowers attended Ruskin's London lectures; he certainly became a great admirer. In its obituary for Gowers, *The Lancet* recorded that he was a constant student of Ruskin's works.[60] Ernest wrote that his father admired Ruskin partly for his style, but mostly for his subject matter. On one occasion, when Ernest was riding in a carriage with his father at Broadstairs, Kent, in the 1880s, his father could not contain his enthusiasm when he spotted his idol:

> We passed an elderly bearded man in a cloak, walking along the grass between the road and the cliff. He stopped the carriage, went up to the stranger, exchanged a word or two with him and shook hands. When he got in to the 'fly' again he said to me: 'Now we shall always be able to remember that I have shaken hands with John Ruskin'.

## Marrying into the Baines family of Leeds

By 1870 Gowers, who had shone as a student, had now graduated MD, been awarded the University Medal, and was ready to embark on his career, already a great achievement for the boy for whom study had been such an isolated and self-driven pursuit. He was, like many other Victorians, moving up from the relatively humble origins of the artisan class, into the new and rapidly expanding professional class. Peterson writes that in the medical world of nineteenth-century London, those who had reached the highest levels of the profession lived and practised among the most prestigious and fashionable members of English society. They often married well, sent their sons to public school and university; they owned carriages, hired servants, and donned the morning coats and top hats that daily bespoke their elevated status:

> Qualifying at age twenty-one, the aspirant to consulting status stayed in London, serving in minor hospital posts, seeking the beginnings of practice, and make what connections and income he could. At twenty-six, he became a Fellow of his College and, with luck, by age thirty he might be appointed assistant physician or surgeon at one of the London hospitals. For most young men this decade was primarily a time of surviving and waiting for the posts that would secure their future as consultants. Promotion to full physician came typically at age forty, and election to Royal College office by age fifty. If senior status in a London teaching hospital is used as an index of success, then for most of the nineteenth century, the inner circle of elites numbered no more than 180—five percent of all London practitioners and just over one percent of medical practitioners in England and Wales.[61]

Gowers never reached the status of his two mentors Jenner and Reynolds, Jenner became Physician-in-Ordinary to Queen Victoria, and Reynolds was appointed Physician to the Royal Household. Nonetheless Gowers was well on his way towards joining the 'elite' five per cent of medical practitioners in London.

In 1870 Gowers was appointed the first Medical Registrar at the National Hospital for the Paralysed and Epileptic, established ten years earlier in Queen Square, Bloomsbury. The next chapters will concentrate on developments in neurology, the genesis of the National Hospital, and Gowers' contributions, before returning to

Gowers' personal life and interests after 20 years in which he focused his energies almost solely on his career. Gowers barely eased his self-imposed work pressures after he graduated with such distinction. By the time he reached the age of 45, he began to suffer debilitating bouts of ill-health, including severe sciatica. His health had probably never been robust. In 1895 he told his new-found friend G. E. Morrison that for the 20 years after he started his career in 1870 'I did not make a single new friend—working always another medical mine'.

Fortunately he found time for courtship. Although he had had a passing flirtation with a girl he met in Coggeshall, and there are fond references in his diary to a girl in Yorkshire, it was not until he qualified and had the prospect of an income that he could contemplate anything more serious. It was Russell Reynolds who introduced Gowers to his future wife, Mary Baines. Reynolds, like Gowers, had been an outstanding but impecunious student. After qualifying in 1852 he had joined his brother Henry, a Congregationalist minister, who had moved to Leeds from Essex three years earlier. The Reynolds brothers were deeply involved in debates over the future of the Congregational Church, and wrote a book on the subject in 1860.[62] Their sister Susannah went to stay in Leeds shortly after Henry's move, and while there she met widower Frederick Baines, ten years her senior. Susannah Reynolds became stepmother to Frederick Baines' three young children, one of whom was four-year-old Mary Baines. When Russell Reynolds also moved to Leeds, in 1852, he established a practice based in Henry's house. Susannah had married Frederick Baines in 1850, and now lived a short walk away from Henry. Reynolds boarded with his sister and her new family while he was in Leeds, so first met Mary when she was a child.

The Baines were well-known Nonconformist liberals. In 1801, Mary's grandfather, Edward Baines, had bought the failing *Leeds Mercury*, a weekly newspaper with a circulation of around 800 copies, and by the 1820s had turned it into one of the most influential and respected provincial papers in the country, with a circulation of over 5000, advocating parliamentary reform, the abolition of the slave trade, the separation of church and state, the extension of civil liberties, and the introduction of universal public education. The *Leeds Mercury* became a leader of Nonconformist opinion. After the 1832 *Reform Bill*, Edward Baines entered parliament as MP for Leeds where he remained until he retired in 1841.

Edward Baines had four sons, of whom Frederick, Mary Baines' father, was the youngest. The eldest, Matthew Talbot, also entered parliament where, under Lord John Russell's administration he became president of the Poor Law Board, and then, under Palmerston, gained a seat in Cabinet as Chancellor of the Duchy of Lancaster. The second son, Edward Baines junior, succeeded his father as editor of the *Leeds Mercury* and became MP for Leeds in 1859. The third son, Thomas, moved to Liverpool, where he bought the *Liverpool Times*, acting as its editor for 30 years. Both through the *Leeds Mercury* and their direct involvement in politics the Baines family became highly influential. Particularly through their in-laws, the Reeds of Hackney, the family were also closely associated with both the London Missionary and the British and Foreign Bible societies.

In 1837 Mary's father Frederick had become one of the partners in the *Leeds Mercury* but he was frequently unwell and spent a good deal of time abroad. He concentrated on the business side of the *Mercury* 'though he also had the ability to write tersely and gracefully'.[63] A number of his children were sent to boarding schools, including Mary who attended a Nonconformist school in Brighton.

Later in life Gowers became friendly with both Rudyard Kipling and Dr Leander Starr Jameson, both of whose names were inextricably linked with British imperialism, and it is worth noting that Edward Baines junior and his brother Frederick, in keeping with liberal sentiment at the time, supported Britain's imperialist expansion, and while the Mercury advocated advanced liberal opinions on most domestic questions, it always supported an 'enlightened and reasonable Imperialism'.[64]

Gowers is unlikely to have met Mary Baines in Leeds, but her strong Congregational background must have had considerable appeal to him. Russell Reynolds had only remained in Leeds for a short time because one of his teachers, the physiologist and physician Dr Marshall Hall, persuaded Reynolds to take over his London practice. Gowers was probably introduced to Mary Baines when she was staying at the Reynolds' family home at Romsey in Hampshire. The couple had much in common and it was a happy marriage in which Gowers compensated for the early loss of his father and his lack of siblings through utter devotion to the family they created. Marrying into such a large, close-knit, and intellectually interesting family must have been a wonderful contrast to his lonely childhood. But Mary remains a shadowy figure because of her self-effacing personality. One of the few glimpses of her was provided by her son Ernest, when he described the lengths to which Gowers would go in his commitment to shorthand:

> He taught it to his children as soon as they were of any age to learn to read and write. When he became engaged he persuaded his fiancée to learn it in order that their love letters might take the form of shorthand postcards, always his favourite form of correspondence. I do not know which was the more characteristic, of my father to make this suggestion or of my mother to comply with it without a murmur.

By the early 1870s Ann Gowers and her son had saved enough money to buy the lease of 50 Queen Anne Street, Cavendish Square. The bulk of the money must have come from the sale of the house Ann's mother had owned in Doncaster. Ann Gowers bought the lease of their new London home from army surgeon John Wordsworth.

In the centre of London's elite medical world, it was a good area in which to start a consultancy, and it was from here that Gowers later practised as a neurologist. Queen Anne Street was close to Harley Street and within walking distance both of UCH and the National Hospital for the Paralysed and Epileptic (in the heart of Bloomsbury). Charles Darwin's brother Erasmus lived in the same street, and Charles Darwin's son Francis, a medical student at the time, was living with his uncle. The physician Edward Liveing lived at number 52 and Marcus Gunn, the ophthalmic surgeon, lived at number 54. Gowers remained there for nearly 40 years. From the time of his marriage in 1875, the house in Queen Anne Street became the family home as well as his consulting rooms.

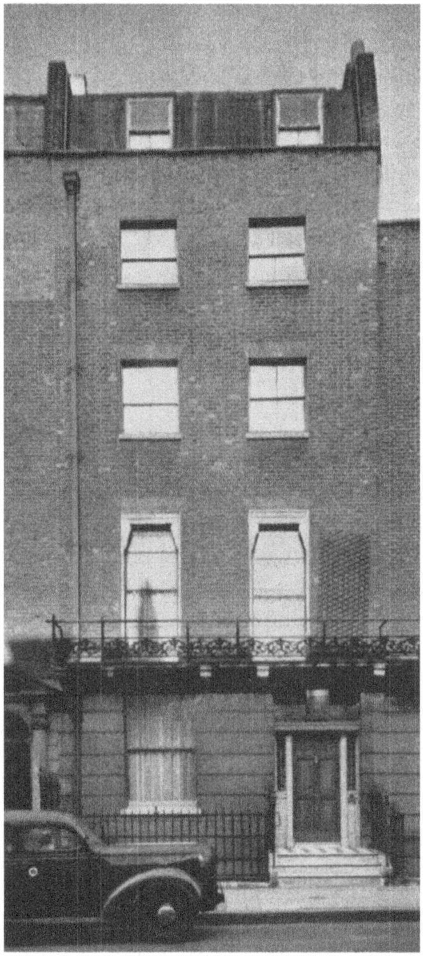

**Fig. 4.11** 50 Queen Anne Street, Cavendish Square, in 1948. From Critchley, 1949.

Chapter 5

# Choosing neurology

Russell Reynolds must have influenced Gowers' decision to specialize in neurology. By 1868 he had already invited his conscientious and able student to contribute to his multi-authored text, *A System of Medicine*.[1] Between 1864 and 1869, Reynolds had also been a physician at the National Hospital for the Paralysed and Epileptic, Queen Square, and knew that the position of medical registrar was about to be created. Whether the new position also influenced Gowers' choice or not, he committed himself to neurology with the same dedication he had shown when he was persuaded to become a medical apprentice and study for his London matriculation.

A brief overview of the significant developments in neurological knowledge may be useful in reminding us of the context within which Gowers embarked on his career and the stage that neurological research and conjecture had reached when Gowers entered the field in 1870. The anatomy and functions of the brain and nervous system were a source of increasing medical interest in the first half of the nineteenth century, but theories about the functions of the brain had first emerged in the ancient world. Galen, the leading medical thinker in Rome from AD 130–200 developed theories about the functions of the nervous system that dominated medical thinking for centuries. He based his untested theories on Hippocrates' four 'humours', and concluded that consciousness and soul were located in the middle ventricle of the brain and that the cerebellum and the fourth ventricle beneath it controlled actions and emotions. Largely through the medical text written by Avicenna of Persia in about AD 1000, translated into Arabic and Latin by Jewish scholars in Muslim Spain, Galen's teaching spread, and survived until the Renaissance.[2] However, European exploration of human anatomy was also constrained until the seventeenth century by a papal edict that held dissection to be sacrilege.

In 1662, Descartes wrote what was tantamount to the first textbook in neurophysiology, placing the brain 'fairly and squarely in control of everything else'. In his *De Homine* he recognized the existence of what would later be regarded as reflex responses and provided a speculative interpretation of their possible mechanism—believing that all motor acts were 'the consequence of sensory energy "reflected" back out of the brain as movement'.[3] In Oxford, Thomas Willis, who first used the term 'neurology', suggested that nerves could intercommunicate peripherally as well as in the brain. Willis made accurate dissections of the brain (having been supplied with bodies through an arrangement with the local hangman) and recognized that nerve fibres, not the ventricles, linked different structures within it. Another significant discovery was the result more of serendipity than scientific method. The wife of the Italian physician Galvani observed that the frogs' legs she was preparing for her husband's dinner twitched when they touched her copper and iron pans, an observation that led Galvani to investigate the electrical basis of nerve excitability.[4]

Towards the end of the eighteenth century, study of the physiology of the nervous system intensified. Franz Joseph Gall, after carrying out neuroanatomical studies in Germany, suggested that different parts of the brain might control specific functions of the body. This introduced the vital concept of brain 'localization' (although Gall's 'phrenology', in which he attempted to specify and map what was controlled, was later dismissed).

After the *Anatomy Act* of 1832, dissection became an accepted practice in British medicine, enabling closer examination of internal organs. Scientific method, with its emphasis on statistical collection and analysis, also became more common in the nineteenth century. This was an area in which Gowers was to excel. Already, as a young man, he had been influenced by discussions with Cornelius Walford of the Statistical Society. As a medical student he had worked for two men, Jenner and Reynolds, who were members of the London Medical Society of Observation. The Society was formed in 1850 to promote accurate pathology and therapeutics by clinical and allied investigation, the value of which was to be estimated by the numerical method. Significantly for their disciple Gowers, this was to be by:

> the collection of records of cases observed by the members, the particulars in every instance (whether observed at the bedside or after death) to be noted in writing at the moment of observation, fullness of detail to be constantly held in view as deeply important, but accuracy alone to be considered absolutely necessary.[5]

Jenner had kept records of nearly 1000 cases of acute continued fever at the London Fever Hospital, records that enabled him to determine the difference between typhus and typhoid fevers. Russell Reynolds, who joined the Medical Society of Observation in 1860, must have led Gowers not only towards neurology, but also reinforced the importance of basing research on an accumulation of accurately observed case records.

Neuroscience and clinical neurology made slow progress over the century after Galvani's discovery of the electrical transmission of nervous impulses. Neuroscience focused on research into the functions of the brain and nervous system, while neurology would eventually become a medical specialty concerned with the diagnosis and treatment of disorders of the brain and nervous system. Clinical neurology not only explored how the nervous system malfunctioned, but also attempted to identify and classify the disorders affecting it. Stein and Stoodley observe:

> The discoveries about nervous function made by the great nineteenth-century clinical neurologists, such as Hughlings Jackson, Charcot, Head and Holmes . . . owed little to electricity, but much to the old-fashioned Hippocratic method of careful observation of symptoms and signs in life, and later correlating them with postmortem revelations about the location of the trauma, tumour or stroke. This classic technique led to the reaffirmation of perhaps the most important neurological concept of all, namely the general principle of *localization of function* within the nervous system.[6]

In Germany, Romberg subdivided clinical neurology into the disorders which either increased or decreased motor and sensory function. His *Manual of the Nervous Diseases of Man*, generally regarded as the first modern neurological textbook, was based on these subdivisions.[7] At about the same time, another German, Hermann von Helmholtz, invented the ophthalmoscope, a diagnostic instrument that was to prove invaluable in neurological, ophthalmological, and general medical practice.

It was on diseases of the brain and spinal cord that physicians such as Gowers began to concentrate. In the 1850s, 20 years before Gowers entered the field, Marshall Hall (Russell Reynolds' mentor) described the 'reflex arc', the nervous circuit involved in the automatic and involuntary activity that results from a stimulus without the brain having time to receive, process, and then send a message to the muscle concerned.[8] He concluded that several neurological disorders, including epilepsy, were caused by the malfunctioning of this reflex arc.[9] In 1855, Russell Reynolds himself wrote a monograph on the diagnosis of diseases of the nervous system, based on a logical classification of neurological disorders,[10] and later an important monograph on epilepsy.[11] In the late 1860s, Hughlings Jackson correlated sites of brain pathology, often syphilitic, with the associated patterns of epileptic seizures, and then reasoned that motor function must also be represented in a localized part of the cerebral cortex.

The discovery of localization had a gradual but profound impact on neurological research, prompting a series of investigations to localize other aspects of brain function in the cortex. Being able to locate the specific sites that controlled speech and movement meant that lesions could also be located in the cerebral cortex of a living patient. It was accurate localization that allowed the first successful brain surgery to be carried out at a time when no technology existed to help locate lesions.

This was the extent to which neurological research had progressed when Gowers began his career in 1870. Although there had been significant advances in both knowledge and practice, neurological diagnosis depended solely on the skill and clinical knowledge of the doctors. There were no diagnostic aids such as X-rays or magnetic resonance imaging, nor even cerebrospinal fluid examination. There was little scientifically based therapy, although many remedies, including bromides and electrotherapy, were in vogue.

## The National Hospital, Queen Square 1860–70

Between 1860 and 1870, two significant, but very different, institutions began to make their name in neurological research: one in London and the other in Paris. The National Hospital, Queen Square, opened in London in 1860; two years later Alfred Vulpian and Jean-Martin Charcot were appointed to the Hôpital de la Salpêtrière in Paris.

When Charcot arrived the Salpêtrière housed around 5000 indigent females. His exploration of the diseases afflicting these women led him to discover and describe a number of neurological diseases and match specific lesions to neurological disorders such as epilepsy, multiple sclerosis, and stroke. His theatrical teaching style drew crowds of observers, and the school of clinical neurology that developed at the Salpêtrière became famous throughout the world. Charcot, recognized as one of the great nineteenth-century neurologists, tends to be known by the general public for his investigations into hysteria and hypnotism (which later included males). Notably, after watching Charcot's demonstrations on hysteria at the Salpêtrière, Sigmund Freud switched his studies from neurological research to medical psychopathology.

The National Hospital for the Paralysed and Epileptic not only provided specialized care for patients (both men and women) with neurological disorders, but, through the foresight and intervention of the Lord Mayor of London, also offered an environment within which to carry out neurological research. The first hospital in the world dedicated specifically to the care of people with neurological illnesses, it owed its existence to Johanna Chandler, a middle-aged woman who lived with her brother Edward and sister Louisa not far from Queen Square. Ten years earlier their grandmother had been paralysed by a stroke, and her grandchildren cared for her at home until she died. This made them realize how little help was available for the care of people suffering from chronic neurological handicap. The Chandlers approached the Lord Mayor, Alderman David Wire, who supported their proposal to raise funds for a specialized hospital. The Chandlers envisaged a 'board and care' home for incurables. Fortunately for neurological research, the Lord Mayor, who was himself partially paralysed, intervened. He insisted that the new hospital should be created for the investigation as well as treatment of nervous diseases. Thus it was originally designated the National Hospital for the Relief and Cure of the Paralysed and Epileptic (generally referred to in later years as either the 'National Hospital' or 'Queen Square').

In the 1860s there were more than seventy small specialist hospitals in London. For example, the London Galvanic Hospital opened in Cavendish Square in 1861, dedicated to the electrical treatment of nervous and muscular diseases. It failed to flourish, but stronger competition came from the London Infirmary for Epilepsy and Paralysis that opened near Harley Street. Founded in 1867 by the German physician, Julius Althaus, it moved to larger premises in Regents Park in 1872, changing its name to the Hospital for Diseases of the Nervous System. A century later, as Maida Vale Hospital for Nervous Diseases, it finally amalgamated with the National Hospital for Nervous Diseases, Queen Square, and the Maida Vale site closed in 1983.

Queen Square is in the heart of Bloomsbury, which was at the time the centre of much of London's artistic and medical life. When the hospital opened its doors to its first patients in 1860, it had eight beds for women, a small outpatient department, and a dispensary. Only potentially treatable cases were accepted. The hospital decided that if, after a probationary period of residence, the case was considered incurable by the treating physician, the patient had to make way for someone whose case was more hopeful. The discharged case would then be followed in the outpatient department, but cared for at home. The majority of patients were treated free of charge.

In 1866 the hospital expanded to include the house next door, 26 Queen Square (purchasing its lease from the artist William Morris), increasing its inpatient capacity to 64 beds. An early plan of the hospital, now occupying these two Georgian houses, shows a ground floor comprising an outpatient waiting hall, a boardroom, consulting room, private office, dispensary, laboratory, a ward with an adjacent day room, and a porter's room. Upstairs were the baths, electrical room, and gymnasium, a padded room, and two more wards. Patients could only 'come indoors' on the recommendation

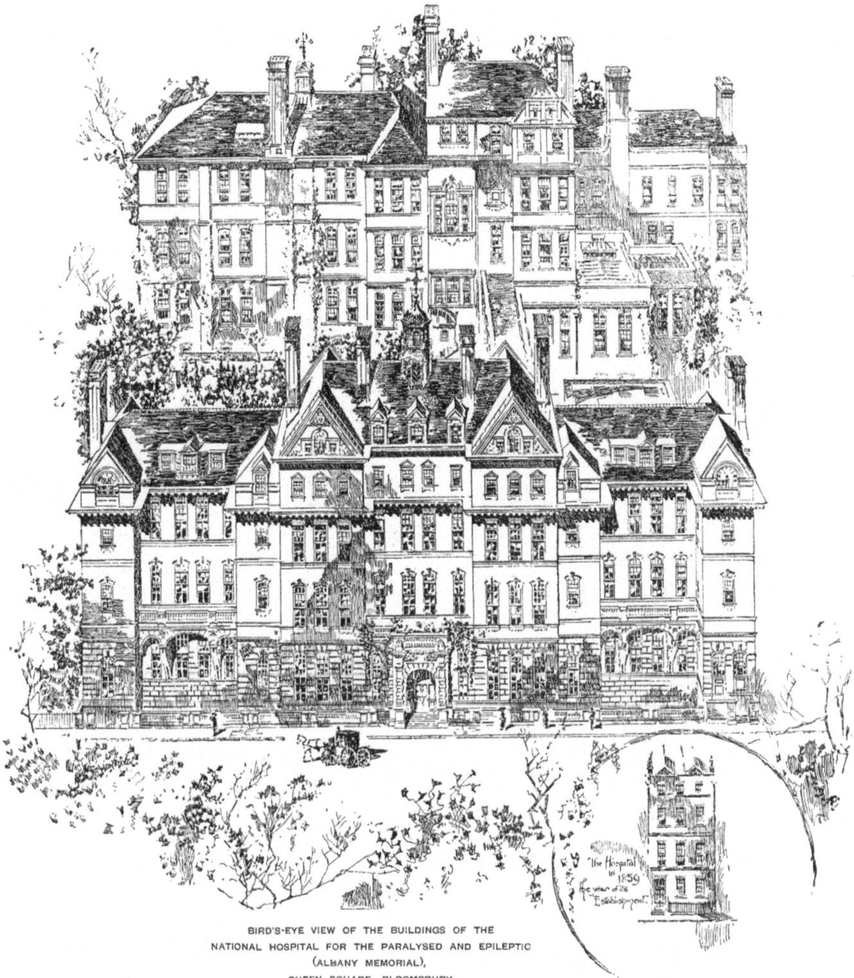
"The Hospital
in 1859
the year of its
Establishment."
BIRD'S-EYE VIEW OF THE BUILDINGS OF THE
NATIONAL HOSPITAL FOR THE PARALYSED AND EPILEPTIC
(ALBANY MEMORIAL),
QUEEN SQUARE, BLOOMSBURY.

**Fig. 5.1** Bird's-eye view of the buildings of the National Hospital for the Paralysed and Epileptic (undated). Image courtesy of the Queen Square Library, Archive and Museum.

of a physician, after they had first been seen in outpatients, and with the final approval of the Board of Management.

Queen Square was the first hospital to institute day rooms. With carpeted floors, flowers, paintings on the walls, and a patients' library, it had a comfortable, almost luxurious atmosphere. However, it was also a hive of activity:

> The life of the hospital was at its busiest, and in every department of affairs the daily routine proceeded with the smoothness of a perfect mechanism. Sir Russell Reynolds had said that for patients of this hospital in a degree transcending everything done elsewhere, there

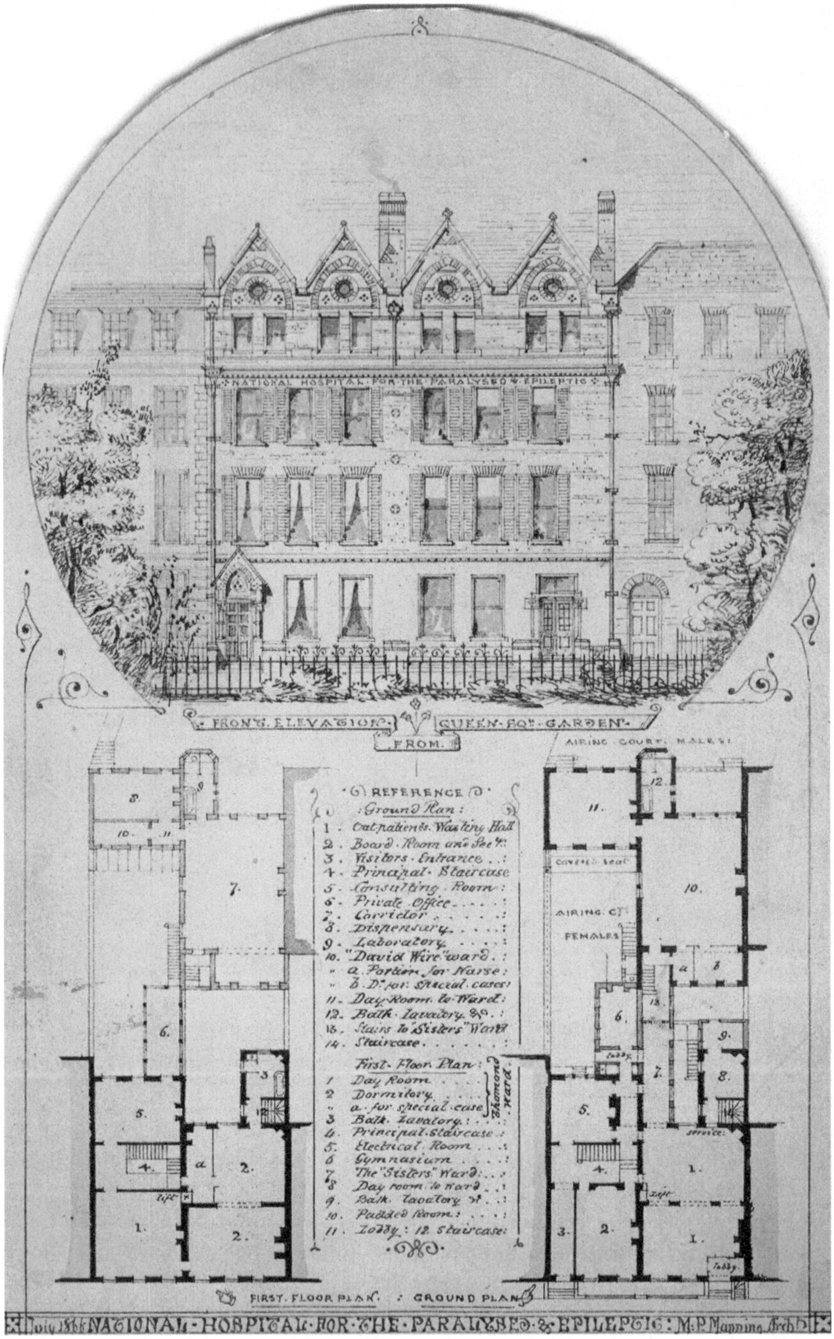


**Fig. 5.2** Floor plan of the National Hospital, Queen Square (undated). Image courtesy of the Queen Square Library, Archive and Museum.

> must be 'treatment, treatment, treatment, always treatment'. The hospital was a veritable workshop bewildering in the complexity of its subtle machinery. Patients were rubbed, stretched, smacked, kneaded, straightened, electrified, hung from tripods on the roof, swathed in bandages, and steeped in sulphur baths. Their torpid muscles were roused by passive movements. They were cased in plaster jackets, weights were attached to their legs, and occasionally they were hypnotized. If after all had been done the stubborn malady won the day in too many instances, it was only because the result striven for lay beyond the reach of human powers.[12]

The outpatient department at Queen Square offered special services that were not available anywhere else in London, or even in Europe. It developed rapidly: in 1870, Gowers' first year at the hospital, over 2000 individual patients, many of them children, made 12,000 visits.[13]

## Initial appointments to the Queen Square staff

The first staff physician was Yorkshireman Jabez Spence Ramskill, appointed in 1859. Ramskill persuaded the Chandlers to include epilepsy in the mission of the hospital.[14] Epilepsy and cases of paralysis became the commonest admissions to the hospital. Significantly, he strongly encouraged the hospital to use bromides to treat epilepsy. Ramskill wrote relatively few original papers but contributed to the literature on aphasia, the management of diphtheria, and lead poisoning. Charles Edouard Brown-Séquard, a Mauritian well connected in the literary and artistic world who had been elected to the Royal Society for his work on the physiology and pathology of the nervous system, was also appointed in 1859, but had left Queen Square well before Gowers joined the staff.

A crucial appointment so far as Gowers would be concerned was that of the subsequently eminent neurologist John Hughlings Jackson, who joined the consulting staff in 1862. Hughlings Jackson was born into a Dissenting family in a small country village outside York and had started his medical training as an apothecary's assistant. He came under the wing of Thomas Laycock at the York Medical School before moving to London, where he rented accommodation for three years in the home of fellow Yorkshireman, Jonathan Hutchinson. Both Ramskill and Hughlings Jackson had followed in the footsteps of Hutchinson, a brilliant clinician and surgeon. It is said that Hughlings Jackson was tempted to focus on 'philosophy', but that Hutchinson persuaded him not to abandon medicine. 'Philosophy' was a term that was used at the time to include some studies that later fell under the umbrella of science: 'natural philosophy' and 'mechanical philosophy' were both part of the Preliminary Scientific curriculum that Gowers studied. It has been suggested Hughlings Jackson's 'philosophy' may have been the science of neurophysiology or abnormal psychology, rather than philosophy as it is understood today.[15] Hughlings Jackson's ideas were also influenced by the evolutionary theories of his friend Herbert Spencer, who argued that societies and organisms exhibited hierarchical divisions, and that increasing size led to increasing complexity and differentiation of function.

When Hughlings Jackson was appointed to the consulting staff he was required to visit the National Hospital twice a day and see outpatients in their homes. Hutchinson and Ramskill encouraged Queen Square to appoint him. Ramskill, who had worked with him at the London Hospital, had a large caseload of patients with epilepsy and hemiplegia. He asked Hughlings Jackson to help him, introducing him to the challenges of epilepsy and giving him a clinical focus. Brown-Séquard, who was also influential in Hughlings Jackson's appointment, on the one hand encouraged Jackson to focus on the study of the nervous system rather than the 'wider observation of disease in general' but also suggested that he should not narrow this focus to epilepsy alone.

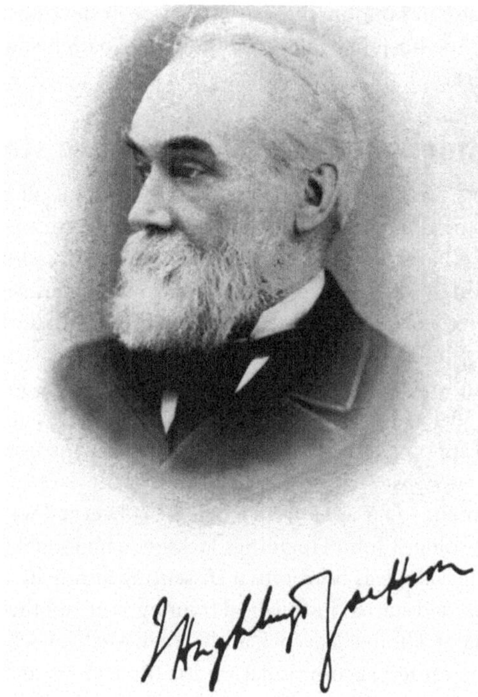

**Fig. 5.3** John Hughlings Jackson. Image courtesy of the Queen Square Library, Archive and Museum.

In 1867, Hughlings Jackson became a member of the permanent staff. The Queen Square history describes some of his strengths and weaknesses:

> Without doubt Jackson is to be regarded as the greatest figure in British neurology. Not only an accurate and shrewd clinical observer he was, above all, a deep thinker with a philosophic attitude of mind. His humility and gentleness were not always conducive towards the recognition of his superlative abilities.
>
> Jackson was modest and tolerant to a fault. His colleagues respected and revered him without perhaps fully understanding his way of thought. They were aware that he was a great and remarkable man, but it took outsiders, and those of a later generation, to realize him for what he was—a genius. In part, this was due to Jackson's inability to express himself

> simply and clearly. He did not lecture well, and he was not a great teacher. As a writer he was obscure. His text was cluttered up with additions, elaborations, amendments, parentheses, qualifications, footnotes, afterthoughts, and asides.[16]

Hughlings Jackson was a grave, kind-hearted, and self-effacing man, with a lively sense of humour. Charles Mercier wrote that not only had he 'the keenest sense of humour of any one I ever knew, but on the utterance of a witticism his face would light up, and he would throw his head back with uncontrolled delight'.[17] He was also a restless man 'whose mind seemed to be in a state of constant conflict between his desire to give pleasure and his fear of being bored or bound'.[18] Younger men such as Gowers and, later on, Henry Head and James Taylor, played a significant role in interpreting and disseminating his ideas, and over the years many of his intuitive insights were proved correct. His undoubted brilliance lay in his ability to construct sophisticated conceptual models of the way the brain works, based on his clinical observations. The evolution of the brain, as Hughlings Jackson envisaged it, ranged up from the centres that were least organized towards those that were most organized, from the simplest up to the most complex, and from the most automatic up to the most voluntary: and thus the highest centres made up the 'organ of the mind'.

Charles Bland Radcliffe succeeded Brown-Séquard in 1863. Radcliffe strongly supported the teachings of du Bois-Reymond, father of clinical electrophysiology and ardent exponent of electrotherapy. Like Ramskill, Radcliffe also promoted the use of bromides in the treatment for epilepsy (Gowers recorded that nearly two tons of potassium bromide were dispensed at the National Hospital in 1899).[19]

Three other staff were appointed in 1864, but did not overlap with Gowers. Edward Henry Sieveking remained at Queen Square for only three years, being persuaded to move to St Mary's Hospital where he maintained his interest in epilepsy and devised an aesthesiometer for assessing sensation. Victor Bazire, a native Mauritian like Brown-Séquard, was appointed in the same year, but died early in 1867 from a cerebral haemorrhage. Russell Reynolds, Gowers' mentor, was appointed physician to Queen Square in 1864. He was not a prolific writer, but was a master of the English language, making his name at the age of 27 with his monograph on epilepsy. It was this monograph that helped him get appointed to the staff of UCH, where he eventually succeeded his friend William Jenner as Professor of the Practice of Medicine at UCL.

In 1867, Thomas Buzzard joined the staff. Born in 1831, Buzzard had been trained at King's College Hospital, qualifying MD in 1855, and then joined the British army staff in the Crimea. Henry Charlton Bastian, also a physician to UCH and later its Professor of Medicine, was appointed to the Queen Square staff, shortly after Buzzard. Bastian, appointed Professor of Pathological Anatomy at UCL in 1867, had been one of Gowers' lecturers. He shared Gowers' fascination with natural history and had published on the flora of Falmouth and a collection of the ferns of Great Britain. He was elected Fellow of the Royal Society for his 1864 monograph *The Anguillulidae*, in which he named 100 new species of free nematode worms. He was a lifelong friend of Herbert Spencer and a strong supporter of the theory of evolution. His first major publication in neurology was on the identification of a degenerated tract in the spinal cord, which was later named after Gowers, whose investigation was more definitive.[20]

In a letter to Gowers many years later, Buzzard described these changes in the staff:

> Almost simultaneously Sieveking resigned (the St Mary's staff put pressure upon him!) and Reynolds also left a few months later. Jackson *ipso facto* became physician and I went up on Reynolds' departure [in 1869].'[21]

Critchley summarized the developments in nineteenth-century neurological science before Gowers became a neurologist:

> When Hughlings Jackson was a medical student, neurological practice was largely made up of epileptics, hysterics and paraplegics. The last group was a heterogeneous one, from which some sort of classification was beginning to shape. With the first descriptions of paralysis agitans ['shaking palsy' now known as Parkinson's disease] in 1817, of disseminated sclerosis in 1837 [*sic.*], and of locomotor ataxy [also known as tabes dorsalis: a form of neurosyphilis occurring between 5 and 20 years after the original infection] in 1847, clearer ideas were possible. Year by year, and in rapid succession, the secrets of the nervous system were yielding to the clinico-pathological researches of the 19th century physicians. William Gowers found himself in the throes of great activity along these lines, and, joining the band of pioneers, soon became conspicuous among them.[22]

One non-medical appointment to Queen Square needs to be mentioned. Burford Rawlings was appointed as the hospital's secretary in about 1865, remaining in the position until 1902. In due course his position was expanded to become 'secretary and general director', and he became embroiled in an acrimonious controversy with the medical staff who wrote letters to *The Lancet*, *BMJ*, and *The Times* because of this concentration of power in the hands of one man, who was an administrator, and not a member of the medical staff. They complained that the institution had become 'practically, and to a great and dangerous extent, in the hands of one man', particularly in the absence of any medical representatives on the Board (Gowers was one of the signatories).[23] A committee of inquiry was established, chaired by Sir Edward Fry, which recommended various changes. Almost immediately after the Fry Report was published in June 1901, Rawlings announced his impending retirement, leaving the hospital in January 1902. This is mentioned here, because after he retired Rawlings wrote *A Hospital in the Making*,[24] published in 1913, which contains some of the few descriptions of the National Hospital in its early days. Despite the bitterness of his departure, his successor recorded that Rawlings had been particularly successful in raising the funds necessary to build and expand the hospital.[25]

By 1870, when Gowers became Queen Square's first medical registrar, there were ten physicians, four of whom had connections with UCH. Four (Radcliffe, Ramskill, Hughlings Jackson, and Reynolds) had moved down from Yorkshire, the county where most of Gowers' relatives on his mother's side lived, and where Gowers himself had not only spent a year as a farmer's apprentice but also his holidays after his father died. Radcliffe, Hughlings Jackson and Reynolds also came from Dissenting families. This Nonconformist ethos (similar to that of the 'Godless institution', UCL) had been reflected in a minute of the Board protesting against anything in the hospital chapel 'of a proselytising or pueseyite [*sic.*] nature ever being introduced into the hospital'.[26] It must have been a congenial environment in which to start his working life.

It was the hospital in which Gowers would concentrate most of his working life, and which provided many of his immediate colleagues. He divided his time between his growing consulting practice (about which scant records survive); his position as assistant physician at UCL, where he also lectured; and his clinical work, his research, and his teaching at Queen Square. He was on the staff at Queen Square for nearly 40 years, and it is with Queen Square that his name is most closely associated.

Many years later, in 1905, Gowers and Buzzard (who was by then 84 years old) reminisced over dinner about their years at Queen Square. The following day Buzzard wrote to Gowers, clarifying issues over which he felt he had been less than lucid, and looked back at some of the early influences both on his own career but also within the hospital:

> From Hughlings Jackson I need hardly say I derived infinite advantage. I always look upon him as my master in neurology. From Reynolds (a great personal friend for whom I had a great affection) I curiously enough, as it has always seemed to me, derived nothing. But when you and Bastian came on the scene you appeared to me to bring into the hospital an atmosphere of scientific precision and method by which I was much struck. I imagine that you brought to us the Jenner influence. Radcliffe and Ramskill were then dominant at the hospital and had they brought in then the sort of colleagues they affected (as we experienced later) what difference it would have made in the future of the hospital. I believe it was a turning point in the fortunes of the hospital. Had the two R's secured their way the hospital would have preserved a decidedly commercial tone instead of developing on the lines which we have watched.
>
> I appreciated the Jenner influence imported because although I had enjoyed large opportunities of studying disease I had never had the advantage of the systematic training which was given at University College. In my youth I had been a clinical clerk to Todd and had appreciated his genius-like qualities and admired him much. But he was not a good teacher, and the training of clinical clerks was never very good. There is a wonderful amount of good to be derived from the association of men eager to learn upon the same staff. A sort of atmosphere is created which reacts upon all though there is no direct teaching.[27]

## Medical registrar and physician's assistant 1870–2

Gowers' official position was medical registrar and physicians' assistant. The reason for creating the position of medical registrar was explained later by Burford Rawlings:

> Lacking proper channels for its dissemination, much of the valuable knowledge obtained in the wards and out-patients rooms was running to waste, and the suggestion of the medical authorities that a registrar should be appointed was at once agreed to. The creation of this office was noteworthy. It was the first step towards investing the hospital with the great reputation as a teacher it long since attained, and the historical importance of the event was enhanced by the appointment to the post of Dr (now Sir) W R Gowers who has delighted to call himself a child of the hospital and whose active association with it has ceased only recently.[28]

Hospital registrars were required to supervise students in reporting medical cases. Gowers also attended the hospital post-mortems. The interest in morbid anatomy had developed slowly in the early nineteenth century, then increased between 1830

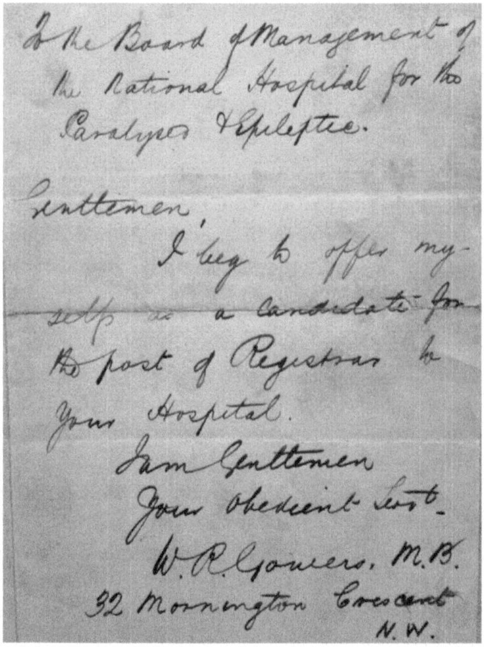

To the Board of Management of
the National Hospital for the
Paralysed & Epileptic.

Gentlemen,
I beg to offer my-
self as a candidate for
the post of Registrar to
your Hospital.
I am Gentlemen
Your obedient Servt.
W. R. Gowers, M.B.
32 Mornington Crescent
N.W.

**Fig. 5.4** Gowers' application for position as medical registrar, 1870. Image courtesy of the Queen Square Library, Archive and Museum.

and 1850. Sir James Paget, who had been appointed curator of the museum at St Bartholomew's Hospital in 1837 and then demonstrator of morbid anatomy, made his name as a pathologist by using his observational powers in surgical pathology.

In his first year, Gowers reported on the outcomes of 500 patients who had been treated at the hospital. He also drew up an inventory of the diagnoses of all the inpatients, which listed 65 epileptics, 26 paraplegics, and 28 hemiplegics. There were also five cases of chorea, five cases of lead palsy, four cases of locomotor ataxia, and four brain tumours.

He reported on a sample of 360 outpatients, classified into: epilepsy and other chronic convulsive affections (216); hysteria (1); melancholia (2); general paralysis of the insane (2); hemiplegia, right (37); hemiplegia, left (22); brain tumour (1); labio-glosso-laryngeal paralysis (1); paraplegia (13); progressive muscular atrophy (2); infantile paralysis (8); locomotor ataxy (3); paralysis agitans (6); facial paralysis (4); oculo-motor paralysis (1); paralysis from lead (5); local spasm (1); chorea (9); writer's cramp (1); vertigo (2); neuralgia (5); other diseases (10).

In the Annual Report in which these appeared, the hospital reported positively on the use of electricity in a 'wide margin of diseases', stating that it would, in appropriate cases, relieve pain, restore voluntary movement, relax spasm, and redevelop wasted muscles. It also reported on the extensive use for both inpatients and outpatients of Turkish, vapour, douche, needle, and sulphur baths.

## Promotion to honorary assistant physician 1872

Gowers' dedicated work as medical registrar was rewarded when he was promoted to honorary assistant physician at Queen Square late in 1872. His referees included the ophthalmologist Dr Richard Liebreich. Liebreich, fifteen years his senior, was also a painter and sculptor. Born in Germany in 1830 he lived primarily in Paris, before moving to London in 1870. He was appointed ophthalmic surgeon to St Thomas' Hospital in 1871. He eventually gave up hospital work to concentrate on painting. Liebreich published the first atlas of ophthalmoscopy, the *Atlas des Ophthalmoscopie*, in 1863, and designed an ophthalmoscope called the 'Liebreich ophthalmoscope'. His reference for Gowers read:

> I have had the opportunity of examining a great number of patients together with Dr Gowers and I am very glad to express the opinion that he is not only thoroughly acquainted with Ophthalmoscopy in general but that he is a very practised diagnostician observing the minutest details and representing them in drawings of remarkable correctness to nature, and also to interpreting very accurately their clinical significance in relation to diseases of the nervous system.[29]

It was Hughlings Jackson, Clifford Allbutt, and Gowers who introduced into England the clinical use of the ophthalmoscope in neurological diagnosis.[30] In 1879, in an appendix to the first edition of his book *A Manual and Atlas of Medical Ophthalmoscopy*, Gowers discussed the commercially available ophthalmoscopes at the time.[31]

Charles Radcliffe also acted as a referee:

> At the present time I know of no one unattached to a hospital who is more worthy to fill this office of Assistant Physician to a hospital than Dr Gowers. Indeed, looking back from a considerable time at the names of the men who have been appointed to this responsible office in the various metropolitan hospitals I fail to find that of a man who can be considered as more worthy. All this I say advisedly after having had for a long time past, in the National Hospital for the Paralysed and Epileptic and elsewhere, abundant opportunities of putting Dr Gowers' worth to the test in every way.[32]

In response to a request for more information he wrote 'Dr Gowers is thoroughly versed in all matters relating to the medical use of electricity'.[33]

Hughlings Jackson reported on Gowers' work as medical registrar:

> I have looked at the cases sent in by Dr Gowers. Those of patients under my care were reported by him without the least assistance from me. Since, or soon after, his appointment as our Medical Registrar, I have left entirely to him the case-taking of most of my inpatients. I may particularly mention that the investigation by electricity and the views expressed on the coordinated convulsions and as to pre-systolic murmur are in no way derived from me.[34]

Gowers had studied under Michael Foster. Born in 1836 Foster, another Dissenter, studied classics at UCL and then went on to the medical school. Between 1867 and 1870, at the invitation of William Sharpey, he was an instructor in physiology and histology. Later he moved to Cambridge and created the Cambridge School of Physiology. He wrote to his former pupil from Cambridge to say how much he was

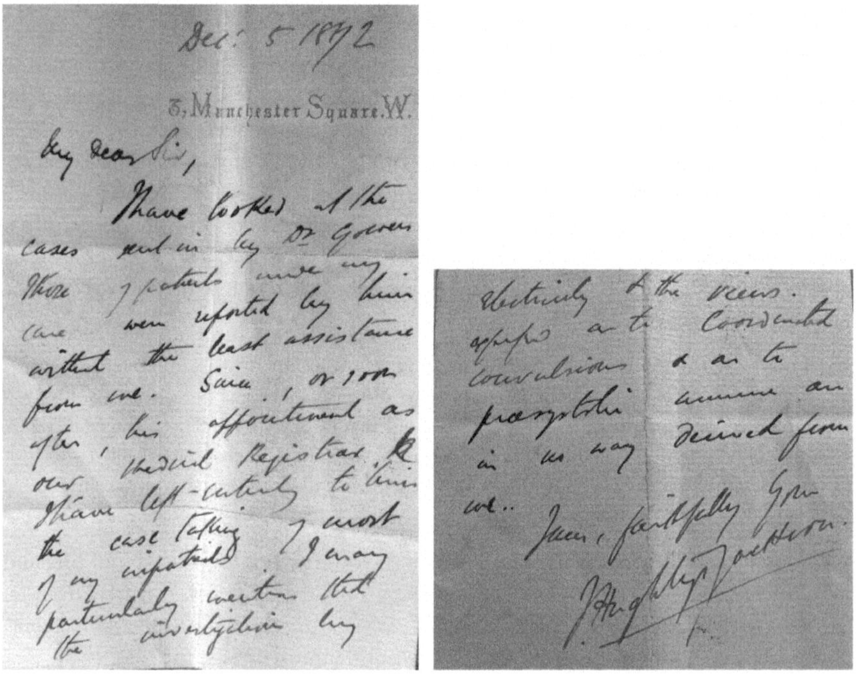
Dec: 5 1872

3, Manchester Square. W.

My dear Sir,

I have looked at the cases sent in by Dr Gowers. Those patients under my care were reported by him without the least assistance from me. Since, or soon after, his appointment as Medical Registrar to our [illegible] I have left entirely to him the case taking of my inpatients. I may particularly mention that the investigation by the

electricity of the viscera. [illegible] as to Coordinated convulsions & as to [illegible] in no way derived from me.

Yours faithfully

J. Hughlings Jackson.

(a) (b)

**Fig. 5.5** Hughlings Jackson reference, p. 1 (a) and p. 2 (b). Image courtesy of the Queen Square Library, Archive and Museum.

'delighted with the way in which you strive to unite in your daily work, Physiology and Practical Medicine'.[35]

Gowers' new responsibilities lay primarily in the outpatient department where he saw his patients in a pokey, ill-equipped room, often shared with a colleague. Here, for 20 years, he interviewed and treated patients:

> Week by week with his characteristic energy and thoroughness, he investigated the patients allotted to him, and when they presented symptoms that threw light on the nature or localization of disease recorded these in shorthand for future study or reference. Thus he collected an enormous body of facts and observations which served him well in writing his celebrated *Manual* and other publications.[36]

## New Queen Square colleagues 1870–90

Few other new physicians of note were appointed to Queen Square in the 1870s. It was not until 1880 that David Ferrier was appointed assistant physician to the hospital. In 1883 he started to urge surgeons to try operating on the brain, and is seen as having played an important role in the emergence of neurosurgery. But Ferrier's greatest strength was physiology. Before he joined the staff at Queen Square, he proved

Hughlings Jackson's theories about the localization of function in the cerebral cortex to be correct when in the 1870s he carried out experiments on the brains of animals in London and at the West Riding Lunatic Asylum in Yorkshire. The asylum was one of the largest and most famous asylums of the Victorian era. Under the directorship of James Crichton-Browne it was a significant institution in the development of psychiatry and the neurosciences in Britain. Henry Maudsley (yet another Yorkshireman from a Dissenting family), who was to become one of the foremost alienists (psychiatrist) of his generation, served for a year as assistant medical officer in 1857 immediately after graduating from UCH. It was at the West Riding Asylum that Ferrier produced the first map of the motor cortex which demonstrated that different functions of the brain were located in different regions of the hemispheres.

In 1880 Charles Beevor was appointed medical resident officer, and promoted to physician in 1882. In 1883 he started to collaborate with the surgeon, Victor Horsley, on research into the minute representation of movements in the cerebral cortex.

Victor Horsley, the most outstanding figure in the development of English neurosurgery, was appointed surgeon to Queen Square in 1886. Two years later, he and Gowers reported in the *Medico-Chirurgical Transactions* the first successful surgical removal of a spinal cord tumour, following an accurate diagnosis by Gowers. A 42-year-old man had developed pain below his left shoulder blade in 1884, which had varied in intensity but had become more severe. In March 1887 the man's legs became progressively weaker and then later he developed spastic paraplegia and urine retention. Gowers diagnosed the presence of a spinal cord lesion at the approximate level of the sixth or seventh thoracic spinal cord segment, probably due to an aneurysm or a tumour. This diagnosis was regarded at the time as a rarity, 'quite beyond the realm of treatment' and a diagnosis 'scarcely ever ventured during life':

> Gowers had already expressed the opinion in one of his papers that a spinal meningeal growth, such as occasionally revealed itself in the autopsy room, was not beyond the powers of surgery, and, indeed, should be more amendable than an intracranial neoplasm. The temptation rose strongly in Gowers' mind to evoke the aid of surgery, a daring project which had never been hazarded. He then invited his old chief, Sir William Jenner, to see the patient; the diagnosis was supported and also what was more important, the idea of a surgical attack. Mr Victor Horsley, then a young surgeon of 30 years, was asked to see the patient, and was afforded the invitation to operate.[37]

Horsley operated at the anticipated level, but then had to open the spinal canal two vertebrae higher, before finding a tumour, which he removed. Horsley and Gowers reported that both leg and bladder functions recovered well (their paper was one of the few in which Gowers collaborated on an equal footing with a co-author).[38]

The survival of an archive of letters between the two men make it possible to discern the relationship between Horsley and Gowers. In the era before the telephone, urgent daily exchanges about cases had to be conducted by letter or telegram, so these were often both frequent and written in great haste. Gowers was aware of the importance of headache and observing optic neuritis ('papilloedema') as one sign of cerebral tumour, and attempted to localize the site of the tumour from focal signs or seizures, but it was clear from his letters that he was always cautious about the precision of his localization when asking Horsley's opinion on whether surgery would be viable. He was clearly

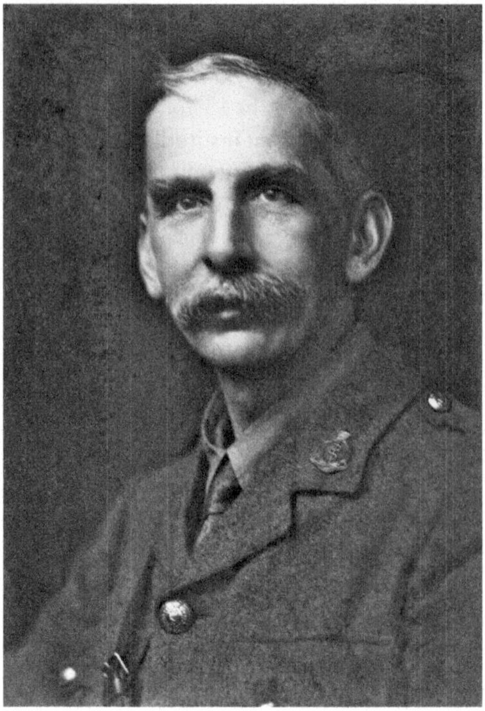

**Fig. 5.6** Victor Horsley. Image courtesy of the Queen Square Library, Archive and Museum.

aware of the need for emergency surgery in cases of raised intracranial pressure. It was often Gowers, particularly in cases of 'tic douloureux' (a nerve disorder that causes a stabbing or electric-shock-like pain in parts of the face), who pressed for surgery while Horsley erred on the side of caution. Gowers would call in at Horsley's house and send messages asking him to operate if he identified a case on the wards, becoming impatient if the surgeon was out of town and did not respond promptly. These exchanges often had to be conducted via terse telegrams. At one point, the decisions became so difficult that Gowers wrote explaining the protocol he preferred:

> I consider it is for a physician to ask a surgeon as a last resort and for the surgeon then to ask the physician for his opinion as to doubtful points both relating to the question of an operation being performed—i.e. merely information to help him in forming an opinion—not to determine it—and perhaps also as to what. If in this case the last comes up I have an idea but I would rather let it come after yours is formed.[39]

But the relationship was generally amicable. In November 1891 Horsley asked if he could use one of the beds allocated to Gowers' patients for a case of his own. Gowers replied that he would agree, but was already being required to reduce the number of beds his patients were occupying because he was not an inpatient physician and was allowed only a small number of beds. He suggested subterfuge: 'Why not have the patient put into one of Dr Ramskills' beds, borrowing it in silence?'.[40]

This was the institutional and intellectual context within which Gowers would spend much of his working life, and which provided the environment in which his research could flourish and he could make his name as a clinician, writer, and teacher. His first 20 years there were spent as a living example of the Victorian ethic of 'work, work, work', in which he had little time for anything but his career.

In March 1874, at the age of 29, he resigned his position as medical registrar:

> Finding that other and increasing engagements render it impossible for me to devote that time to the duties of the first Medical Registrar which is necessary for their efficient discharge I must beg to resign into your hands this appointment which I had the honour to receive four years ago.[41]

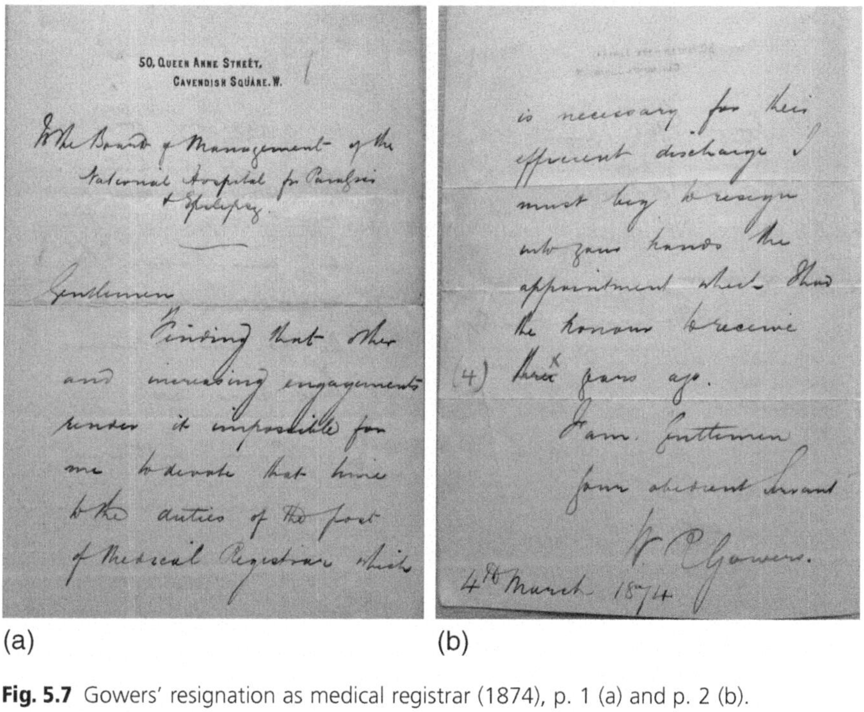

50, Queen Anne Street,
Cavendish Square. W.

1

To the Board of Management of the National Hospital for Paralysis & Epilepsy.

Gentlemen

Finding that other and increasing engagements render it impossible for me to devote that time to the duties of the post of Medical Registrar which is necessary for their efficient discharge I must beg to resign into your hands the appointment which I had the honour to receive (4) three years ago.

I am, Gentlemen
your obedient Servant
W. R. Gowers.

4th March 1874

(a) (b)

**Fig. 5.7** Gowers' resignation as medical registrar (1874), p. 1 (a) and p. 2 (b). Image courtesy of the Queen Square Library, Archive and Museum.

He was already making a name for himself within his profession, and found himself fully occupied with his clinical work, research, teaching, and writing.

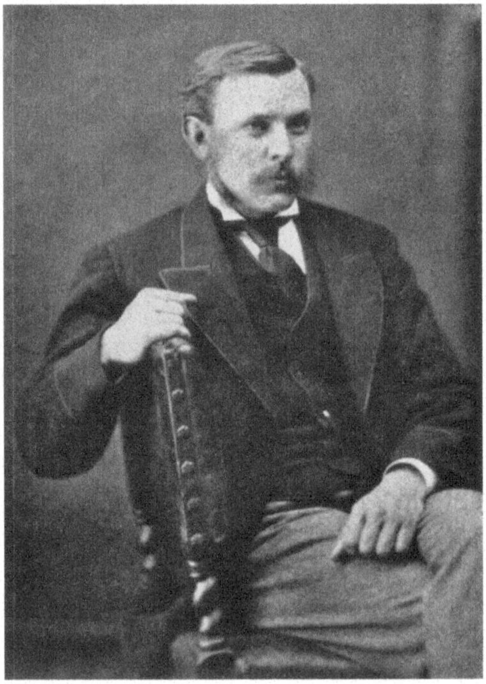

**Fig. 5.8** Gowers aged 29 (1874). Image courtesy of the Queen Square Library, Archive and Museum.

## Chapter 6

# Gowers and clinical diagnosis

Gowers himself wrote that the 20 years from 1870–90 were devoted almost entirely to his work. He made few new friends although, as described later, he was always a most dedicated and thoughtful father. Before the story returns to more personal aspects of his life, however, it must focus on the quality of his work and the achievements that made his name as a neurologist—as a clinician, a researcher, and a teacher.

When Critchley wrote his biography of Gowers he gave it a strictly chronological structure. However, this seemed potentially cumbersome here, given that there is now so much more information about his private life. The neurological chapters that follow move generally from Gowers' day-to-day clinical work, to the research that emerged from his practice as a clinician, concluding with his more formal pedagogical purpose, particularly looking at his *Manuals* and his university lecturing.

Fortunately he was working in a stimulating scientific research environment at Queen Square, in which he could develop his skill as a clinician, and it was in the clinical setting that Gowers first began to make his name both as a diagnostician and also as a teacher.

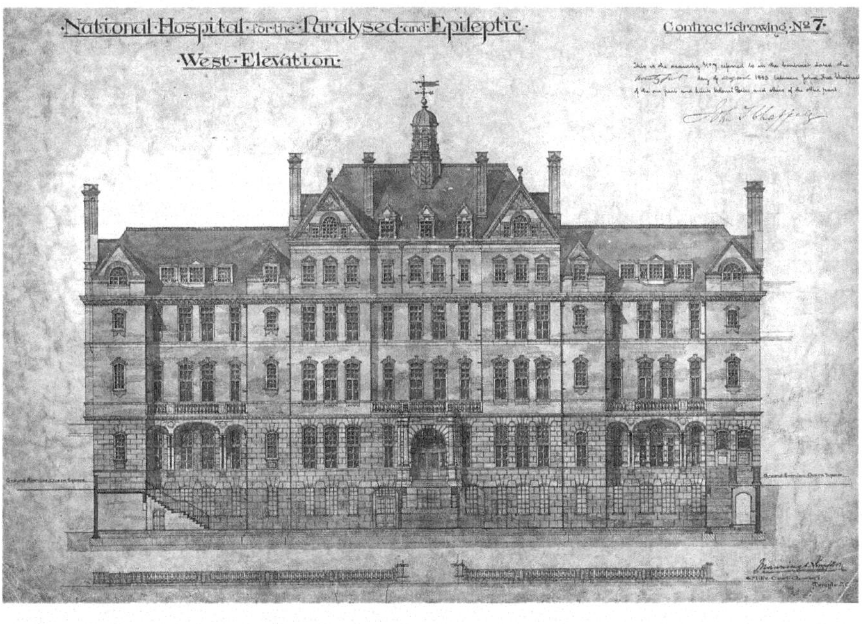


**Fig. 6.1** National Hospital (1883). Image courtesy of the Queen Square Library, Archive and Museum.

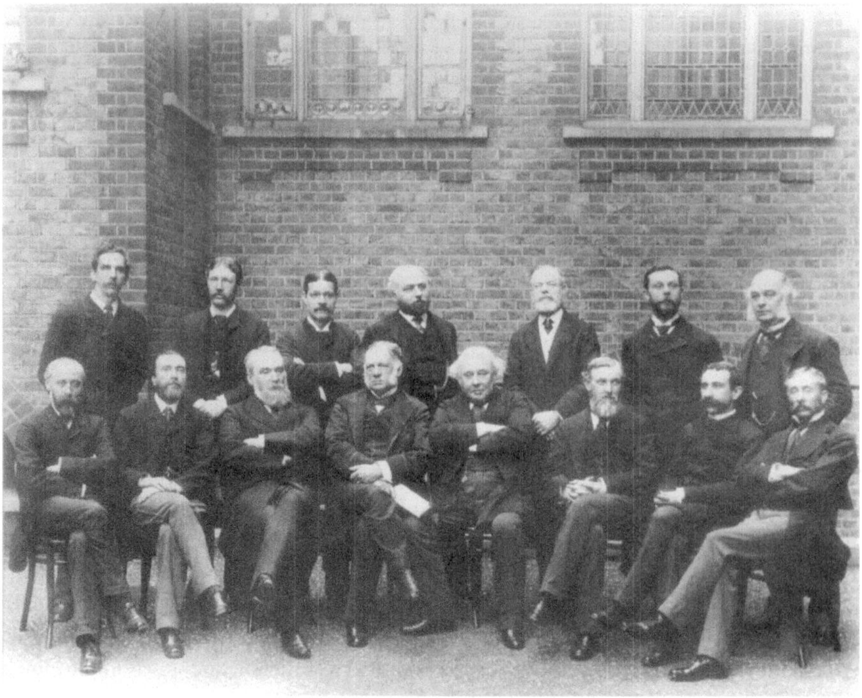

**Fig. 6.2** Queen Square consultants (1886). Back row, left to right: Horsley, Beevor, Cumberbatch, Thomas Buzzard, Brundenall Carter, Ormerod, Adams. Front row, left to right: Gunn, Bastian, Hughlings Jackson, Ramskill, Radcliffe, Gowers, Semon, Ferrier. Image courtesy of the Queen Square Library, Archive and Museum.

As a diagnostician Gowers always advised his students of the risks of allowing preconceptions to lead to false conclusions, and provided the following advice:

> The method you should adopt is this: Whenever you find yourself in the presence of a case that is not at once and completely familiar to you in all its details, forget for the time all your types and all your names. Deal with the case as one that has never been seen before, and work it out as a new problem sui generis, to be investigated as such. Observe each symptom and consider its significance. Then put all the symptoms together and consider the meaning of their combination, especially whether there is any one part of the nervous system at which disease might cause them all.[1]

He made seminal contributions to the art of diagnosis. He introduced the clinical methodology for distinguishing between upper and lower motor neuron lesions, a robust division that has stood the test of time and is the starting point for determining the precise level at which the pathway controlling movement is affected by disease. Early in his career he identified that it was the lower motor neuron which made the ultimate connection with the muscle, and later wrote in the first edition of his *Manual of Diseases of the Nervous System*:

> It is worthwhile to consider for a moment the whole motor path, from the cortex of the brain to the muscles. We may consider it as composed of two segments, an upper and a lower. Each consists of a ganglion cell above, a nerve fibre, and the terminal ramification of the latter. The upper cerebrospinal segment consists of the cortical ganglion cell and the pyramidal fibre, which proceeds from the cell, passes through the brain and cord, and ends by dividing into the spongy substance of the anterior cornu. The lower 'spino-muscular' segment consists of the spinal ganglion cell, and the fibre proceeding from this, passing through the anterior root and nerve trunk to the muscle, where it divides and ramifies on the muscle fibre. The elements of the two segments do not probably correspond in number. Each cortico-spinal element is connected with many spinal-muscular segments. It will be found that this conception of the motor path conduces to clearer ideas of many phenomena of disease.

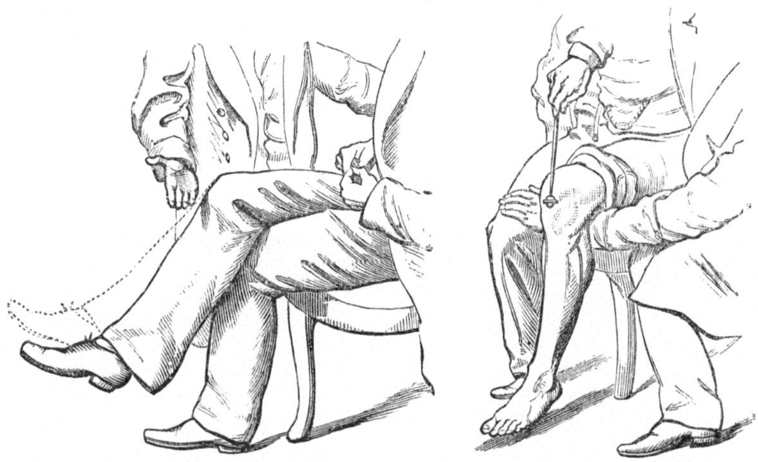

FIG. 1.—THE KNEE-JERK.
The dotted line indicates the movement which follows the blow on the patellar tendon.

FIG. 2.—THE KNEE-JERK.
Method of obtaining it when it is not readily produced in the ordinary way.

**Fig. 6.3** Illustration of the knee-jerk in the *Manual of Diseases of the Nervous System*, 1st edn, Vol. 1, p.12, figs 1 and 2 (London: Churchill, 1886). Courtesy of Mr Alexander Scott.

In 1879 Gowers reported to the Medical and Chirurgical Society of London his ingenious experiments on the knee-jerk. He had tied a revolving drum to a patient's foot, tapped the tendon below the knee cap (the patella) with a hammer, and recorded the movement of the foot using a pen attached to the drum. This allowed him to measure the delay between the hammer tapping the patellar tendon and the moment the leg muscle contracted. His measurements supported his theory that the knee-jerk was a spinal reflex.

Amongst the neurological signs Gowers elicited at the bedside were: the presence of optic neuritis; the reactions of the pupils to light; reflex withdrawal of the foot on

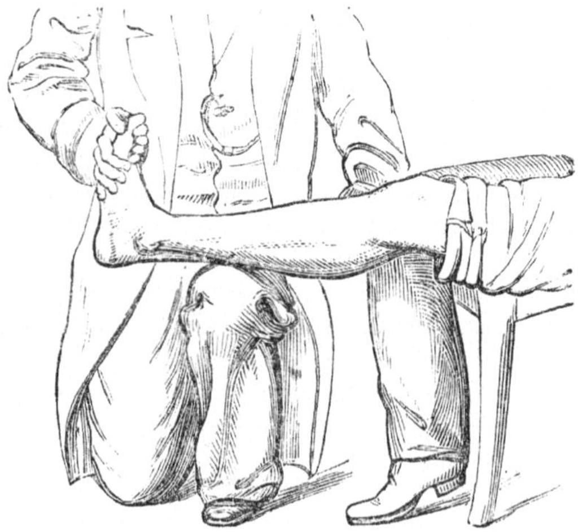

FIG. 3.—METHOD OF ELICITING THE FOOT-CLONUS.

**Fig. 6.4** Illustration of the method of eliciting the foot-clonus in the *Manual of Diseases of the Nervous System*, 1st edn, Vol. 1, p.13, fig. 3 (London: Churchill, 1886). Courtesy of Mr Alexander Scott.

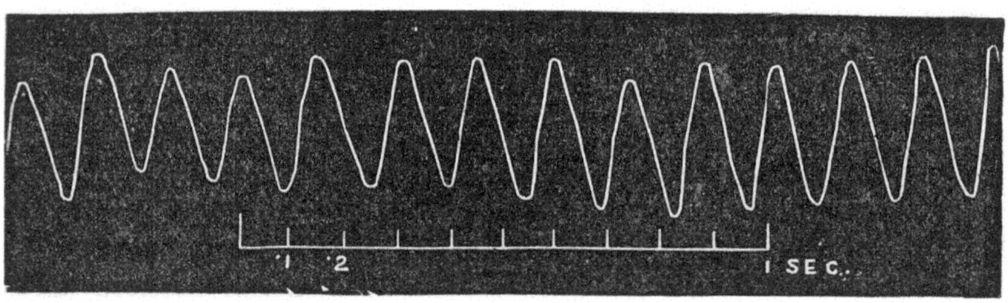


**Fig. 6.5** Illustration of tracing of the foot-clonus in paraplegia, in the *Manual of Diseases of the Nervous System*, 1st edn, Vol. 1, p. 13, fig. 4 (London: Churchill, 1886).

stimulation of the sole (known as the 'plantar reflex' before the extensor plantar response was described in 1896); other skin reflexes such as the gluteal, abdominal, and cremasteric; and the knee- and ankle-jerks. He also recorded the presence of involuntary rhythmic jerking movements of the ankle (clonus) and of the eyes (nystagmus). He used a tug on the pubic hair to diagnose hysterical coma (according to Critchley, Gowers was taught this particular trick when he was an apprentice, demonstrated by an old Coggeshall doctor). He tested the patient's strength by assessing voluntary movement of individual muscles, sometimes assisted by electrical stimulation, and tested grip by using the dynamometer, and applied simple tests, such as asking the patient to draw a straight line on a piece of paper, to assess coordination. He tested light touch with the feather end of a quill pen, and two-point discrimination with Sieveking's aesthesiometer (a graduated bar with two points, one moveable and the other fixed, to allow a value to be recorded for the threshold of tactile discrimination). He reported in his *Manual* figures for different parts of the body including 1.5 mm for the tongue, 3 mm for the fingertips, and 75 mm for the upper thigh. The sharper end of the quill pen was used to test pain, test tubes containing hot and cold water to test temperature sensitivity, and weights to test what was known as 'muscle sense' in the ataxias.

Critchley described Gowers on his ward rounds in his later years:

> He visited his wards more often than his colleagues, perhaps three times a week. Seated by the bedside he would carefully read the case-notes made by his assistant. Once again he would go over the points in the history, elucidating, elaborating. His own examination would follow—full, detailed, but without the tedious slowness of some other neurologists. A clinical point, or an unusual symptom or sign would attract his attention. He would perhaps send for a copy of his *Manual* to verify an observation. Often he would produce his pocket-book and made some shorthand memorandum which at home would be amplified and indexed for later reference. . . . Aided by an adequate knowledge of neuropathology as it stood in his day, and by a thorough grounding in neuroanatomy, he interpreted his observations scientifically.[2]

Gowers' 'obsessional perfectionism', continued Critchley, 'burned with that hard gem-like flame which in later years could not fail to bring success'. As a diagnostician 'he relied on close application, keen observation, a brilliant memory, a methodical system of case-recording, and painstaking physical examination'. He was always alert to the risks of misdiagnosis: accurate observation could lead to the right diagnosis, but there was always the risk of error, as he explained in a lecture on 'Mistaken diagnosis':

> Gentlemen,—It is always pleasant to be right, but it is generally a much more useful thing to be wrong. If you are right, all that you do, as a rule, is to confirm your previous opinion, your previous habits of reasoning and your previous self-esteem. But if you are wrong you generally gain in knowledge and gain perception of the way in which your method of diagnosis needs improvement, and the influence on self-esteem is not likely to do you harm.[3]

He gave the example of a patient who presented himself in out-patients when Gowers was pressed for time and was unable to carry out a full sensory examination. The patient was an 'oil and colour' merchant who handled tints (which contained arsenic). The man complained of a three-year history of impotence, numbness in his extremities, and pains in his muscles, and twitching in his muscles that increased when he walked. When tested, he was found to have no ankle-jerks, but he was able to stand upright with his eyes closed. Gowers suspected that syphilis was the source of the problem and prescribed arsenic as the remedy. He wrote in his notes how much he hated these rushed consultations, but that the patient had come from far away and Gowers felt he could not turn him away.

As instructed the patient returned five weeks later and Gowers related to the audience an aphorism which flashed before him from his old teacher, Jenner, who had once said: 'Gentlemen more mistakes are made by not looking than not knowing'. As Gowers was about to examine the man's legs he saw, to his consternation, what were classical signs of chronic arsenic poisoning: darkening and bumpiness of the skin.

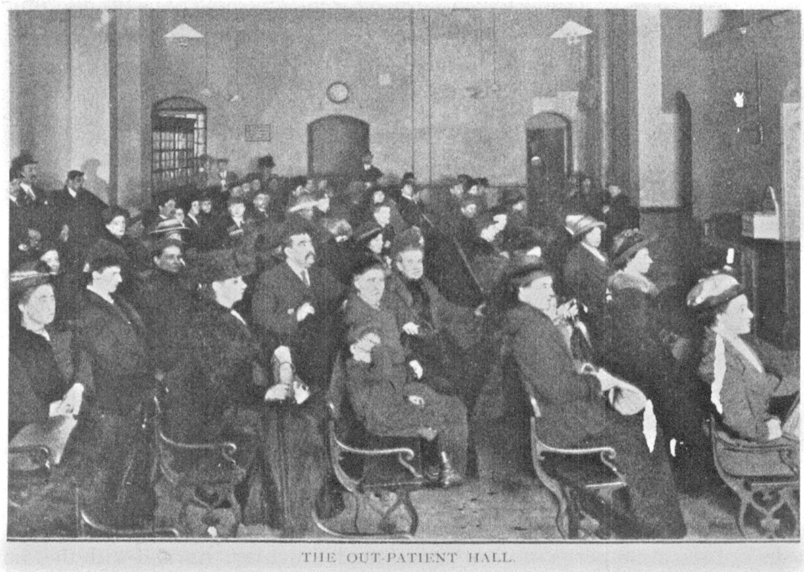


**Fig. 6.6** The outpatient hall, Queen Square (undated). Image courtesy of the Queen Square Library, Archive and Museum.

It emerged that not only had the man been exposed to arsenic through his work, but he had also taken it during the first year after his symptoms emerged. Gowers immediately stopped the arsenic and prescribed potassium iodide. The man's symptoms failed to improve, and Gowers thought this was probably caused by the iodide bringing the arsenic into the blood from the tissues, causing further irritation. He sent the patient to a colleague who was an expert on arsenic poisoning. The three lessons Gowers drew from the case were: always examine the patient from top to toe; never rush a consultation; and, finally, seek further expert advice if treatment is ineffective.

Herbert Brown described witnessing at UCH one of the best instances he saw of Gowers' outstanding diagnostic skill, one which had, he believed, never been equalled before and of which Gowers himself was 'justifiably very proud':

> The son of the chief hall porter at the hospital was seriously ill with paralytic symptoms, the detail of which, if I ever knew them, I have forgotten. This was in 1881, when I was house-physician to Sidney Ringer, and I have a vivid recollection of the case, for I had the privilege of giving the anaesthetic (chloroform). Gowers' diagnosis was an abscess in the temporo-sphenoidal lobe of, I think, the left cerebral hemisphere. Gowers diagnosed its exact location, and pointed out to the surgeon—Rickman Godlee—the exact spot in which to introduce a trocar; as the stylet was withdrawn, pus was evacuated, and a small drainage tube was introduced. The patient made a rapid and complete recovery.[4]

On a case of chronic lead poisoning, Gowers said:

> I was told that it seemed to be a case of 'simple neurasthenia'. I looked casually at the bed-card and at once my eye was caught by the record of his occupation 'Painter'. I looked

> from the bed-card to his gums, and there I saw written in equally distinct characters the record of the effect of his occupation—in a conspicuous lead-line'.[5]

Gowers liked precision in diagnosis and the language used to describe symptoms. His antipathy to the word 'neurasthenia' is an example. It had first been coined by the American physician George Miller Beard in 1869 to describe a wide range of psychological and physical symptoms including fatigue, irritability, headache, dizziness, anxiety, depression, and intolerance to noise. Beard attributed these symptoms to the stress of 'modern life and urbanization'. Gowers commented on the speed with which the term had been adopted:

> It is a contribution to the medical nomenclature which we owe to our transatlantic brethren, and it attained universal use with the utmost celerity. The concise and concrete character of the word gives it a satisfying definiteness. This depends to a large extent on its classical and somewhat graceful sound. Not only is it graceful to the ear, but it is graceful to the mind of the patient who suffers and longs to know from what, who longs to have a name for that which he, or more often she, feels must be a more definite malady than is suggested by the commonplace designation of 'nervous weakness'.[6]

'You may use it to collect the symptoms of the case under a general designation' Gowers wrote, 'but do not let it cover them as a cloak'.

## Clinical lectures at Queen Square

Gowers started teaching informally in 1873, after he was appointed an assistant physician, and his teaching clinics soon became 'thronged with physicians from all over the world standing in the gangways and straining the capacity of the accommodation'.[7] Sir Gordon Holmes, one of Gowers' successors at Queen Square, had an elderly patient who had been one of Gowers' pupils. This student had visited Queen Square and been invited into the outpatient room by Gowers, who started to discuss enthusiastically the symptoms of a case he had just seen. When the student left, Gowers invited him to come again and bring some colleagues with him. This was the beginning of outpatient postgraduate teaching at the hospital.[8] Gowers' reputation spread rapidly and his outpatient room was soon crowded with doctors. In 1879, Buzzard and Hughlings Jackson instituted regular Thursday afternoon clinical lectures at Queen Square, at which Gowers often lectured, and the hospital soon expanded its clinical teaching in outpatient and inpatient practice to four days a week.

Critchley describes the 'brilliance' of Gowers' out-patient teaching:

> Gowers was able to combine teaching with out-patient consultations, and he set the practice which has been followed ever since. He was not aware beforehand of what cases were attending and he saw the patient for the first time in the presence of a critical and admiring audience. He took the history, examined the patient, and afterwards discussed the nature of the case, the differential diagnosis, prognosis, and treatment. There was no set talk; no questions or answers. The whole performance was a type of thinking aloud which could be witnessed profitably by medical men however skilled or experienced.[9]

Between 1887 and 1896, a total of 2500 students and practitioners attended the National Hospital clinical demonstrations, which had an average attendance of ten visitors each session. The hospital rapidly earned a reputation in medical circles for providing one of the best opportunities in Europe for clinical instruction in the diagnosis and treatment of nervous diseases. Gowers was one of the brightest stars in its galaxy of talent. He continued his outpatient clinics at Queen Square until 1893, by which time he was exhausted from overwork.

Holmes and Critchley both described Gowers' formal lectures and teaching style. Holmes wrote:

> It was, however, in his formal lectures that he excelled as a teacher. These, which almost invariably presented new observations or carefully reasoned conclusions, were carefully prepared and delivered in a slow high-pitched voice which compelled attention from even the least interested.[10]

Critchley suggests that Gowers' lecturing technique inspired others to emulate him, establishing a style of 'neurological didactics' that outlived him:

> Gowers was pre-eminently a virtuoso—stimulating, arresting, informative. Like other great Victorian figures he had more than traces of the showman in his technique. It was Gowers who inspired the tradition of neurological didactics—and after his day something of the same genre was continued by Risien Russell, by Collier and by Kinnier Wilson.[11]

If clinical cases were to be shown, careful arrangements were made beforehand with his house physician. 'Gowers was well aware of his skill as an instructor, and was even guilty of a certain justifiable vanity in respect of his powers of attractive large audiences.'[12]

## Gowers' clinical notes at Queen Square

Gowers' clinical case notes in the Queen Square archives cover the years 1879 to 1911, some of the earliest recorded are in the same volume as those of his chief, Hughlings Jackson (for whom he carried out pathological examinations of a number of fatal instances of brain tumour).[13] Each set consists of a brief outpatient sheet, bound together with the inpatient notes. The inpatient front sheet includes the patient's personal details, admission and discharge dates, duration of illness, treatment, diagnosis, as well as the name of the physician, house physician, and clinical clerk. The continuation sheets consist of treatment cards, fit charts, temperature recordings with pulse and respiration records, weight, and urine analysis. Visual field charts, clinical and post-mortem drawings, and occasional photographs are included. Correspondence with other doctors and patient follow-up letters were added as postscripts. The notes were bound each year with an index. In later years notes for male and female patients were bound in separate volumes. From the late 1880s, microscopic tissue examinations appeared as an addendum to the macroscopic pathological reports.

More than thirty volumes dedicated to Gowers' own inpatients also provide an insight into the case mix that provided the raw material for his *Manual*. The commonest diagnoses were epilepsy, spinal cord disease, strokes, functional nervous disease (including hystero-epilepsy), neurasthenia, cerebral tumours, insular sclerosis (multiple or disseminated sclerosis), chorea (irregular, spasmodic, involuntary movements of the limbs and facial muscles), and neuromuscular disorders. The secondary neurological consequences of syphilis accounted for one in ten admissions, and cases of paralysis agitans, the ataxias, tics, and tremors were also admitted. Laboratory investigations consisted of a few basic blood and urine tests. In 1891, cerebrospinal fluid examinations were introduced.

The notes provide an insight into the case material and treatments available in the early days of the hospital. Gowers saw a 22-year-old woman in outpatients who complained that she had suffered headaches and had been unable to walk for some months. He diagnosed a cerebellar tumour and wrote in the notes that she must be admitted as soon as possible. However, the patient died. Her case notes show Gowers' post-mortem drawings of an upper mid-brain tumour pressing on the left side of the cerebellum.

Some notes are written in Gowers' longhand, giving as much detail as is found in modern patient files. When commenting on a particular case recorded by his house physician, Gowers occasionally lapsed into shorthand.

Critchley noted that in the early case records the emphasis fell on diagnoses which by 1949 were becoming less common, while other disorders familiar by 1949 were recorded infrequently. Appearing more frequently in Gowers' day were angular curvature of the spine, hystero-epilepsy, and myelitis. Although already identified, disseminated sclerosis was diagnosed relatively infrequently.[14] Diffuse cerebral arteriosclerosis was rarely recorded:

> Haemorrhage, and acute softenings of the brain were, of course, clearly visualized, but the manifold symptoms of the hypertensive and of the arteriopath were inadequately described under the conceptions of anaemia and hyperaemia of the brain.[15]

## Inventing diagnostic aids

The mid-Victorian entrants into the medical profession were not necessarily welcomed by the older hands. J. F. Clarke, reminiscing in 1874, complained, tongue-in-cheek:

> Many practitioners of the present day are not contented with pursuing the 'even tenor of their way' to eminence and success. Each and every one is anxious to be original and a discoverer. Thus, one identifies his name with some therapeutic 'discoveries'; one finds the dung of a toad, judiciously administered, an infallible remedy for consumption; whilst another declares from a 'large experience', that the 'thin white curd of asses' milk' is an universal panacea. Young surgeons who have yet to 'gain their spurs' 'invent' all kinds of imaginable instruments. One, who has never seen a gunshot wound, may modestly give to the Profession an improved bullet extractor, to be procured only of Weiss or Coxeter. Another, who probably has never performed ovariotomy, introduces a new 'clamp', or something else, to 'arrest haemorrhage'; whilst another, less ambitious or more 'modest,' contents himself with parading a new kind of tweezers for extracting superfluous hairs.[16]

Gowers was one young doctor who turned his hand to inventing new devices, but in his case these were diagnostic aids, or other devices to make his daily life easier. Gowers was always an enthusiastic inventor. The first evidence of this was the hookah he designed while still at Coggeshall (badly slicing his finger in the process). His son described his passion for what Victorians would have referred to as 'tweaks' or 'dodges':

> He was at great pains to acquire the art of writing legibly, whether in shorthand or in longhand, when on rail or road. He could not bear to waste time. Railway carriages were shockingly lighted in those days, and he had made a candle-lamp of his own design with a rubber pad that would adhere to the carriage window. ... Before the days of main electricity he lit his dining room with a battery in the sideboard, which was effective while it lasted but did not last long. Before the days of telephones he equipped his house with a system of speaking-tubes terminating in an exchange of his own devising in his consulting room.

Gowers' enduring interest in accurate diagnosis led him to devise several diagnostic instruments, the first in the 1870s, and he sometimes arranged for these to be manufactured by Hawksley's in Oxford Street. He designed the instruments for his own use, but some were adopted by his contemporaries, and his blood cell counting apparatus and his haemoglobinometer were still to be found in clinical laboratories more than a generation later.

His first attempt at devising an instrument for general, rather than his own use, was a 'safety hypodermic syringe', which he described in 1872. This was a simple means of preventing an accidental overdose. The piston of the syringe was fitted with a metal collar, screwed into a position that prevented it from being drawn back further than the level required to deliver the designated dose.[17] However, Critchley writes that there was no evidence that this, the first of Gowers' devices, ever became popular.

Five years later, in 1877, he devised a haemocytometer.[18] He had been working in Professor Burdon Sanderson's laboratory at UCH and 'secured for himself a considerable degree of fame for persuading Hawksley's to devise a modification of Hayem's haematometer'.[19] His instrument came to be widely used for some years as a convenient tool for counting the number of red cells in a given volume of blood. At the time the instrument was devised the only available method for carrying out these counts required the use of one particular manufacturer's microscope which had a special eyepiece. With this microscope the red blood cells were counted in a glass cell of known volume incorporated in a microscope slide. Gowers' refinement was to have the cell on the slide made to a carefully controlled depth of 0.2 mm, to have manufactured a pipette with an exact volume into which blood from a prick made in the fingertip was drawn up, and to have had manufactured a mixing chamber of known volume which contained a diluent. The blood from the pipette was added to the diluent in this cell on the microscope slide, a cover slip was positioned over the glass cell and held onto the surface of the slide by spring clips. The floor of the cell had 0.1 mm squares etched into it. The blood cells which gravitated to the floor of the cell could then be counted using any available microscope, and their number in a given volume of blood calculated after correcting for the effects of the dilution. Years later, Gowers added further subdivisions etched into the floor of the cell to make the counting process easier.[20]

In 1878 he devised a method he claimed to be as exact, simpler, and more convenient than any yet made for estimating the level of haemoglobin in the blood. He demonstrated this haemoglobinometer to the Clinical Society of London, an event reported by both *The Lancet* and the *BMJ*. Having established how a 'standard' level was determined, the apparatus was described by the *BMJ*:

> The apparatus consisted of two tubes in a small stand, both tubes of the same diameter. One contained the standard which, for stability, was glycerine and gelatine tinted with carmine and protocarmine to the exact tint of the dilution of normal blood (1 in 100). The other tube [with a capacity of 20 cubic mm] was graduated. A capillary tube holding 20 cubic mm., a bottle with a pipette, stopper, and a guarded needle completed the apparatus. In use, a drop or two of distilled water was placed at the bottom of the graduated tube; the 20 cubic mm of blood were then measured and mixed with the drop of water; more water was then added until the tint was the same as that of the standard. The amount of water added, indicated by the numbers on the divisions, showed the percentage of colour, i.e. haemoglobin, compared to the normal.[21]

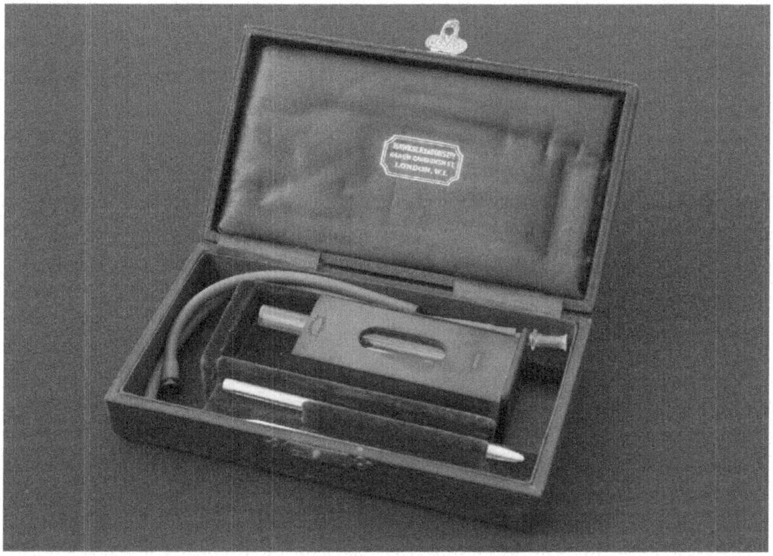

**Fig. 6.7** The Gowers' haemoglobinometer. Welsh Museum of Health and Medicine.org

In Gowers' apparatus, the tube containing the blood to be measured was mounted vertically, parallel to the tube containing the standard, to make it easier to compare the colours in the two tubes.[22] The brief reports in the *BMJ* and *The Lancet* describing Gowers' 1878 demonstration comprised 'the modest debut of the famed Gowers' haemoglobinometer, which remained for over twenty years the standard technique in haematology, until modified later by Haldane's instruments'. It was still being used, and referred to as the Haldane-Gowers haemoglobinometer, in the 1940s.[23]

Sometime before 1879 Gowers also devised a way to measure sugar in urine by mixing the urine with an equal amount of liquor potassae and boiling it in the upper part of a test tube. The depth of the colour change provided him with a reasonably reliable measure of the glucose content.[24]

Gowers also persuaded a London manufacturer named Pillischer to produce an ophthalmoscope in which the weaker lenses were arranged at the centre of the rotatable disc containing the lenses, with the stronger and less often used lenses on the periphery. The lens disc could be moved between two pivot positions in the head of the instrument. In this way, Gowers created a smaller, more manageable instrument than those previously available, but still containing an adequate range of lenses. This instrument was not mentioned in later editions of *Medical Ophthalmoscopy*, possibly because other designs had become commercially available.

Gowers continued to devise diagnostic tools throughout his life, especially to help him in his private practice. In 1904, to make it easier for the patient to exert maximum power of grip in reasonable comfort, and for measurements made on different instruments to be compared more reliably, he modified the design of a widely used dynamometer to make it easier for patients to hold while the strength of their hand grip was recorded. He arranged for each individual instrument to have its scale standardized and its graduations marked.[25]

In the same year he designed a 'triple-wick' candle to help him use an ophthalmoscope in patients' poorly lit homes. Unlike modern ophthalmoscopes which have an electric light source built into the instrument, those in Gowers' time consisted only of a set of lenses suitable for bringing into focus the retina at the back of the eyeball, and other parts of the eyeball. Light was directed into the eye provided by an independent source.

Gowers described the problem thus:

> At a patient's house it is generally difficult, and often impossible, to obtain a suitable light for making observations. This is especially the case when a light for the ophthalmoscope is needed. An ordinary electric lamp simply gives the image of the incandescent wire on the retina unless the lamp glass is ground to a degree that dims the light. A common candle throws only its own small image on the fundus. Every efficient portable electric lamp is heavy and uncertain in its action, and the best lamp of all—a paraffin lamp with a broad wick—is not only cumbersome but soils whatever is near it to a degree that is at last insupportable. A serviceable light I have often obtained by cutting away with a knife one side of two pieces of candle, so as to bring their wicks near enough together for the flames to blend. This suggested the idea of a three-candle wick.[26]

When all three wicks were lit, Gowers' triple-wick candle provided a stable and uniform source of light for examining the retina (the Queen Square library still has his own triple-wick candle).

Ever the inventor, the last of his instruments appeared in 1909. Gowers had a special ear speculum constructed to help examine the eardrum. It had a magnifying lens inside, with a metal ring holding it in an oblique position, thus providing a magnified view of the ear drum.[27]

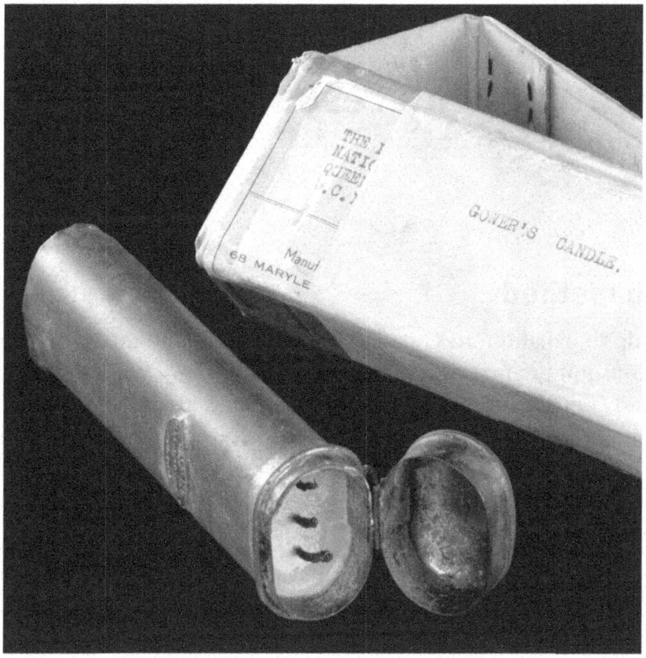

**Fig. 6.8** Gowers' own triple-wick candle. Image courtesy of the Queen Square Library, Archive and Museum.

The *BMJ*, noting the centenary of Gowers' birth, summed up 'one of the greatest clinicians and teachers of clinical medicine of the nineteenth century':

> Few, alas, are left among us who saw Gowers in action as a clinical observer and teacher, but for these few the recollection of his clinical acumen, the fruit of a vast experience stored in his mind in orderly fashion and ready for instant recall, and of the inspiring quality of his teaching, is imperishable. There still lives among neurologists, handed down by those who were his colleagues or his pupils, a store of legends of his astonishing diagnostic skill and insight and of those forceful personal qualities in which the Victorian generation of physicians was so rich.
>
> The lesson of this is that at the very foundation of sound medical practice lies a wide and deep familiarity with its material: the patient and his illness. Nothing can replace this, nor can all the ingenuity of the laboratory, nor the penetration of the skiagram, provide a substitute for direct observation at the bedside, the clinic, or the consulting room, and the unceasing contemplation of this direct experience. The complete physician, in fact, must be a connoisseur of clinical material, and not the least factor in the acquisition of this measure of skill and intuition is the careful and systematic recording of what has been observed. It is necessary to stress these points in view of the increasing reliance by doctors upon the special methods of the numerous and too autonomous departmentalists, and of the increasing tendency of the student to regard note taking as a form of drudgery.[28]

Chapter 7

# Gowers the researcher

## Research method

Gowers made shorthand notes on all his cases, and maintained a systematic filing system. He was not the first doctor to use shorthand—Gowers himself pointed out that in the early nineteenth century a Dr Sheppard of Canterbury was using shorthand for his case notes, and noted that a Dr J. H. Gladstone FRS had used it for scientific work since 1846. Gowers used his shorthand as an essential research tool throughout his working life. He described this many years later when he was trying to persuade others of its merits:

> In every science that rests on observation, the need for written record is absolute. No memory, whatever its capacity, can be trusted. Immediate record alone can make observation effective. That which is secured by the use of shorthand, even at low speed, is this: in a given time there can be twice the amount of record that is possible with longhand, and yet twice the time in which to observe. For the greater amount of record, observation must be more minute, more precise. Description at once reveals unsuspected uncertainties, and the greater the amount of record the more accurate is the observation, the more valuable is the result. The effect of the use of shorthand is, and must be, on the quality of scientific work so far as observation is concerned.
>
> Nor is it alone a matter of quality. Many of the facts observed are changing, passing. In these the effect of the use of shorthand is not merely qualitative; facts can be described which longhand could not possibly record. It must be remembered that shorthand enables, when necessary, not twice, but three and four times the amount of record and thus transient phenomena can be adequately described which would elude entirely the slow pursuit of longhand, however abbreviated. The difference is thus absolute; observations can be secured that would otherwise be lost. These facts are true of our work as a branch of natural science. I emphasise them because the statements are true of every science which rests on observation, and in all natural sciences the art we advocate would of necessity increase the capacity of every worker, and augment the value of his work.[1]

Anecdotes about Gowers' passionate advocacy of shorthand in later life have tended to overwhelm the logic of his argument. In an age before tape-recorders, typewriters, or computers, shorthand offered the most effective data collection tool available. The compression it offered, an additional benefit in record keeping, is demonstrated by his 1862 apprentice diary in which over 50,000 words are contained in a book roughly the size of a modern iPhone.

It is refreshing that Gowers' obituary in the *Journal of Nervous and Mental Disease* recognized that the 'prodigious amount of material at his disposal' was obtained not only from his masterly power of observation but also his ability to record in shorthand.[2]

In an article about the National Hospital, Queen Square, Critchley noted that as a clinician Gowers recorded punctiliously.[3] This view was endorsed by P. G. Easton in a letter to the *BMJ*:

> One asset of Sir William's that was not mentioned was his outstanding skill in shorthand—and I have no doubt that this unusual accomplishment was a great help to him in his wonderful career.[4]

This methodical recording made it possible for him to base his 1881 Gulstonian lectures about the causes of epilepsy on first-hand evidence derived directly from the study of 1450 patients seen at the National Hospital. His knowledge of the available literature also allowed him to spot inconsistencies and assess their significance.

Critchley observed that by 1879 Gowers had developed his own technique in medical writing and research:

> He differed from some of his contemporaries—[Hughlings] Jackson and Bastian for instance—and from others who were to be his colleagues a little later—Ferrier, Horsley, Risien Russell, Semon—in that he did not indulge in philosophical conjecture nor compile data from the published work of others. ... Although he doubtless read much and used references as required, he relied almost entirely upon his own clinical or clinico-anatomical experiences.[5]

Gowers frequently repeated to his children Thomas Carlyle's aphorism that 'genius is an infinite capacity for taking pains'. He demanded the same standards of others as he set for himself. Ernest Jones, who in later life translated and promoted the works of Freud, was a 25-year-old recently qualified doctor when he worked under Gowers' exacting guidance on a research project in 1904. Gowers suggested that he carry out a piece of research on hemiplegic stroke in order to attempt to document the relative frequency of various accompanying clinical features that might help physicians make the clinical distinction between brain haemorrhage and cerebral thrombosis. Jones was first instructed to peruse all the English and French literature available on the subject, and then go through the casebooks of UCH back to its foundation in 1830, and finally to ascertain more cases by visiting the local borough infirmaries.[6]

Once at Queen Square, Gowers rapidly began to accumulate a large collection of cases. It was not long before he was ready to start publishing his findings. However, his earliest papers, written in the 1870s, did not break new ground. Critchley writes:

> He was feeling his way, as it were, through the labyrinth of nervous disorders. The manifold syndromes of spinal and cerebral disease lay around, but few at that time had clear ideas as to the morbid anatomy of many of the clinical pictures. Even the normal morphology of the nervous system was imperfectly recognized, while neurophysiology was a *terra incognita*. In these first few papers Gowers showed himself still *in statu pupillari* and in the process of clarifying his ideas by putting them on paper.[7]

Despite the cautious start, the years 1870–90 were Gowers' most productive. Critchley described 1879, in particular, as Gowers' *annus mirabilis*, because, in addition to shorter papers, four important original works were either written or published: lectures on epilepsy, *Epilepsy and Other Chronic Convulsive Diseases*; a monograph on *Pseudohypertrophic Paralysis*; an address, *Diagnosis of Diseases of the Spinal Cord*; and his *Manual of Medical Ophthalmoscopy*. 'Four masterpieces thus saw the light, each of which was the product of detailed and careful research, and all of them broke new ground.'[8] His contributions to neurological research were recognized by the hospital board in 1880 when they promoted him from assistant physician to the physician for outpatients.

## Epilepsy

Although epileptic seizures were described a little over 3000 years ago,[9] and were regarded as expressions of physical illness in the Hippocratic writings *On the Sacred Disease*,[10] there were few advances in the scientific understanding of the disorder until the nineteenth century, when the number of publications dealing with scientific features of the disorder rapidly increased. Gowers was a prominent figure among the writers of these publications.

In 1874 Gowers wrote 'Cases of convulsion in organic brain-disease', his first article about epilepsy, the disorder which preoccupied him throughout his professional career.[11] The last was his Hughlings Jackson lecture on 'Special sense discharges from organic disease', published 36 years later, in 1910.[12] In the intervening years he published two editions of a monograph *Epilepsy and Other Chronic Convulsive Diseases*,[13] chapters on epilepsy in each of the two editions of Part 2 of his *Manual of Diseases of the Nervous System*,[14] nine papers dealing with various aspects of epilepsy, and another book entitled *The Borderland of Epilepsy*,[15] based on papers published late in his career.

When Gowers joined the staff at Queen Square there were two main competing theories about the site where epileptic seizures were generated: in the lower brainstem (situated close to top of the spinal cord), or in the cerebral cortex (the intricately layered covering of the hemispheres of the brain).

In the early nineteenth century it was generally thought that epilepsy manifested itself as: (1) tonic–clonic seizures in which the patient becomes unconscious and has convulsions over the entire body (grand mal, haut mal); (2) tonic seizures (widespread more continuous muscular spasms); and (3) minor lapses of consciousness or absences (variously called petit mal, leipothymia, or partial epilepsy). The consensus was that generalized seizures arose from the medulla oblongata (the lowest part of the brainstem).[16] In 1833, after working out the mechanism of the reflex arc, Marshall Hall had suggested that increased activity in the afferent component of the arc (the incoming sensory nerve), increased activity in the central component of the arc (situated in the spinal cord and the brainstem), that led to an excessive output of activity into the efferent, or outgoing, motor nerve section of the arc producing the convulsions that occurred on both sides, i.e. generalized seizures.[17] Convulsions from increased afferent arc activity were Marshall Hall's 'eccentric epilepsy'. The results were similar if overactivity arose in the spinal cord or brainstem, but Marshall Hall called these 'centric epilepsy'. However, this idea could not, in its own right, explain loss of consciousness. Marshall Hall suggested that perhaps the overactivity of the brainstem caused spasm of the muscles of the neck and the larynx.[18] The sufferer lost consciousness because the spasm obstructed both breathing and the return of blood from the brain. If Marshall Hall's theory was correct, patients suffering grand mal seizures should have lost consciousness after their convulsions began, which was not the case based on clinical observation.

Sixteen years later, Todd suggested that epileptic fits arose in the cerebral hemispheres, where paroxysmal overactivity caused loss of consciousness. Bilateral convulsions would occur if this overactivity spread from the hemispheres to the brainstem. Todd also noted a link between lesions on the surface of the brain and convulsing on the opposite side of the body. However, he argued that convulsing on one side of the body, associated with known brain pathology, though it resembled true epilepsy, was a different phenomenon. True epilepsy had no detectable structural pathology, and was a disease in its own right.[19] In the mid-1850s Russell Reynolds and Delasiauve also asserted, independently, that epilepsy was a distinct disorder and had no detectable cause, and this idea became generally accepted.[20,21] In 1860 Brown-Séquard suggested that overactivity of the brainstem during seizure activity spread stimulated the medullary vasomotor centre, causing brain artery spasm. This explanation was more convincing than the one that Marshall Hall had proposed, because the spasm would have caused loss of consciousness earlier than would obstructed breathing.

By 1861, Russell Reynolds had developed a concept of how generalized tonic–clonic convulsive seizures originated in the brainstem.[22] This was supported by animal experiments carried out in Germany in which bilateral convulsions had been induced by inserting needles into the dorsal part of the rabbit pons immediately above the medulla oblongata.[23] By the late 1860s, therefore, it was becoming increasingly accepted that epilepsy arose in the brainstem, even though this did not easily explain non-convulsive epileptic seizures which involved loss of consciousness, nor did it explain changes in behaviour or sensation that accompanied some seizures.

In 1870 Hughlings Jackson published evidence that one-sided convulsions originated in a specific 'localized' part of the cortex of the opposite cerebral hemisphere. He also deduced that motor function might be localized in the cerebral cortex, and began to argue that genuine epilepsy also originated in the cerebral cortex rather than the brainstem. Charles Bland Radcliffe put forward another theory: that a temporary decrease in activity in an unspecified part of the brain might release the normally inhibited ability of muscles to contract, and thus lead to convulsions.

When Gowers was developing his ideas about epilepsy, the rival theories about the primary site in which epileptic seizures were generated, the brainstem or the cerebral cortex, were still a matter of controversy. At first he generally supported Hughlings Jackson's ideas on the mechanisms underlying seizures, but Critchley suggests that whereas Hughlings Jackson was interested in 'the more recondite' problems of its pathophysiology, Gowers was concerned 'with the bricks and mortar of the subject, and he set out patiently to observe phenomena and to collect facts, rather than to weave speculative webs'.[24]

Throughout his career Gowers held that epilepsy was a disease in its own right. However, particularly in his later publications, he shifted ground far enough to concede that an 'organic epilepsy' caused by organic brain disease, such as meningitis or a tumour, could exist where structural pathology existed in the brain, so long as the pathology was no longer active.[25] Gowers, therefore, believed that epilepsy involved a narrower range of manifestations than had been described earlier and has been accepted since.

In 1879 Gowers' achievements were beginning to be recognized by his peers. He was elected a Fellow of the Royal College of Physicians in 1879 and, as the youngest recruit, was invited to deliver the 1880 Gulstonian lectures. The topic he chose was epilepsy.[26] In preparation for these lectures Gowers analysed his 1450 cases of genuine epilepsy by their characteristics, the clinical features of their seizures, what appeared to provoke them, and their underlying preconditions (as far as these could be determined). He deliberately excluded any cases that might be caused by organic brain disease such as tumour, meningitis, syphilis, or other coarse organic disease, as well as all cases of convulsions that followed hemiplegia. He also excluded 'simple hysterical attacks, unattended by distinct loss of consciousness'.[27] Even though his 1450 cases may not all have been his own patients, the fact that Gowers could accumulate so many examples of the disorder over one decade indicates its prevalence in London at the time.

In 1881, he expanded these lectures into *Epilepsy and Other Chronic Convulsive Diseases.*[28] In this monograph he dealt with the disorder variously called 'true', 'genuine', 'essential', or 'idiopathic' epilepsy, rather than the more inclusive modern category of 'epilepsy'. However, he also included sections on 'unilateral convulsive epileptiform seizures', and 'hystero-epilepsy' (a phenomenon that was of great interest to Charcot and his colleagues at the Salpêtrière).

By this time it was becoming accepted that the essential component of epileptic seizures was not convulsing, but loss of consciousness. Partly as a result of this, auras, with distortions of vision, hearing, smell, taste, and altered mental states, were being recognized as signs of impending convulsive seizures, and also as epileptic events in their own right even in the absence of convulsions. Hughlings Jackson had already written about these, and Gowers covered them in some depth in his *Epilepsy and Other Chronic Convulsive Diseases*. Some of these phenomena had also already been described in detail by Théodore Herpin in his *Des Accès Incomplets d'Épilepsie*[29] (published posthumously), but Hughlings Jackson claimed only to have become aware of the book in the 1890s, so it seems likely that Gowers did not know of it either, at least when he wrote his book in 1881.[30] Gowers provided an overview of the drugs employed to manage epilepsy, making it clear that he preferred to use potassium bromide.

Critchley wrote that Gowers' *Epilepsy and Other Chronic Convulsive Diseases* was still seen as a classic in 1949:

> The introduction of luminal [phenobarbitone] in about 1914 and of diphenyl hydantoinate in 1936, are practically the only great therapeutic advances in the subject since his time; while pathophysiology remained but little advanced until the application of electroencephalography just before the last war. For any purely clinical consideration of the subject Gowers' monograph was, and still is, unsurpassed, and it is a grim irony that so many modern neuropsychiatrists hasten into print upon some aspect of the disease, without preliminary reference to the writings of Gowers.[31]

The greatest and most enduring importance of Gowers' book lies in his interpretation of the genesis of epileptic seizures. He had concluded that Hughlings Jackson's notion was the most satisfactory of the competing theories. He argued that the suggestion that the discharge of nerve cells began in the brainstem could not explain the 'aura' that patients with epilepsy experienced, a sensation that might occur either alone or sometimes before bilateral convulsing. It would be better explained if discharges began in the sensory regions of the cerebral cortex. He appears to have envisaged the possibility that events in the brainstem might play some subsidiary role in producing attacks. He mentioned, without comment, Radcliffe's idea[32] that convulsing was the result of decreased brain activity, although Russell Reynolds had earlier dismissed the notion as improbable.[33]

When supporting Hughlings Jackson's explanation, Gowers expressed those ideas more simply and also offered another, significant refinement to his colleague's theories. Hughlings Jackson had suggested that an epileptic fit was a manifestation of spontaneous or induced overactivity of nerve cells in the cerebral cortex, as a result of their functional instability. He believed that any additional motor and sensory manifestations of the epileptic seizure could be caused by the spread of the overactivity from the site of its local origin in the brain. The spread, he argued, could also explain loss of consciousness in the seizure. The temporary paralysis that followed some fits could be caused by exhaustion of those parts of the brain made to over-function by the seizure discharge.

Gowers suggested that the nervous system might have an inherent resistance (more or less equivalent to the later idea of inhibition) which tended to prevent both the initiation and the spread of the activity of an epileptic seizure in the brain. A sudden local loss of resistance could start a seizure discharge, with the degree of local resistance around the discharge then modulating its spread. Loss of consciousness during seizures could be explained if the spreading discharge inhibited function in strategic sites elsewhere in the brain.

Gowers argued that if local inhibition of the motor area of the cortex continued after a seizure had ended, temporary inability to move one side of the body (the post-epileptic hemiplegia described by Todd) could be explained. Gowers' theory of resistance was not entirely original, and he may have absorbed the idea from Radcliffe's publications in the 1850s and 1860s. Handfield-Jones had also used the idea in 1873 to explain some of the motor features of Parkinson's disease,[34] and Gowers' colleague at UCH, Sydney Ringer, professor of therapeutics, had written an article in which he raised the possibility of inhibition in epilepsy; however, Ringer was concerned mainly with its possible role in producing migraine headaches.[35]

Gowers shifted little in later years from the intellectual stance he took in 1881. In 1900 he dealt in some detail with the manifestations of minor epilepsy.[36] By the time the second edition of *Epilepsy and Other Chronic Convulsive Diseases* was being prepared (with the assistance of James Collier and Victor Horsley) he had data from some 3000 cases to analyse, which he embellished with material from the more recent literature.[37] In some of his papers published between the two editions, and also after the second edition, he touched on questions such as insurance and epilepsy,[38] epilepsy and heredity,[39] and whether women with epilepsy should marry.[40]

Towards the end of his career, Gowers returned to the theory of inhibition, reinterpreting it against advances in physiology, and taking into account developments in the microscopic anatomy of the central nervous system.[41] Ultimately, in 1906, he located the most probable site of inhibition as being between the axon terminal of one neuron and the dendritic process of another to which it was functionally connected. He did not know at the time that transmission across this synaptic gap was chemically mediated. He suggested that inhibition of the transmission of an incoming nerve impulse arriving at the site was probably achieved by a dynamic but mechanical process: that the dendrites retracted away from the axon terminal, thus widening the synaptic gap. So unless the incoming stimulus was particularly strong, it could not easily traverse the synaptic gap.[42] His suggestion became known as 'Gowers' theory of sleep' depending on a temporary and periodic dendritic retraction.[43]

Although his theory was later derided, Gowers appears not only to have emphasized the notion of epileptic seizures being produced by loss of inhibition, but to have correctly predicted the site where it was likely to occur.

## *The Borderland of Epilepsy*

One of Gowers' last publications was *The Borderland of Epilepsy*, published in 1907.[44] The title captured and has continued to hold the imagination of future generations of neurologists. Gowers' concept of a 'borderland of epilepsy' acknowledged a clinical reality, and the idea it embraced provided a framework within which to produce an interesting and informative description of a number of related commonly occurring disturbances which frequently lead to diagnostic confusion. The book covered a range of disorders later collected together under the generic rubric of 'funny turns' including vagal and vasovagal attacks, vertigo, migraine, and parasomnias.

In the second half of the nineteenth century, knowledge about the range of symptoms that could occur in epileptic seizures had increased rapidly, mainly through the publications of the Swiss physician Theodore Herpin[45], Hughlings Jackson,[46] and Gowers himself[47] (including his lecture on minor epilepsy). While Gowers' findings were based on clinical observation alone, his conclusion that borderland disorders were, in fact, not related to epilepsy has since proved to be correct, although it can still sometimes be hard to differentiate between epilepsy and 'funny turns'.

*The Borderland of Epilepsy* provides a fascinating insight into Gowers' bedside technique, richly illustrating his strengths both in listening closely to what his patients were telling him and then faithfully recording their stories. In his writing he then attempts to answer the questions they pose. For example, he concludes that although people frequently faint at the sight of blood they never do so if it is merely portrayed. The richness of his narrative reflects the extent to which he is absorbed by the experience the patient has described to him.

### Fainting

Gowers emphasized the difficulty in distinguishing fainting from certain varieties of minor epilepsy in which consciousness is either impaired or lost, without any convulsions, and with no clear history of a warning 'aura'. However, he did not consider the problem of diagnosis in cases where patients suffer convulsions after fainting. He had a reasonable idea of many of the cardiovascular processes that are now known to cause fainting, and pointed out that while a patient usually experiences warning symptoms before fainting, occasionally these may be absent. Gowers speculated that there must be a mechanism which suddenly halts the activity of nerve cells in the part of the brain controlling consciousness, and that it might be explained by the sudden retraction of dendrites away from their junctions with the axons of other neurons, as this could prevent the communication of nerve cells to, and within, the centre responsible for consciousness.[48]

## Vagal and vasovagal attacks

Gowers suggested that the term 'vagal attacks', though unfamiliar, seemed 'a useful designation for prolonged seizures, the symptoms of which consist chiefly in disturbance of some of the functions of the pneumogastric' (thoughtfully adding his customary definition, reminding the reader that 'the vagus is the nerve through which respiratory and gastric sensations are felt').[49] His description differed somewhat from the modern vasovagal syncope (the 'simple' faint).

He described prolonged disturbances, lasting between ten and thirty minutes, that appeared to indicate disordered function of the vagus nerve. The symptoms could appear as discomfort seeming to arise from the stomach, lung, or heart, and could involve a sense of impending death. The extremities were pale and cold, and there was occasionally slight tightening of muscles. The sufferer did not lose consciousness, but might appear to be thinking slowly and find breathing difficult. The disorder, he noted, was more frequent in women. Gowers concluded that this might sometimes be an 'extended' epilepsy. However, while he may have been correct in some instances, these days such disturbances would probably more often be diagnosed as anxiety-related panic or hyperventilation attacks. He also described 'partial syncope' in which the only manifestation was temporary loss of sight (he made no reference to his own temporary loss of sight when helping Dr Giles in Coggeshall, which may well have fallen into this category).

## Vertigo

Gowers rejected the term 'giddiness' used as 'a popular synonym for vertigo' to describe the phenomenon on the grounds that it originally meant 'light-heartedness', whereas vertigo, which meant 'turning' was more precise. He distinguished between a 'subjective' and 'objective' vertigo, but included in his definition of the latter more than the pure rotational vertigo that gives the sensation of spinning.

He discussed 'aural vertigo' at some length, and again characteristically described the tests he used and gave precise definitions of his terms:

> In the cases described, hearing was tested up to 2000 vibrations by C tuning forks. By 'middle C' is meant that between the treble and the bass, 256 vibrations. The precise number varies with the pitch, and is easier to remember if we call it 250. The C within the treble is $C^1$, 500 vibrations, and that within the bass $C_1$, 125 vibrations. Above $C^3$, 2000 vibrations, hearing is tested by Galton's whistle, and recorded by the number of vibrations, which are indeed convenient for lower notes. Tinnitus is a symptom of great importance, as evidence of labyrinthine irritation; the world 'continuous' is used in opposition

> to 'pulsating,' and 'constant' is employed in the sense of persistent. The sound of steam escaping from a kettle is continuous, but may or may not be constant.[50]

However, while he knew about the peripheral vestibular apparatus in the inner ear and was aware that dysfunction of the semicircular canals could cause vertigo, Gowers appears to have been unfamiliar with the connections of the vestibular system in the brainstem. He knew that Ménière had described the effects of haemorrhage into the peripheral labyrinth, and referred to one patient who had been diagnosed by Wilks as suffering from Ménière's disease. Gowers did not cover disorders such as vestibular neuronitis (first identified in 1924) or paroxysmal positional vertigo, though he did describe patients being woken from sleep by experiencing vertigo, and also suggested that brief loss of consciousness could occur in vertigo caused by inner ear disturbance.

Gowers agreed with Hughlings Jackson that vertigo was an expression of disordered motor function, and also suggested that some instances of vertigo were epileptic.

## Sleep disorders

In *The Borderland of Epilepsy*, Gowers considered night terrors, sleepwalking, and narcolepsy. Narcolepsy, with its sudden lapses into sleep, he wrote, could be confused with the unconsciousness of epileptic seizures if there appeared to have been no convulsions, there had been no auras, and there was no history of excessive daytime drowsiness. He did not recognize that if there was no history of narcolepsy, the phenomenon of cataplexy (abrupt falling provoked by sudden laughter or anger while conscious) could easily be mistaken for an epileptic drop attack.

## Migraine

Chapter 5 of *The Borderland of Epilepsy* covered migraine. Interest in migraine had been awakened in Britain in the 1870s with the observations of Airy[51], Liveing,[52] and Latham[53], and with Liveing's influential idea that the disorder occurred as result of 'nerve storms' in the brain. Gowers did not explore the question this raised of a possible relationship between migraine and epilepsy:

> Some surprise may be felt that migraine is given a place in the borderland of epilepsy, but the position is justified by many relations, and among them by the fact that the two maladies are sometimes mistaken, and more often their distinction is difficult.[54]

His exploration of migraine in *Borderland* focused mainly on the problem of differentiating between migraine attacks whose aura phase began with alterations of sensation that spread from a local site at the periphery of the body, and focal sensory epileptic seizures with their much faster progression. Gowers also described some other preliminary manifestations of migraine that could conceivably have been regarded as epileptic.

In the first edition of Volume 2 of his *Manual* Gowers had already devoted 19 pages to the topic of 'paroxysmal headache or migraine'.[55] More than a century later, the account in the *Manual* of the clinical manifestations of migraine still contains (with the clearest explanation) almost all one would expect to find in modern, exhaustive descriptions of the condition—although the underlying mechanisms of the disorder are now better understood, and its treatment has changed. Gowers began his account in the *Manual* with an elegant *de facto* definition of the disorder:

> Migraine is an affection characterised by paroxysmal nervous disturbance, of which headache is the most constant element. The pain is seldom absent and may exist alone, but it is commonly accompanied by nausea and vomiting, and is often preceded by some sensory disturbance, especially by some disorder of the sense of sight. The symptoms are frequently one sided.[56]

Thus he perceived migraine not simply as a matter of headache but as a disturbance of the nervous system whose most frequent manifestation was headache. This may be why he devoted considerable attention to the disorder's sensory manifestations:

> The characteristic feature of the symptoms is their paroxysmal character. During the intervals, most patients are free from any symptoms of nerve derangement, although a few suffer from slighter headaches of a different character, occasional or continuous. The precise elements that make up the paroxysmal seizure vary in different cases, and often even in the same individual. Headache ... is the most constant, and is very seldom absent; next in frequency are nausea and vomiting, then some disturbance of vision, affection of speech, disturbed sensation in the limbs, and vaso-motor derangement, while the least common are motor symptoms in the limbs. The frequency of the vaso-motor derangement will be variously estimated, however, according to the phenomena included in the term, and if a simple change in frequency or tension of the pulse, or in the colour of the face, is included, this disturbance becomes one of the most frequent features of the attacks.[57]

Migraine attacks, Gowers suggested, might be provoked by 'excessive brain work', fatigue, excitement, digestive disturbances (particularly related to diet), visual impressions, bright light, or changes in the intensity of ambient light. Slight warning symptoms could occur before the actual migraine attack, including a heavy head, somnolence, and slight headache. His description of the headache itself shows great empathy with migraine sufferers:

> The headache is not only the most constant symptom, it is also the most distressing ... It varies very much in degree, but is very seldom trifling. Often it has a characteristic course, uniform in the same patient; it begins gradually, slowly increases to a considerable degree of intensity, and after a variable time it subsides, sometimes slowly, sometimes rapidly. It is usually an acute pain at the onset, and may remain so throughout, or may assume a duller character as it spreads. Movement, noise, and light usually increase its intensity. ...
>
> In most cases the headache begins one side, and in many it is confined to one side; in others it becomes general. ... When the pain begins at one spot it most frequently is in the temple, and is confined at first to a small area that can be covered by the tip of the finger. In other cases it begins in a small spot on the forehead, or in the forehead and eyeball, seldom in any limited area at other parts of the head. When thus limited at first, it seems generally superficial, but often has a boring character, as if some instrument were being forced into the skull.[58]

His clear exposition largely completed the process, begun by Tissot in 1780, of educating others about the clinical pattern and behaviour of the malady.[59] Yet he did not include some of its clinical characteristics. For instance, Gowers did not provide a clear description of the intolerance to light frequently associated with attacks, though he wrote that light made the headache worse. Although he described the site and severity of migraine pain, he said little about its character. In particular, he did not mention the 'throbbing' character of the pain. However, throbbing is generally overlooked in nineteenth-century migraine literature and was barely mentioned in Liveing's monograph.[60] Gowers did not describe frequently recurring migraines that could merge into a state of continuous headache, sometimes persisting over a long time. Nor did he mention some of the potential complications of the disorder, perhaps because, as a consultant, he did not follow typical individual migraine sufferers over time.

In other publications Gowers provided even more detailed accounts than in the *Manual* of the disturbances of visual and bodily sensation encountered in migraine, in particular the sensory symptoms which needed to be differentiated from the sensory effects produced by cortical epileptic discharges arising in, or spreading into, the brain's sensory mechanisms.[61]

When Gowers speculated about the anatomical origins of migraine attacks he carefully weighed the rival theories of the time, in particular the vascular and neural theories. The vascular theory itself involved two rival hypotheses. In 1861, Du Bois Reymond[62] argued, on the basis of his own appearance when he had migraine attacks, that the headache was the result of spasm of the arteries in the head caused by the sympathetic nervous system overacting. In 1867, Möllendorf put forward his contrary theory: that the headache was due to dilation of the cranial arteries.[63] In 1872, Latham put forward a reasonably persuasive hypothesis, that the migraine aura was the effect of vasoconstriction of brain arteries, and that the subsequent dilation of the extracranial vessels caused the headache.[64]

The original neural theory suggested that migraine was a form of neuralgia of the scalp. However, in 1873 Liveing concluded that it was best explained by the existence of a 'nerve storm' in the brain. Liveing's interpretation proved popular in the later nineteenth century, partly because it could explain how migraine attacks could be evoked by triggers like emotion, or emerging from darkness into bright light, which vascular theories could not.

Gowers, influenced both by the fact that migraine attacks could be triggered by psychological tension, and by the recent discovery of localization of function in the cerebral cortex, tended at first to side with the neural theory. Later, however, when writing on 'the curious sensory symptoms that constitute the premonition of attacks of migraine',[65] or prodromas, he seemed to support the vascular theory, particularly because it might explain the type of migraine aura which involves changes in body surface sensations as well as visual disturbances. He was also conscious that the extent of the disturbance of the visual fields in some migraine auras could not easily be explained unless both visual cortices were involved, and was more easily explained by a decreased blood flow in the area supplied by the basilar artery than by any single localized brain disturbance.[66] The competing hypotheses of Gowers' day have not yet been entirely resolved.

It is interesting to note that Gowers frequently suggested the regular oral intake of glyceryl trinitrate for the long-term management of migraine. This seems a rather curious recommendation when the substance can be used to induce attacks in people prone to migraines.

## Syphilis and the nervous system

In 1889 Gowers estimated that 13 per cent of the male population of London was affected by syphilis. Whether or not this figure was accurate, syphilis was not only prevalent, its effects were often devastating and long term. Gowers wrote about neurosyphilis on a number of occasions between 1877 and 1906. The spread of syphilis to the nervous system was an important cause of neurological disability in the Victorian age. But, at least in the early stages of Gowers' career, the full extent of its ravages on the nervous system was not recognized. Gowers earned a reputation as an expert on the disease and his advice, together with that of Buzzard and Reynolds, was sought in 1895 when Lord Randolph Churchill was dying of 'general paralysis of the insane' as a result of syphilis.[67]

To follow Gowers' publications chronologically is to watch the course of medical knowledge about neurosyphilis unfold.

### Theories about syphilis before 1863

Before 1863, syphilis was generally thought to be responsible for particular patterns of lesions involving parts of the external and internal surfaces of the body and the bones, but there was no clear evidence that the disorder involved internal organs. In 1863, Samuel Wilks, pathologist and physician to Guy's Hospital, described the syphilitic lesions that he had found in the brain and the various organs within the chest and abdomen during autopsies.[68] Before Wilks' paper, it had been thought that the brain could only be involved as a consequence of lesions that originated in the skull bones extending inwards. Wilks showed that syphilitic lesions could also develop in the brain surface membranes within the skull. These lesions evolved into 'gummas', soft tissue growths, which might sometimes invade the brain substance and gradually die, becoming increasingly caseous (or 'cheesy') as they aged. Wilks noted that similar processes could involve cranial nerves and, at the spinal cord level, could lead to external compression of the spinal cord. He also noted the presence of syphilitic nodular lesions in the intracranial arteries. This important work earned Wilks his election as a Fellow of the Royal Society, and stimulated a more intensive investigation of the pathological changes underlying the clinical manifestations of syphilis, including those involving the nervous system.[69]

Gowers became caught up in this exploration in the 1870s when he was a medical registrar and *de facto* pathologist at Queen Square. He did not achieve any particularly novel findings, as later discoveries demonstrated, but his pathological observations provided early verification of the discoveries of others. The combination of the findings from his data and his clear exposition helped inform English-speaking readers of the range of neurological illnesses that could be caused by syphilis. Writing in 1889, he explained that he wanted 'to render more definite the knowledge that already exists, and not to bring new knowledge into existence'.[70]

## Visceral syphilis

Gowers' first publication on syphilis described a demonstration of specimens he gave before the members of the Pathological Society of London in 1877.[71] He showed a gumma (a small soft tumour), apparently originating in the dura (the outermost of the three membranes covering the brain and spinal cord) and invading the underlying cerebral cortex along the penetrating blood vessels. He believed that all of the intracranial gummas that he had seen had originated in the pia mater (the innermost of the three membranes). He reported his second specimen as a great rarity: a tumour arising from the dura in a case of congenital syphilis. The third specimen was a large frontal lobe gumma; a separate cerebellar gumma; and multiple nodular enlargements of cerebral arteries, including one nodule that encircled a middle cerebral artery. Most of the arterial nodules appeared to originate outside the adventitial (outermost) coats of the vessels, but there was one nodule that encroached on the arterial lumen (inner cavity). Gowers' report implies that the specimens involved abnormalities that were then regarded as relatively novel.

In the light of modern knowledge, this novelty becomes clearer in Gowers' next paper on neurosyphilis, which appeared at much the same time as the first edition of Wilks' *Lectures on the Diseases of the Nervous System*.[72] Wilks might have been expected to maintain his interest in syphilitic afflictions of the internal organs, but scarcely expanded beyond the neurological manifestations he had first discussed in 1863. He did not mention syphilis as the cause of general paralysis of the insane, referring to it only as occasionally causing 'locomotor ataxy' (also called 'tabes dorsalis', or simply 'tabes'), the form of neurosyphilis that occurred some time after the original infection and which caused severe stabbing pains in the legs and trunk and an unsteady gait. Even by 1886, Wilks remained sceptical that the two might be connected.[73] In Reynolds' 1879 *System of Medicine*, Charles Bland Radcliffe wrote about locomotor ataxia[74] and Henry Maudsley about general paralysis of the insane[75] without syphilis being considered as a cause of either.

## Syphilitic neuroses

In his 1879 paper on syphilitic neuroses, Gowers explored a wider range of disorders that might possibly be caused by syphilis.[76] The term 'neurosis' had been introduced into medicine a century earlier by William Cullen to describe a disease of the nervous system the pathological basis of which was then unknown (rather than the modern usage describing varieties of psychological disturbance).[77]

Gowers divided neurological diseases into those where: (1) the primary change was intrinsic to the nervous system itself and originated in its nerve cells, their fibres, or the interstitial tissue (these were his 'neuroses'); and (2) diseases originating in the bones, vessels, and membranes of the nervous system, and neoplasms (disorders which Gowers termed 'adneural diseases'), and which might produce secondary changes in the nervous system itself. Syphilis of the nervous system was mainly adneural, manifesting itself in chronic meningitis, syphilitic disease of blood vessels, and syphilitic growths. Suspicion had been growing that primary neural diseases, or neuroses, might be caused by syphilis. Gowers examined this hypothesis, basing his arguments primarily on his experience at Queen Square.

Although he accepted that focal epileptic seizures are often the result of adneural syphilitic disease, Gowers wrote that he had no evidence that acquired syphilis could cause 'idiopathic epilepsy' (the term he used at the time).[78] However, he had found some cases in which congenital syphilis appeared to be responsible for seizures with the characteristics of idiopathic epilepsy. He had no evidence to suggest that chorea or paralysis agitans (Parkinson's disease) might have syphilitic aetiologies. Following Fournier, who first suggested that syphilis might cause primary neural disease (a neurosis),[79] he deduced that general paralysis of the insane was probably caused by syphilis. He knew that constitutional (secondary) syphilis might be followed by generalized muscular atrophy, and that similar wasting and weakness might rarely follow syphilitic spinal pachymeningitis. Syphilitic infection, he argued, might occasionally cause primary lateral sclerosis of the spinal cord. Fournier had noted that tabes dorsalis could be preceded by syphilis, a view with which Gowers agreed. However, Wilks pointed out that the most conspicuous pathological findings in tabes, sclerosis of the posterior columns of the spinal cord, could also arise from syphilitic adneural disease compressing the spinal cord.[80]

Gowers observed that the onset of syphilitic adneural diseases was rarely delayed by more than eight or ten years from the initial syphilitic lesion. Primary manifestations of neural syphilis tended to appear after distinctly longer intervals. Further, antisyphilitic therapies that were often successful in treating adneural syphilitic manifestations did not appear to delay the course of primary neural disorders caused by syphilis.

Thus, as early as 1879, Gowers identified a more extensive range of neurological manifestations of syphilis than his more senior London colleagues appear to have accepted. Time would prove him correct. However, without abandoning the concept, Gowers did not use the term 'adneural' in later publications. From 1879 onwards, his articles were concerned primarily with aspects of the primary neural consequences of the infection that had recently been identified, and he appeared to be more interested in tabes than in general paralysis of the insane, possibly because those afflicted with the latter were more likely to find their way into the hands of 'alienists' (later called psychiatrists). There was, of course, the almost inevitable contemporary mention of the effects of adneural syphilitic manifestations, mainly gummas, in Gowers' later publications.

## Lettsomian lectures on syphilis and the nervous system

In 1881 Gowers explored further the link between previous syphilis and tabes, citing French authors, particularly Fournier[81] who had found the two associated in some 80 per cent of tabes cases. In contrast, certain German authors (he cited Westphal, Remak, and Bernhardt) had noted it in only up to 25 per cent of their cases. Gowers thought the Germans' lower rate might be explained by their use of retrospective data;

evidence of the link might not have been looked for when the older statistics were being collected.

Gowers also noted that the reaction of the pupils to light in tabes sufferers was impaired, and also in general paralysis of the insane and other patterns of syphilitic disorder. At a time when statistical analysis in medicine was relatively new, Gowers noted that in his (limited) data the association between previous syphilis and tabes occurred with a similar frequency in his public patients seen at Queen Square and his private patients, though syphilis was less frequent in the latter. He therefore argued that syphilis probably played a causal role in producing tabes. It might have been safer simply to note that his data did not refute that interpretation. He also recorded again that the anti-syphilitic remedies of the day (mercury and potassium iodide) did not appear to be effective in treating tabes.

Gowers' Lettsomian lectures were published in 1889 in the January issues of *The Lancet*.[82] It had by that time become clear that syphilis was a transmissible infectious disease but it was not known what organism caused it, and there were no laboratory diagnostic tests available. Instead of basing his analysis of neurosyphilis on the site of origin of the pathological process, he now emphasized that some of the macroscopic neuropathological changes were inflammatory and inherently non-specific. Other changes involved abnormal tissue formation and were more specific: for example, gummas, changes in the arterial wall, and chronic dural pachymeningitis. He viewed histology as diagnostically unreliable, and expressed the hope that 'the progress of bacteriology may supply us with a conclusive criterion'.

He explored the range of neurological disorders that might be caused by syphilitic infection, speculating that a peculiar distribution of lesions might help to determine whether or not particular patterns of pathological change were caused by syphilis in cases with a past history of the disease. He specifically mentioned disseminated subacute myelitis and inflammations of multiple nerve roots, both occurring in individuals with earlier syphilitic infections. However, he concluded that he did not have enough evidence to determine this. Nor was he certain whether syphilis could cause acute meningitis.

He considered the question, not yet fully settled, of whether syphilis could cause delayed-onset degenerative disorder intrinsic to the cells of the central nervous system. He admitted that the only good evidence for the relationship between the two, particularly in the case of tabes, was 'numeric'. By that time he had collected 170 cases of tabes, with 55 per cent having definite evidence of previous syphilis and a further 14 per cent having a history of a 'sore' of uncertain nature sometime in the past. He therefore concluded that tabes was a delayed complication of syphilis. He was well aware of the connection between the Argyll Robertson pupil (a pupil that 'accommodates but does not react to light') and syphilis and felt the disease might also cause primary optic atrophy. However, he was unsure whether it could produce primary muscular atrophy or whether this occurred alone or in combination with signs of dysfunction of the lateral columns of the spinal cord. Gowers was attracted by Strümpell's suggestion (1883–4) that the syphilitic 'virus' could produce a neurotoxin which persisted in the sufferer's body and slowly affected the primary neural elements of the nervous system.[83]

In 1899 Gowers explored the relationship between tabes and general paresis (slight paralysis) of the insane in a separate paper, by that time believing that the causal relationship between syphilis and tabes dorsalis was an established fact, and that if tabes and general paralysis of the insane coexisted in the same person the tabetic manifestations tended to appear later than those of the general paralysis.[84]

## Prognosis and treatment of syphilitic diseases of the nervous system

In 1903, Gowers explored the prognosis and treatment of neurosyphilis.[85] He carefully related the prospects of functional recovery, after the nervous system was involved, to the nature and stage of development of whatever syphilitic pathological process existed at the start of the treatment. Inflammatory disturbances often responded well to potassium iodide or mercury, so long as they were provided early enough. Potassium iodide by itself, he wrote, was often enough to achieve any improvement possible, though occasionally mercury proved more effective. Since the treatments did not appear to destroy the organism responsible for the disorder, Gowers argued that continuous anti-syphilitic therapy was less useful than repeated courses of treatment at intervals. The main effect of the two treatments was to reduce inflammation. After the inflammation, however, repair of the previously inflamed tissues might lead to fibrosis which could then shrink, occasionally injuring local neural elements. He argued that if syphilitic endarteritic areas encircled a blood vessel, the shrinkage of the healing fibrotic lesion might narrow the artery to a significant extent and perhaps even obstruct it. When the syphilitic manifestations were degenerative or toxic, as in tabes and general paralysis of the insane, the available syphilitic treatments could not be expected to help.

## 'The nature of tabes' and 'The pain of tabes' (1905)

In 1905, Gowers gave two lectures on the slow degeneration of the spinal cord that is associated with syphilis, known as 'tabes', the Latin word for wasting or decay. The connection between tabes and previous syphilis had now been established, and he was interested in the altered physiological mechanisms producing its symptoms. Although the most conspicuous pathological change was in the posterior columns of the spinal cord, particularly in the medial parts (Goll's tracts), Gowers recognized that these changes followed degeneration of the posterior roots of the spinal nerves. He also knew that the corresponding peripheral nerves showed degenerative change; the whole peripheral sensory neuron was affected. In his papers he grappled with two separate issues: the pains that people with tabes had to endure, and the mechanism of their 'ataxic gait'.

He described in detail the various patterns of pain experienced by patients with tabes, and concluded that, since seemingly superficial 'lightning' pains were experienced in areas of the body's surface that were insensitive to painful stimuli, these pains must be transmitted to the brain through pathways that conveyed touch sensation. The pains probably arose in degenerating sensory nerve endings at the periphery of the body. He was unsure of the site of origin of the rather longer-lasting pains that seemed to arise more deeply within the body, and speculated that they might originate within the spinal cord. Given what was known about sensory physiology at the time it was a reasonable interpretation, and showed, as in some of his later publications, that he was aware of contemporary developments in physiology.

Aware of Sherrington's work on spinal reflex mechanisms, he produced a more convincing explanation for the ataxia of tabes:

> ... we cannot doubt the reality of the spinal mechanism nor can we doubt that it depends chiefly on the afferent muscle nerves. It must be disordered in tabes, in which these nerves are so conspicuously impaired. Even when the impulses produced in them are merely delayed, as we so often find to be the case with the nerves of the skin, we can easily conceive the effect of such delay in causing disorder. Each impulse would arrive just too late to excite the due contraction, and just in time to disturb the action which its absence induced. In the derangement of the spinal mechanism I think we may perceive one cause of the ataxy of tabes and, perhaps, that which determines its peculiar character.[86]

Gowers could not explain the altered process in more detail. He reasoned that the posterior column nerve fibres probably terminated in the cerebellum (which coordinated motor activity initiated in the motor areas of the cerebral cortex with sensory input from the muscles). Therefore the damage to the posterior column in tabes probably disturbed the cerebellar coordination of motor acts. As a result the ataxia of tabes involved both cerebellar and spinal cord components.

Gowers explained the mechanism by which previous syphilis led to tabes using the selective neurotoxin hypothesis that he had mentioned 15 years earlier. However, his new hypothesis was more convincing. The earlier neurotoxic idea did not easily explain the onset of tabes many years after the original syphilitic process had become inactive. Neurotoxin produced by the organism that caused syphilis should have ceased to act long before tabes appeared. Gowers therefore suggested that the syphilitic organism, while still active, had produced changes in some (unspecified) body component which not only persisted, but also produced some substance with selective neurotoxic properties, leading to progressive damage to neural elements.

Gowers' 1905 lecture on 'The nature of tabes' shows him at his best, interpreting clinical phenomena against both established and recent scientific knowledge, and filling in gaps in the story with shrewd and well-founded deductions which later research often proved correct.[87] It is also interesting that Gowers noted that between the time of his lecture and the publication of its text, other researchers, Metchnikoff and Roux, had announced that they were investigating an organism, the *spirocheta pallida*, as the possible cause of syphilis.

## 'The dystrophy of tabes and the problem of trophic nerves' (1906)

In 1906, in his final paper solely devoted to neurosyphilis, Gowers discussed 'the dystrophy of tabes' and the problem of trophic nerves.[88] By 'dystrophy' he meant changes such as the grossly deformed joints that could develop in the disorder (Charcot's joints), recurved knee joints, perforating ulcers that could occur on the feet, muscle wasting, and keratitis (inflammation of the cornea of the eye). His focus had also moved beyond neurosyphilis to consider issues such as the occurrence of underdeveloped limbs in both congenital hemiplegia and after poliomyelitis in early life. He surmised that changes in sensory innervation were probably responsible, particularly in relation to tabes, but produced no all-embracing explanatory hypothesis.

For nearly three decades Gowers' publications on syphilis had remained at the forefront of the exploration of one of the major causes of neurological disability in the Victorian era. He had thought his way through the disturbed physiology that must have been involved, and had, through his publications, continued to keep his contemporaries in the English-speaking medical profession aware of the advances being made in understanding what was, at the time, a distressingly common and debilitating disease.

## Diseases involving the basal ganglia (the 'dark basement' of the brain)

### Paralysis agitans

When at the peak of his teaching, Gowers had no equal at Queen Square and a number of his clinical demonstrations focused on a group of diseases now believed to be due to dysfunction of the grey matter in the basement of the brain (later referred to as the basal ganglia). The commonest of these was Sydenham's chorea (St Vitus's dance), rife amongst children in the slums around the hospital. There was also a veritable epidemic of writer's cramp (then known as 'scrivener's palsy') amongst the growing army of middle-class clerks in the civil service.

Gowers lectured and wrote extensively about these two conditions, but arguably his main contribution to the contemporary field of movement disorders was his description of paralysis agitans in the first edition of the *Manual*. The eighteen pages in which he discusses the malady begin as follows:

> Paralysis agitans, or Shaking Palsy, is a disease of the second half of life characterised by the symptoms indicated by its name, muscular weakness and tremor, and also by muscular rigidity. The symptoms usually commence locally and gradually, but tend to spread and to become general. From the fact that it was first fully described by Parkinson in 1817, it has been called 'Parkinson's disease' but the name, which he gave it of 'shaking palsy', is both apt and adequate.[89]

He then proceeds to describe his personal observations on 50 men and 30 women who had come under his care. The description is augmented by his own sketches illustrating the characteristic simian body posture and the hand and foot deformities frequently present in the later stages of the illness. Half of his patients had presented when in their fifties and, intriguingly, only three cases had presented for the first time over the age of 65. He emphasizes the heterogeneity of the clinical features of the disorder and the variability of its course, making it impossible to provide an accurate prognosis for the individual patient at the time of diagnosis. Nevertheless, he states that in the classical presentation the malady starts in one arm and then spreads to the contiguous leg before crossing to involve the other arm, and then the leg, over the next one to four years. He confirmed a coarse slow tremor present at rest due to the alternating contraction in opposing muscles that most commonly affected the fingers and hand as a classical hallmark of the disease, but also noted that it involved the leg, jaw, eyelids, and lips. He likened the hand oscillations to the rhythmical movements of 'Orientals beating small drums', and observed that the tremor was exacerbated by cold weather and was sometimes still present in the lighter stages of sleep. Another original finding was that tremor sometimes lessened as stiffness and slowness increased in a limb. He also described a slightly faster distinct tremor in some patients, present only when the hands were outstretched or in action. He emphasized the blurred borderlines between some cases of isolated tremor and the shaking palsy.

> Senile tremor often commences on both sides, paralysis agitans almost always on one. There is not, however, any sharp demarcation between the two affections, and it is difficult to say in which category some cases should be placed.[90]

Gowers also recorded the frequency and amplitude of tremor, measured on a rotating drum device, to illustrate the differences between the involuntary movements seen in paralysis agitans and those occurring in insular sclerosis (now known as multiple sclerosis), general paralysis of the insane, hysterical tremor, and tremor following a stroke.

Even more significant than his full description of the characteristics of the tremor, Gowers closely scrutinized the 'poverty of movement' first noted by James Parkinson in 1817, and concluded that the dextrous movements were not only feeble, but that there was a slowness of initiation. Irrespective of the severity of the disease, some power always remained in the limbs. Gowers believed that the associated muscular stiffness compounded the slowness, and that it was this feature of the disorder that led to the bleak outlook. Fatigue, motor restlessness, and depression were common, and some patients presented with rheumatic limb pains. There were frequent complaints of feeling hot and experiencing profuse perspiration, even in the winter, and leg oedema occurred in the later stages of the disease.

Gowers concluded, from a review of the available anatomical literature, that no convincing structural lesions had been found in the brain or sympathetic ganglia, but he felt that heredity was an important aetiological factor in about fifteen per cent of cases and that a loss of nutritional vitality in the dendrites involved in motor function was the likely cause. Not until 1917 would Konstantin Tretiakoff demonstrate that the pigmented nerve cells of the locus niger were severely damaged in 'maladie de Parkinson'.

Gowers considered possible predisposing influences, and was intrigued that a number of his cases had occurred after a severe emotional trauma, or in individuals suffering chronic anxiety. In 1904 he revisited this idea in his chapter on the disease in Allbutt's *System of Medicine*:

> The influence of fear is indeed the only fact in the causation that can be called intelligible. Its direct effect is on the motor centres, to induce the movement necessary for escape, which seems to have made the term 'movement from' a name for all such peculiar mental states ... If that movement be impossible, tremor results, and thus we have the word to 'tremble' as a synonym for fear. He who trembles is said to be 'paralysed by fear', and he is, in fact, for the moment suffering from 'paralysis agitans'. The sudden tremor of alarm

> has indeed been known to persist and to assume all the characteristics of the malady now under consideration.[91]

Gowers considered paralysis agitans to be the least amenable to therapeutic agents of all the diseases of the nervous system involving a loss of vitality and a degeneration of cells and tissues (abiotrophies) but recommended Indian hemp, arsenic, small doses of strychnine, opium, and one-eighth of a grain of cocaine as useful symptomatic treatments. His experience with belladonna and physostigmine was less favourable, and he stated bluntly that electrotherapy was ineffective.

## Writer's cramp

Gowers used the term 'occupational neurosis' to describe a spasm caused primarily by the act of writing 'which has been excessive in degree', and sometimes associated with a tremor or contortion of the hand.[92] He conceived of writer's cramp as a dilapidation of the writing centre in the motor cortex due to faulty penmanship and workload. He noted that it was prevalent amongst males, because fewer women were engaged in occupations involving a large amount of writing (Charles Dickens' novel Bleak House describes the legion of solicitors' clerks engaged in copying legal documents in the never-ending case of Jarndyce and Jarndyce). Gowers advocated re-education with a freer style of writing employing the shoulder and upper arm to move the quill across the page; later in his career he also discussed the importance of trying to alleviate associated anxiety. He observed that this appeared not to affect people who used shorthand or wrote on a blackboard. Attempts to learn to write with the other hand were sometimes successful, but he warned that the disorder could affect the previously unaffected side too. He also described cases in which the disorder spread to involve other dextrous activities over time and cause considerable pain and contortion of the hand.

Writer's cramp may have been a subject close to his heart. A rough word-count of the two volumes of the *Manual* comes to approximately 810,000 words. No wonder he wrote his first drafts in shorthand. Nonetheless the final version still had to be transcribed into longhand.

## Sydenham's chorea (St Vitus's Dance)

Gowers' lengthy description of Sydenham's chorea in the *Manual* is a *tour de force*. More than 120 children and young adults were admitted under his care at the National Hospital, making him a leading authority on the disorder for which the cause remained elusive. In 1878 in two articles, 'On some points in the clinical history of chorea', he suggested that in some patients there may be an incoordination of the limbs above and beyond what one would expect as a result of the involuntary movements and that there was an increased electrical irritability in the limbs.[93] In the second article he noted that true hemichorea was very unusual as there was nearly always some additional milder involvement of the other leg. He also reported that convulsions could occur, either during the acute attack or some years later despite apparent full recovery. Three years later he described five children with what he termed paralytic chorea in which weakness of one arm predominated.[94] As the weakness lessened, chorea would often become more apparent in the affected limb before the disease abated. Gowers was well aware of the link with inflammation of the heart in many of his cases.[95] Interestingly, he devoted very little space to Huntington's chorea, whereas today it would feature much more prominently than rheumatic chorea, now virtually eradicated from the developed world by improved public health measures and antibiotic therapy.

### 'Athetosis' and post-hemiplegic disorders of movement

In 1871 Hammond had described a unilateral sinuous writhing movement disorder with abnormal posturing following cerebral haemorrhage, and coined the new term 'athetosis'. In 1876 Gowers described his findings on eighteen cases mainly of children and young adults with abnormal movement disorders following a stroke, and argued that Hammond was not describing a new disease entity or even a new physical sign. In the paper he drew on a careful study of his own cases and on the earlier clinical and pathological observations of Charcot and Weir Mitchell. He suggested that damage to the grey matter of the central ganglia of the brain, including the corpus striatum and the thalamus, was important in causation. His paper included exquisite drawings of the abnormal 'fixed limb' postures.[96]

## Other movement disorders

Under the broad section of 'general and functional' diseases, Gowers also provides lively descriptions in his *Manual* of other movement disorders, including spasmodic torticollis, habit spasms (tics), tremors, and other occupational neuroses including hand cramps associated with seamstresses, telegraphists (using the Morse Code machine), smiths, painters, artificial flower makers, turners, watchmakers, masons, sailors (from rope-pulling), compositors, letter sorters, money counters, and musicians (particularly piano players, violinists, harpists, and drummers), descriptions which can still be read with benefit today. Dubini's electric chorea, Friedrich's myoclonus multiplex, and saltatoric spasms no longer hold a place in contemporary nosological classification of movement disorders but probably represent diverse myoclonic syndromes and psychogenic movement disorders.

Gowers also describes a case of a 10-year-old boy Sydney M, who had been admitted under his care to the National Hospital on 5 October 1886 with clumsiness on eating and who had progressed rapidly to a helpless bed-bound state with pyrexia and emaciation.[97] Gowers noted a sardonic smile, severely slurred speech with swallowing difficulties due to involuntary tongue movements, and a difficulty in closing his mouth. He also had severe asymmetrical contortions and spasms of the limbs. The boy died in hospital in *status dystonicus* six months after the onset of the disease. Post-mortem examination revealed cirrhosis of the liver, but no structural lesion of the brain was detected, even after microscopy. The family history was of note, in that an older brother, admitted to Queen Square seven years earlier, had died of some form of paralysis. Two years later the boys' 15-year-old sister was admitted with a similar disorder. Examination revealed pathological laughter, involuntary tongue protrusion with the subsequent development a few weeks later of writhing involuntary movements of the right leg soon spreading to involve the other limbs. Hyoscine hydrobromide was of mild symptomatic benefit but, like her brother, she went downhill rapidly and died after a five-month illness. Pathological examination of her brain revealed some minute pits in the white matter and there was cirrhosis of the liver. Gowers also refers to a similar case in a 10-year-old boy reported by his colleague Ormerod, in which autopsy had revealed softening in the outer part of the lenticular nucleus and in the pons with cirrhosis. Gowers concluded that this was a hitherto unrecognized disease almost certainly caused by a non-syphilitic, blood-borne toxin. In 1911 Kinnier Wilson, one of Gowers' former assistants, reported a further member of the same family in his doctoral thesis. The following year, in his seminal paper published in *Brain*, 'Progressive lenticular degeneration', Wilson reported the clinico-pathological findings of six cases.[98] This disorder later became known as Wilson's disease, a rare autosomal recessive disorder due to the abnormal handling and transport of copper. Gowers' careful observations must have whetted his young clinical assistant's appetite to solve the mystery.

## Disseminated sclerosis

The present-day neurologist may be surprised that Gowers should have devoted only a little less than one per cent of the pages of the first edition of his *Manual* to the topic of disseminated (or insular) sclerosis. He did return to it in 1909 in an article in the *Phonographic Record*, but this material would have had a limited readership.

However, during our search of archival material at Queen Square, a manuscript of an unpublished clinical lecture that Gowers gave in 1895 came to light. In it, Gowers used clinical details of a fairly advanced case of disseminated sclerosis as a basis for distinguishing between the disorder and hysteria. He also discussed what was then known of the pathology of the disorder, but on the whole the lecture added very little to what was already available in his *Manual*.[99]

Gowers' relative neglect of the topic, and his failure to emphasize the course of the disorder over time, reflected what little was known. The structural pathology of the disease had been recognized in the 1830s,[100] but it was some years before the clinical manifestations of the pathological changes were clarified by Charcot, whose lectures on diseases of the nervous system were not translated into English until 1877.[101] The patterns of evolution of the disorder from its initial stages were not well recognized, nor were the mechanisms causing it yet understood.

## Primary diseases of muscle

Gowers took an early interest in a range of primary muscle diseases, adding to knowledge about them at a time when they were often seen as falling outside the province of the clinical neurologist. Over the years he wrote on diseases of skeletal muscle, or myopathies, on several occasions, and published papers on pseudo-hypertrophic muscular dystrophy, distal myopathy, and polymyositis.

### Pseudo-hypertrophic muscular dystrophy

His interest in this disorder started when he was an apprentice in Coggeshall, triggered by a case of pseudo-hypertrophic paralysis: of the ten children in a family living near

Dr Simpson's surgery, four boys were afflicted by a strange disorder of locomotion, with wasting of some muscles and enlargement of others, and all had hypertrophied tongues.[102]

Gowers was 29 in 1874 when he and Lockhart Clarke described the illness of a 14½-year-old boy who had died of pseudo-hypertrophic muscular paralysis. The paper featured Gowers' own drawings of the microscopic appearance of the muscle and spinal cord pathologies found at autopsy. Gowers and Clarke recorded changes in the spinal cord, a feature not usually reported in earlier autopsies.[103]

Cases began to turn up at Queen Square. Clifford Allbutt brought two more to Gowers' attention; William Adams, his orthopaedic colleague, brought him 18 other cases to examine. When one patient died he was able to study the morbid anatomy of the case. Critchley wrote that the young registrars at Queen Square—Newman, Sankey, Sturge, and Broster—all helped him, allowing him to study what was a little-known affliction, and to make it the subject of a lecture to the UCH students visiting Queen Square.[104]

In 1879 the lecture was published as a series of parts in the July issues of *The Lancet*, then J. & A. Churchill published it as a small monograph. The monograph reported on 23 cases of the inherited myopathy 'pseudo-hypertrophic muscular dystrophy' collected by Gowers from various sources, and 220 cases drawn from the literature.[105] Gowers' compassion for his patients shows in his opening remarks:

> The disease is one of the most interesting and at the same time most sad, of all those with which we have to deal: interesting on account of its peculiar features and mysterious nature; sad on account of our powerlessness to influence its course, except in a very slight degree, and on account of the conditions in which it occurs. It is a disease of early life and of early growth. Manifesting itself commonly at the transition from infancy to childhood, it develops with the child's development, grows with his growth—so that every increase in stature means an increase in weakness, and each year takes him a step further on the road to a helpless infirmity, and in most cases to an early and inevitable death.[106]

He reviewed the existing literature on the disease, focusing in particular on the cases Meryon described in 1852 (the first time the disorder that carries Duchenne's name was described in England), and those described by Duchenne in 1869.[107] Duchenne had recorded the typical fatty infiltration in specimens of affected enlarged muscle (obtained using a 'harpoon' biopsy). Gowers noted that microscopic abnormalities had been found in the spinal cord as well as in the affected muscles in a minority of instances. He had found that, out of his own 23 cases, 18 occurred in males. The five females were much more mildly affected than the males. It seems possible that he may have seen some female carriers, but did not understand its genetic inheritance. He reasoned that the condition was not a manifestation of progressive muscular atrophy and felt it was unlikely to be caused by an affection of sympathetic or trophic nerves. He preferred to regard the disorder as a primary disease of muscle.

Many years later he returned to the topic of pseudo-hypertrophic dystrophy, in particular dealing with its hereditary transmission, in lectures on myopathy in 1902,[108] on heredity in 1908,[109] and on myopathy and syringomyelia in 1909.[110]

## Distal myopathy

In 1902 Gowers presented a lecture on 'myopathy and a distal form'. He started by describing two cases of pseudo-hypertrophic muscular dystrophy and an instance of facio-scapular muscular dystrophy (the Landouzy–Dejerine syndrome). He then described a syndrome which in the French medical literature is still called the 'syndrome de Gowers'. He described what he thought was a unique instance of a 12-year-old boy who experienced the insidious onset of foot drop, followed later by weakness of both hands. The weakness progressed until he was 18 years old, which was when Gowers examined him. His calves were relatively big, the muscles of the front of his left lower leg were wasted, his handgrip was weak, and his forearms and hands were slender. The sternal parts of the sternomastoid muscles in the front of his neck were very wasted and the clavicular heads of these muscles were absent. Both sides of the tongue were wasted, and there was some weakness of the upper face. There was no mention of any altered sensation or delayed relaxation of contracted muscle, i.e. myotonia. There were no microscopic studies of the affected muscles. Gowers was convinced that the diagnosis was not peroneal muscular atrophy. Whether or not he described a genuine new entity is arguable. However, Steinert did not describe myotonic dystrophy until 1909, seven years after Gowers' report, and the distribution of muscle involvement in Gowers' patient appears to have been consistent with a stage in the evolution of myotonic dystrophy.[111]

## Polymyositis

In 1899 Gowers described a case he had diagnosed as polymyositis.[112] He started by analysing the disease mechanisms underlying polyneuritis, and went on to argue that polymyositis was similar to polyneuritis, but an underlying rheumatic disorder produced a 'poison' which affected body muscles diffusely, rather than attacking peripheral nerves. This hypothesis assumed that this poison could also affect the peripheral nerves, though to a lesser extent. In his paper, Gowers described one instance of polymyositis that had occurred in a 36-year-old woman. Her disorder had already reached a burned-out stage, with widespread muscle wasting and weakness, and extremely severe stiffness. The disorder had been developing progressively over a couple of years, and she had had a rash on her hands and arms. Sensory and sphincter function were normal. Gowers' diagnosis was made entirely on clinical grounds, without microscopic confirmation. The existence of the rash would now be taken to indicate that this could have been a case of dermatomyositis that had reached an inactive stage. Unfortunately, Gowers supplied neither references nor a literature review, concluding that the condition was very unusual.

# Neurophysiology

When Gowers began his neurological career in 1870 the macroscopic anatomy of the nervous system was reasonably well established, though aspects of the internal structure and of the connections between various parts had yet to be discovered. Knowledge about the physiology and biochemistry of the nervous system was still in its infancy, but physiological knowledge was rapidly increasing. Particularly in the earlier stages of his professional career, Gowers involved himself in original neurophysiological investigations. But throughout his life he continued to offer perceptive interpretations of clinical phenomena as new information about physiology emerged.

## Anal sphincter innervation

In 1877 he recorded pressure changes in the lumen of the anal canal and rectum in three patients suffering faecal incontinence. One had anaesthesia of the whole area innervated by the sacral plexus but no evidence of spinal cord injury. The other two had thoracic-level damage to their spinal cords. The anal sphincters were found to sustain mild contraction in the basal state, and relax if the rectum was distended by means of air injected into it. After a short delay the pressure was released, then gradually returned to its original level. The external anal sphincters remained relaxed through this procedure; only the internal sphincters appeared to respond when the rectum was distended. Gowers concluded that the sympathetic innervation of the rectum and anal canal remained relatively intact, so that a reflex response to rectal irritation persisted though the lesions that existed had inactivated the remainder of the innervation of the ano-rectal region. Gowers' findings were considered sufficiently interesting to be presented to the Royal Society on his behalf by his colleague the Jodrell Professor of Physiology at UCL, J. Burdon-Sanderson.[113]

## Eyelid movement

Two years later, in 1879, Gowers examined the movements of the eyelids.[114] He pointed out that while the lower lid tended to become lower when the eyes looked down, there was no muscle to make the lid lower. The only muscles that could move the lids were the levator palpebrae superioris, which could lift the upper lid, and the orbicularis oculi which, when contracted, would draw the lids together. To explain how the lower eyelid dropped, he identified the different curvatures of the cornea, at the front of the eyeball, and the remainder of the eyeball. Gazing straight ahead, the eye was positioned so that the lids tended to sit at the junction between cornea and the remainder of the eyeball. The greater curvature of the cornea tended to raise or lower the respective eyelids when the eyeball was rotated up or down. When the eyeball was rotated upward by the action of the superior rectus muscle, there was, as well as the effect of the cornea, a linked active contraction of the levator palpebrae superioris that raised the upper lid. If the levator palpebrae superioris was paralysed, the upper eyelid would droop. When it was intact, but the orbicularis oculi was paralysed, if an effort was made to close the eyes the upper lid would droop because contraction of the orbicularis was somehow linked to an involuntary mechanism which caused the levator palpebrae to relax.

Gowers argued that separate mechanistic centres probably existed linking weak and strong contraction of the orbicularis oculi muscle to the levator palpebrae superioris muscle. Gowers tried to interpret his observations of the relatively neglected topic of eyelid, as distinct from eyeball, movement. In so doing, he appears to have concluded that mechanisms must exist in the central nervous system which linked the actions of functionally related muscles. He returned to this idea several times in later publications.

## Eye fixation

Gowers' interest in eye movements was revealed in another article in *Brain* in 1880: a 'Note' examining the mechanisms that allowed someone to fix their eyeballs on a target while moving their head. He suggested this was the result of a combination of reflex and voluntary components.[115] He had studied a patient with possible advanced amyotrophic lateral sclerosis with severe rigidity. The subject was asked to look at an object some distance to the side of where he was currently looking. His head turned quickly towards the new target, but his gaze remained temporarily locked where it was, and then slowly transferred to the new target. Gowers' hypothesis was that there was a reflex from the retina which held the external ocular muscles contracted, locking the eye where it was. Normally, this could be immediately overridden by the will, allowing the gaze to be rapidly transferred from one target to another, but in his patient the disease process had interfered with the mechanism linking the will to the centre that controlled eye movement. This may have been an early report of delayed latency of saccadic eye movements as is seen in corticobasal syndrome with intact vestibular ocular reflexes, but Gowers mistakenly assumed the response depended on intact vision.

## Tendon reflexes

In 1879 Gowers also studied the phenomenon of two tendon reflexes: the patellar tendon reflex (of Erb) or the knee phenomenon (of Westphal), and Erb's 'Achilles tendon reflex', also called 'Westphal's foot phenomenon' (the ankle-jerk).[116] Gowers was using the term 'knee-jerk' for the former at least by 1882.[117]

> At the meeting of the British Association at Cambridge I was talking with Professors Clifford Allbutt and Westphal about the error of the term 'tendon reflex'—which Westphal (who first pointed out the importance of the symptom) had always avoided. He preferred the name 'knee-phenomenon'. I asked, 'Why not call it the "knee-jerk"?' Clifford Allbutt so emphatically approved the term that I took the first opportunity of setting it going, and its use immediately became universal.[118]

Gowers studied reflex responses both in normal subjects and in patients with disease that affected the reflexes. He noted that it was only comparatively recently that a tendon reflex had been accepted as a neural reflex, rather than a direct contraction of muscle produced by a sudden tap on its tendon.[119] In his study he used measurements from a rotating drum (see Chapter 6) on which the time course of muscle tension change could be recorded.The interval between tapping the patellar tendon and the muscle jerk was consistent with nerve conduction at a velocity of 33 metres a second, a value that Helmholtz had previously estimated. On this basis, Gowers concluded that the knee-jerk was a neural reflex. However, he also thought that he could see an earlier small muscle response before the main jerk, and he took this to be a direct response of muscle to the tap on its tendon. When he turned to the ankle, he studied the repeated jerking of clonus, and its repetition rate, rather than single jerks.

The interval between a tap on the Achilles tendon and the initial muscle jerk was too short, in his view, for the response to involve a spinal reflex. He therefore thought clonus was a local direct muscle response to sudden extension of its tendon. He suggested that clonus resulted from a continuing muscle vibration set up by the initial tug on the tendon. When he studied knee clonus he found its recorded rate was slower than that of ankle clonus, and therefore suggested that the clonus at the two sites might be mediated through different mechanisms.

Gowers based the interpretation of his observations on his belief that nerves conducted at a velocity of around 33 metres a second, and the accuracy of his measurement may have been limited by the characteristics of his recording system. Nonetheless, the mere fact that he used the tools and techniques of the experimental physiologists of the day to carry out this study demonstrates his intellectual curiosity, versatility, and energy.

Interestingly, in the second edition of *The Diagnosis of Diseases of the Spinal Cord*, published in 1882, Gowers changed his interpretation of the nature of the knee-jerk. He now suggested that it was a local muscle response produced by an abrupt increase in muscle tension when the patellar tendon was tapped and momentary elongated. Thus he thought that neither the knee-jerk nor the ankle-jerk was a true reflex but both were local muscle responses activated by muscle stretch. His argument depended on the measurement of the interval between tendon tapping and the onset of the induced jerk, on nerve conduction velocity having its published value of around 33 metres per second, and on Tchirjew having shown in experimental animals that the knee response could still be elicited by tapping the patellar tendon even though the complete nerve supply to the tendon had been interrupted surgically. He remained of that opinion in 1885 and 1895.[120]

In 1903, he raised a problem about the speed of nerve conduction.[121] Was it 33 metres per second, as had originally been reported, or was it the more recently reported value of 66 metres per second? Waller replied, indicating the difficulties of establishing when the onset of detectable muscle contraction occurred. Waller's view was it was more likely that the speed was close to 66 metres per second.[122] Gowers may have realized that, if Waller was right, his own interpretations of the nature of muscle reflexes might not hold, though he appears not to have written anything further on the subject.

It appears that Gowers stopped carrying out his own experimental studies after the late 1870s, as he started to use the results of other neurophysiologists when trying to explain how the nervous system functioned.

## Miscellaneous aspects of neurophysiology

Gowers published a series of papers in 1890 in which he discussed the mechanisms controlling various brain functions. He dealt successively with four issues. (1) The way the cerebellum used its input from the direct spinocerebellar tracts, the posterior columns (probably), the vestibular system, and the motor cortex, to produce coordinated voluntary movement and posture maintenance. (2) The fact that nerve cells did not simply go into action only when required, and otherwise remain quiescent, but, particularly in the case of neurons involved in sensory functions or in maintaining posture and muscle tone, were continuously active, with their degree of activity varying with the functions they were stimulated to subserve at different times. (3) The matter of automatic reflex coordination in which contraction of one muscle is accompanied by the relaxation of muscles whose contraction would oppose the action of the contracting muscle (one of his favourite themes). (4) Muscular adaptation and hypnotic catalepsy, where he hypothesized that hypnosis cut off lower-level mechanisms from the influence of higher ones, resulting in excessive responses to stimulation.

Gowers drew on his observations of the consequences of surgery for trigeminal neuralgia to demonstrate that taste sensation was conveyed from the tongue to the brainstem in the lingual nerve and then in the maxillary division of the trigeminal nerve.[123] Horsley's removal of the trigeminal root led to loss of taste on the same side of the tongue. Unfortunately, Gowers did not appear to know of Wrisberg's nervus intermedius, carrying the taste fibres into the brainstem, which presumably was damaged by the surgery, but his use of clinical observations to interpret physiology testifies to the integrity of his method.

## Lumbago

When his lecture on lumbago appeared in print, Gowers had been suffering back pain for many years. He hinted with some feeling that he was troubled by the disorder and after describing its clinical features went into the question of how the pain was produced, his discussion spilling over into a consideration of the pain of muscle cramp. By this time he was aware of the existence of the muscle spindles situated in the fibrous tissue between interfascicular locations. Previously, he had difficulty in explaining the origin of the afferent limb of the reflex arc because he could not easily see how nerve endings in muscle fibrous tissue could respond to sudden stretch of muscle fibres. The spindles gave him a receptor from which afferent impulses could arise, though he did not know that the spindles also had a motor nerve supply. He was forced to conclude that muscle pain arose from the spindles, but at least he had raised questions that had eluded others, and had tried to answer them in the light of knowledge at the time.[124]

Critchley describes 16 January 1904 as the veni vidi vici of the word 'fibrositis' into medical technology.[125] Gowers stated that it was particularly frequent in ladies of unblemished character and also in members of the clergy (perhaps delineating it from the lightning pain of tabes dorsalis). The condition is now termed fibromyalgia and considered a functional somatic syndrome by many authors.

## Nystagmus

In 1908, nearing the end of his professional life, Gowers wrote on nystagmus. His paper was not so much an analysis of the various patterns of nystagmus that are seen clinically, but a discussion on how nystagmus involved the contraction of one external eye muscle and the simultaneous relaxation of the muscle with which its function was paired in opposition. This was the old idea of reciprocal innervation that so often exercised him, now confirmed by evidence from Sherrington but with an added element: that the increasing stretch of the opposing muscle would increasingly trigger its reflex contraction, with reciprocal innervation then causing the originally contracting muscle to relax. Thus he could explain the repeated cycle of involuntary bidirectional eyeball movement that produces nystagmus.

## Conclusion: the significance of Gowers' research

Gowers' neurological research interests were almost entirely driven by his chosen clinical speciality and his determination to understand physiologically and anatomically the neurological phenomena he observed at the bedside. Although he must have seen many psychiatric illnesses in his private practice he was never attracted to investigate hysteria or neurasthenia. Careful observation and scrupulous recording of his findings at the bedside underpinned his clinical method, supplemented where possible by physiological measurement and interpretation in the light of contemporary knowledge of physiology and anatomy. Gowers appreciated that statistics were an essential component of medical research and did his own statistical calculations when needed. This further illustrates his grasp of the scientific method, and his ability to apply it in his investigation of the neurologically ill.

## Chapter 8

# Gowers the writer and lecturer

Gowers was not only a great diagnostician; he also stood out amongst his contemporaries through the quality of his lectures, his research publications, and his textbooks. The close attention Gowers gave to his patients, and the meticulous records he kept of each case, provided the raw material he drew on to develop the hypotheses in his research papers. His lectures were based primarily on his own research; the lectures, in turn, were often published. Well after he had established his reputation as a writer, he explained his underlying principle:

> In general it is a mistake to publish single cases. Far better to work up single points or publish a special case after working up its points comparatively. Nothing pays except that which gives some new suggestion. The great thing is to create a feeling in the reader—I must not miss anything else this man says.[1]

His mastery of clear English matched his 'virtuoso' performances as a lecturer. It was as important to him to pass on medical knowledge as to add to it:

> The formula of Gowers' contributions to neurology may ... be described as the recognition of a number of salient, novel and important clinico-pathological features culled from his experience. These would be worked up and elaborated, and perhaps other cognate observations from the literature would be incorporated. In this way a short paper, or maybe a clinical lecture would take shape. This would then be published in one of the medical periodicals. Later the subject would be re-examined; modifications would be made, and new data added. Then the contribution would appear in book form, his publishers always being the firm of Churchill, and perhaps run to two or more editions. In this way Gowers secured a very wide audience.[2] Critchley, p. 31.

Several of the works published by Churchill were also published in the United States, often by Blakiston of Philadelphia, making them almost simultaneously available to American readers. It was acceptable practice for the same lecture series to be published in both *The Lancet* and the *BMJ*, then be published by J. & A. Churchill as a book, and finally also be published in an American edition.

Gowers published his medical articles and lectures in *The Lancet*, the *BMJ*, the *Medical Times and Gazette*, the *Medico-Chirurgical Transactions*, the *Transactions of the Clinical Society*, *Transactions of the Pathological Society*, and the *Clinical Journal*. He also published a few papers in *Nature* and the *Proceedings of the Royal Society* and *Review of Neurology and Psychiatry*, and was a frequent correspondent in the columns of *The Lancet* and the *BMJ*. He also published papers in shorthand in the *Phonographic Record of Clinical Teaching and Medical Science* (some, but not all, were articles published elsewhere). Like Charcot, he drew most of the illustrations himself.

His son Ernest earned a reputation of his own for his clear written English. His civil service training manual, *Plain Words: a Guide to the Use of English*[3] became an instant best-seller when it was published in 1948, and towards the end of his life he revised Fowler's *Modern English Usage*. He described his father's style:

> In literary style, as in art, he had a marked natural aptitude which he cultivated assiduously. His lectures and books are in admirable English. Possibly he was a little more free with rhetoric than present-day taste thinks proper, but that is the only criticism that can be made. He knew how good his English was, and was justly proud of it. In this, as in his shorthand, his sense of craftsmanship would not let him be content with anything but the best of which he was capable. He took infinite trouble.[4]

As a young man, Gowers had contributed to Russell Reynolds' *A System of Medicine*, and also contributed articles on 'Blood' to its 1877 and 1879 editions. In 1875 he translated into English Pagenstecher and Genth's *Atlas der pathologischen Anatomie des Augapfels.*[5] His potential as a writer was recognized in 1876 when he was invited to edit the section 'Central nervous system' for the eighth edition of Quain's *Elements of Anatomy*, a book which had become the standard textbook in English-speaking countries since its first edition appeared in 1828.

Jones Quain had been the professor of general anatomy at University College from 1831 to 1836. Thomas Sharpey and Jones Quain's brother Richard, and Allen Thomson, and John Cleland jointly authored several editions of *Elements of Anatomy*. John Marshall, surgeon and teacher of anatomy, helped to produce the 1848 5th edition. The 7th edition appeared in 1867, edited by Sharpey, Thomson, and John Cleland. In 1872 Sharpey first enlisted Gowers' help. He wrote to Thomson (by then professor of anatomy at the University of Glasgow) relating a conversation that he had had with William Longman whose firm, now holding copyright for the textbook, was planning an 8th edition.

> I explained that you & I had recommended a rearrangement of the subjects in a new Edition. One part to contain Histology & the structural & physiological anatomy of the viscera—the microscopic anatomy of the teeth—the organs of sense—and all development &c. the other part to contain the bare descriptive anatomy with the descriptions abridged. That with your approval and by desire of Walton I had urged Dr Gowers to eliminate flaws [?] & condense the Second part & that he had been some time employed on it—& that whatever else was done I trusted he would receive suitable remuneration—this Mr L [William Longman] promised.[6]

## *A Manual and Atlas of Medical Ophthalmoscopy*

The first important book Gowers published was his *Manual and Atlas of Medical Ophthalmoscopy* published in May 1879. In 1877 Hughlings Jackson had paid tribute to his skills when referring to a paper by Gowers on Bright's disease:

> I would draw the attention both of ophthalmic surgeons and physicians to some minute ophthalmic observations by Dr Gowers in certain cases of Bright's disease.[7] Dr Gowers is so good an ophthalmoscopist, and, above all knows so thoroughly well the varied healthy appearances of the normal fundus oculi, that I should accept these minute observations of his as being as precise and as exact as it is possible for such difficult observations to be.

Helmholtz invented the ophthalmoscope in 1850, nearly 30 years before Gowers published his *Manual and Atlas of Medical Ophthalmoscopy* in 1879.[8] This was not the first English-language monograph on ophthalmoscopy. Clifford Albright had published a monograph on the same topic eight years earlier, at John Hughlings Jackson's suggestion. However, it did not appear in a second edition.[9]

Gowers, like many of his contemporaries, published with J. & A. Churchill. John and Augustus Churchill had joined their father, John Spriggs Morse Churchill, the first great English medical publisher, in his business at 11 New Burlington Street, London in 1855. Churchill senior had been about to start a medical apprenticeship when he became diverted into publishing. He built up his business by identifying the need for textbooks for the expanding medical profession, and providing 'attractive, cheap, and well-illustrated manuals by competent authors'.[10] His first book of this type was Erasmus Wilson's highly successful *Anatomist's Vade Mecum* published in 1840. J. & A. Churchill continued to be the leading English medical publisher throughout Gowers' career. It was not until 1972 that the medical lists of J. & A. Churchill, E. & S. Livingstone, and Longman were amalgamated; the Churchill Livingstone imprint is now owned by the Elsevier publishing house.

The method of reproducing illustrations in medical texts developed gradually through the Victorian era. The 1828 edition of Quain's *Anatomy* had no illustrations. The 1836 edition included illustrations by Erasmus Wilson, but Wilson's large plates were sold separately, either in black and white, or hand tinted.[11] In 1848, the fifth edition of Quain, edited at UCL by William Sharpey and Richard Quain, was illustrated, 'but not generously'.[12]

In 1858, five years before Gowers became a medical student, Gray's *Anatomy* appeared. Gray, who died at the age of 34, only three years after his *Anatomy* was published, wrote the text and Henry Vandyke Carter provided the striking woodblock illustrations. Gray's *Anatomy* set a new standard in medical textbooks, but Gray's lack of attribution of his sources, and apparent dependence on Quain, earned him a scathing review in the *Medical Times and Gazette* for what, after careful comparison, was deemed to be an unscrupulous use of Quain's text.[13] So while Gowers would have known of Gray's *Anatomy*, UCL may have favoured Quain as the anatomy text for its students.

*A Manual and Atlas of Medical Ophthalmology* was Gowers' first publication with Churchill. The book was based on his experience in the wards of UCH and Queen Square. The first edition ran to 352 pages, including 125 devoted to 50 case histories. There was an appendix dealing with ophthalmoscopes; two sets of chromolithographic plates; sepia drawings of the optic fundus; and drawings of the histology of the retina and optic nerve. It contained detailed discussion of the types of pathological appearance of the optic disc and the surrounding retina and of the retinal blood vessels; and described those associated with the neurological and general medical diseases recorded in the literature or encountered in Gowers' own experience.

Gowers wrote that his primary aim was to publish a series of illustrations (see Fig. 8.1) accompanied by descriptions of the cases from which they were made; however, he thought that a systematic overview of the subject would make the illustrations and notes more useful:

> The cases described were met with in the course of his medical work, and he took great care in securing the utmost possible exactness in his illustrations. Some of the plates are in colour, but more are autotype reproductions of sepia drawings, probably used for the first time in medical works. His chief object was to fix the attention on changes of form rather

> than alterations in colour, which, important as they are, very often mislead the inexperienced. He believed that if the illustrations were studied with the aid of the descriptions prefixed to them the absent colours of the sepia drawings would not be missed by those accustomed to the use of the ophthalmoscope. Where changes of tint are of predominant importance chromo-lithography was employed for the illustrations. The illustrations, which are a striking feature of the book, were all drawn by Gowers himself.[14]

At the time of the first edition, the ophthalmoscope was still finding its place in medical and neurological practice; although many ophthalmic surgeons were more familiar with it, the significance of all the abnormalities they were able to see was still unclear.

Gowers discussed current controversies about the mechanism responsible for producing optic neuritis (which at the time generally referred to papilloedema rather than its current meaning of inflammatory disease of the optic nerve), and the difficulty in deciding whether it was evidence of intracranial disease or of local inflammatory processes. He had carried out many post-mortem pathological examinations of eyes that he had also examined with the ophthalmoscope during the patient's life. He correlated the histology in unstained material with the ophthalmoscopic appearances he had recorded. However, to explain the origin of some, he suggested pathological processes that later proved to be incorrect. For instance, he attributed perivenous haemorrhages in the retina to 'degeneration of veins' (whatever he meant by that). There were minor inconsistencies in the book, such as mentioning possible micro-aneurysms associated with diabetes, but not discussed in his formal description of the ophthalmoscopic abnormalities that had been recorded in diabetic patients. The review in *The Lancet* noted some careless editing in the first edition, criticism that the perfectionist Gowers would undoubtedly have taken to heart.[15]

The book proved popular, and a second edition appeared as soon as 1882. In later editions (1890 and 1904) Gowers' Queen Anne Street neighbour, the ophthalmic surgeon Marcus Gunn, became joint author. The 50 case histories and the material on ophthalmoscopes were omitted from the third edition and the histological illustrations interspersed through the text. The book was roughly the same size as the first edition, but included considerably more descriptive text set out in the same basic arrangement. It still contained remarkably little about multiple sclerosis. However, the interpretation of the diagnostic significance of optic neuritis was beginning to become clearer, and the text recognized that early onset visual loss was likely to be associated with inflammatory conditions in the nerve but not with disc swelling from raised intracranial pressure.

In retrospect, it is a little regrettable that *A Manual and Atlas of Medical Ophthalmoscopy* did not contain more correlation between visual field appearances and the changes seen on ophthalmoscopy. Nevertheless, for a book to run to four editions over a quarter of a century, at a time when knowledge in the area was growing rapidly, testifies to its popularity and practical value for ophthalmologists and physicians. Critchley notes that this book earned Gowers a reputation in Europe.

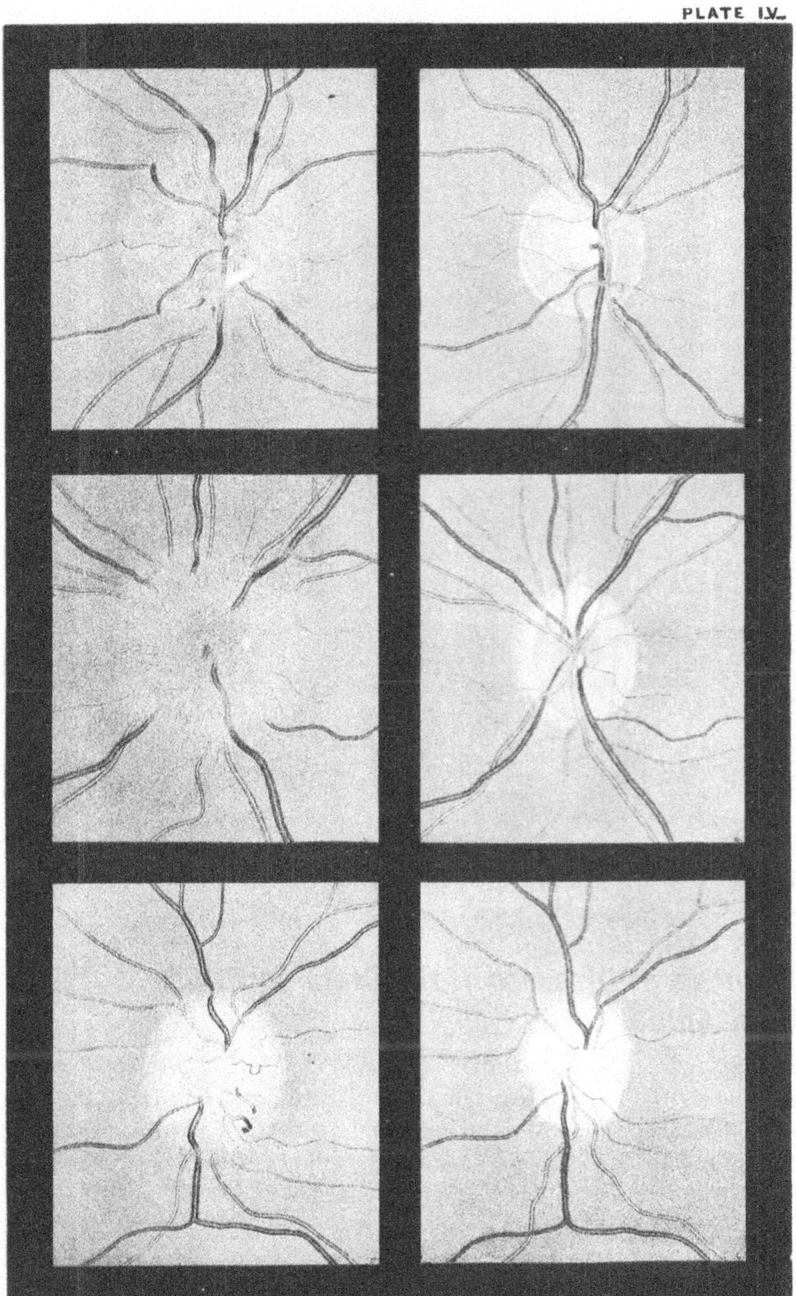


(a)

**Fig. 8.1** (a) Optic neuritis from cerebral syphiloma. From *A Manual and Atlas of Medical Ophthalmoscopy*, 1st edn, plate IV, opposite p. 326, fig. 3 (London: Churchill, 1879).

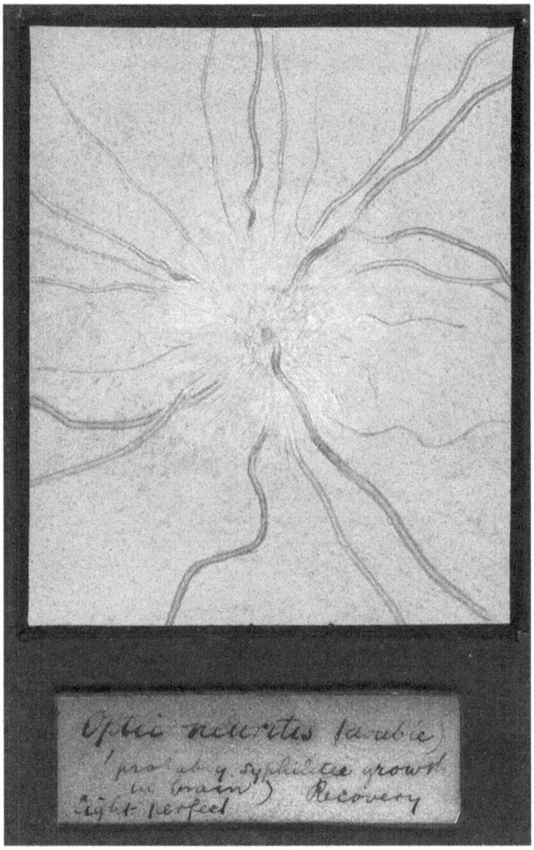


(b)

**Fig. 8.1** (b) Gowers' original drawing of middle section on l.h. of (a). Image courtesy of the Queen Square Library, Archive and Museum.

## *Diagnosis of Diseases of the Brain and of the Spinal Cord*

In 1879 Gowers published a series of papers in the *Medical Times and Gazette* dealing with the diagnosis of diseases of the spinal cord, based on a lecture he had given to the Medical Society of Wolverhampton. In 1880 the lectures were published by J. & A. Churchill as a small book, with slightly modified editions appearing in 1881 and 1885.[16] American editions also appeared in 1881 and 1885.

Critchley wrote that this book was of unusual interest 'for in it are several features which were novel, but which became established as part of the ordinary doctrines of neurology':

> In the first place there appeared an illustration, which is now universally utilized, showing the relations of the spinous processes, the vertebral bodies and the segments of the spinal cord. Gowers himself drew the original picture from dissections which had been prepared for him at UCH by a young demonstrator of anatomy named Victor Horsley.

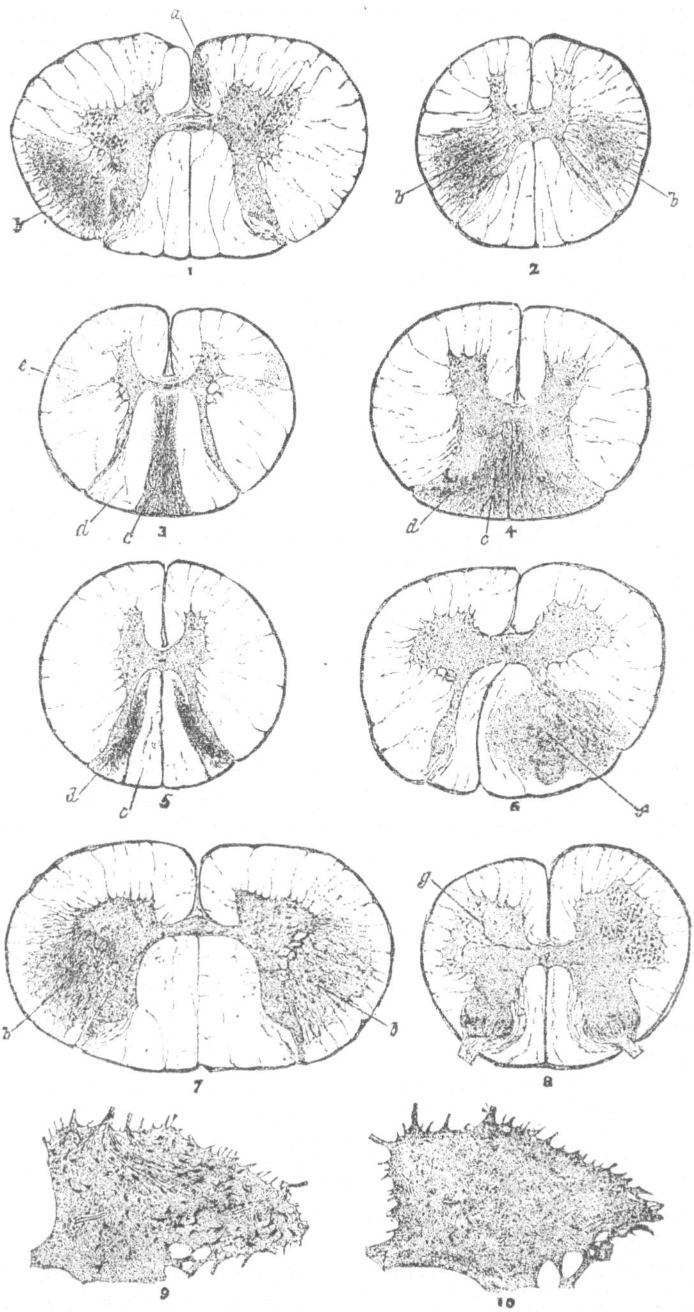

**Fig. 8.2** Important lesions of the spinal cord. From *Diagnosis of Diseases of the Brain and Spinal Cord*, plate, p. 282 (New York: William Wood, 1885).

> Secondly, the author referred almost casually to the presence of degeneration which he had found in the anterolateral region of the cord above a crush injury. This is the first and quite modest mention of the direct cerebellar column that is associated with the name of Fleschig, which today bears the name of Gowers' tract [Critchley appears to have made an error here: Gowers detected the indirect cerebellar tract, not the direct one]. Indeed, we owe this particular term to the perspicacity of Bechterew who detected this original observation in the monograph. ...
>
> The third feature of interest which these lectures hold is the advent of the expression 'knee-jerk' into the literature. Hitherto this clinical test had been referred to in a variety of ways, e.g., the patellar reflex, the Westphal phenomenon, and so on. It is strange that such an essential tool in neurological nomenclature as the term knee-jerk should have made its debut in so unostentatious a fashion. ...
>
> The fourth feature of this monograph is the introduction of the word 'myotatic', from the Greek *Tatikos*, extended. He disliked 'tendon reflex' as a term because the response depended upon a muscle reflex irritability, or more accurately, a 'myotatic irritability'.[17]

Gowers' monograph on the spinal cord was followed in 1885, by *Diagnosis of the Diseases of the Brain*, a series of lectures he had given at UCH.[18] A second edition of *Diagnosis of Diseases of the Brain* appeared in 1887[19] (between the two volumes of the first edition of his great *Manual of Diseases of the Nervous System*). His two works on neurological diagnosis were brought together in *Diagnosis of Diseases of the Brain and of the Spinal Cord*, published by Churchill in 1884,[20] and in the United States by William Wood & Co. in 1885.[21]

Gowers was highly productive in 1879: he also published a paper in *The Lancet* on 'The diagnostic value of so-called tendon reflexes'.[22] Gowers' last separate publication on neurological diagnosis, a lecture on 'General principles of the diagnosis of diseases of the nervous system', was published in *The Lancet* in 1892.[23]

Neurologists reading these works today may get a sense that they are looking at earlier, occasionally flawed, forerunners to the neurological diagnostic manuals of their professional youth. It is hard for the reader not to wonder why clinical and diagnostic methods, now commonplace, have not been mentioned. However, there were virtually no ancillary investigations available in the 1880s: X-rays and cerebrospinal fluid examination were at least a decade away; ophthalmoscopy was a relatively new tool, the revelations of which were not fully appreciated, and, while visual field charting was possible, Gowers did not seem to give it as much attention as later became usual.

Galvanic and Faradic electrical stimulation were used to assess lower motor neuron and muscle function. Even the range of tendon reflexes so widely employed in present-day clinical examination was largely confined to the knee-jerk, though Gowers employed what must have been a relatively insensitive variant of the ankle-jerk elicited by a tap on the front of the shin while the ankle was held in dorsiflexion. There was more emphasis on testing for clonus in the lower limbs, particularly at the ankle, the latter in preference to eliciting the ankle-jerk, at least when testing for it by the method Gowers described. He also mentioned the possibility of obtaining reflex muscle contractions from tapping on muscle tendons in the upper limb (at the lower end of the radius and behind the elbow). However, his account gave the impression that examination of the tendon reflexes was a relatively recent addition to the neurologist's diagnostic toolkit, that its possibilities were not yet fully explored, and that, apart from the knee-jerk, tendon reflex testing was not yet fully accepted into the physician's diagnostic repertoire.

At the time when Gowers was writing, more use seemed to be made of observing reflex contraction of nearby muscles evoked by local stimulation of the skin (by stroking), though many of these responses were capricious and difficult to observe. Some of these cutaneous reflexes are still in use, such as the abdominal and cremasteric (inner thigh) reflexes; others, like the gluteal, epigastric, and scapular, no longer seem to be in common use, though they did provide a previous generation with indications of the approximate level of spinal cord pathology. Babinski's extensor plantar reflex was unknown before 1896: the plantar response mentioned in the literature through the 1880s was withdrawal of the whole leg from a painful stimulus applied to the sole of the foot.[24] Although Gowers mentioned eliciting the extensor plantar response in 1909, he did not seem fully convinced of its diagnostic usefulness.

The interpretation of the examination of sensation in the 1880s and 1890s was limited by the incomplete knowledge of the distribution of the dermatomes, the courses of the sensory pathways within the spinal cord, and by uncertainty as to the tracts mediating particular senses.

Gowers did not codify the clinical examination of the nervous system as some of his Queen Square successors did, notably Gordon Holmes[25], but the rudiments of their approach can be found in his accounts of the relevant anatomy, the physiology-based explanations of neurological phenomena and testing methods, and the recognition that clues about their pathologies could be deduced from the course of the disease, and in the anatomical sites of disturbance.

## Manual of Diseases of the Nervous System

These publications were followed by the volumes which firmly established Gowers' enduring reputation. After the lapse of more than a century, the name William Richard Gowers is primarily remembered in neurological circles for his *Manual of Diseases of the Nervous System.*

The first edition appeared in two volumes, published by J. & A. Churchill in 1886 and 1888. Volume 1 dealt with 'Diseases of the nerves and spinal cord', and Volume 2 with 'Diseases of the brain and cranial nerves, and general and functional diseases of the nervous system'. The two volumes of the second edition followed in 1892 and 1893. The third edition of Volume 1, co-edited with James Taylor, appeared in 1899. Gowers worked on a third edition of Volume 2, but this was never published, although parts of a manuscript marked with his proposed corrections survive in the Queen Square archives. An American version of each edition was published by P. Blakiston Son & Company of Philadelphia.

Gowers drew most of the 374 illustrations; there were also a few photographs. Gowers not only taught himself to draw from instruction books, but having great natural talent became an accomplished amateur etcher.[26]

Etching, his son recalled, was one of Gowers' own skills, 'well suited to his precise and detailed style, and he became an enthusiastic and prolific etcher'.[27] However, the majority of the illustrations in the *Manual* were printed from blocks prepared from Gowers' original drawings by the Typographic Etching Company, using a phototype process. Some of the illustrations in the *Manual* were simple line drawings of patients, many others were highly detailed pathology cross-sections. Gowers also used a few sketches from photographs provided to him by other people, with the sources acknowledged in the text.

There were 463 pages in Volume 1 (1886 edn) of the *Manual*. Volume 2 (1888), which dealt with diseases of the brain, had 975 pages (which had increased to 1050 by the time of the 1898 American edition). The third edition of Volume 1 (1899) had grown to 692 pages, reflecting the accumulation of knowledge over the intervening 13 years. Between them, the final editions of each volume contained about 810,000 words.

Gowers' preface to the first edition explained his motives for writing the book:

> This volume contains the first part of an attempt to give an account of diseases of the nervous system, sufficiently concise to be within the compass of the time-pressed student or busy practitioner, and yet adequate in its outline of a subject which has become wide and deep beyond any other part of medicine.

In the preface to the second edition, he explained his approach:

> I have endeavoured ... to present to the reader the lessons learned by observation rather than the details of the cases observed—to subordinate, as far as possible, theory to fact, the speculative to the practical, and to employ hypothesis only where it is indispensable for the proper grasp of facts.[28]

A number of Gowers' original drawings for the first editions of both Volume 1 and Volume 2 came to light in the Queen Square archives in the course of our research for this biography. The following series of paired illustrations shows these drawings with their equivalent in the *Manual*. The illustrations from the *Manual* are all scans of figures in the J. & A. Churchill first edition. Gowers' own drawings are reproduced courtesy of the Queen Square Library, Archive and Museum.

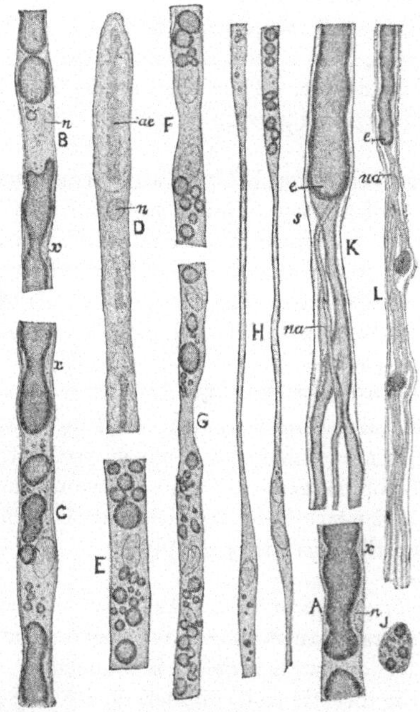

FIG. 28.—A–J. Degeneration of nerve-fibres (osmic acid and carmine staining). A, from sciatic of rabbit four days after section; B, C, same, fifty hours after section; D, a fibre stained with carmine only, to show the axis-cylinder; F, G, fibres from pigeon three days after section; H, two fibres from pneumogastric of rabbit six days after section; J, a lymphatic cell from inter-fibrillar connective tissue, containing globules of myelin that it has taken up; *n*, *n*, nuclei; *x*, *x*, constrictions of the myelin produced by the growth of the protoplasm; *ac*, axis-cylinder. K, L, regeneration of nerve-fibres: K, from pneumogastric of rabbit, seventy-two days after section; L, from sciatic of rabbit ninety days after section; *e*, rounded end of white substance of central end of nerve; *s*, sheath; *na*, new axis-cylinder; in L are two globules of myelin remaining from the degeneration of the old fibre.

(a)

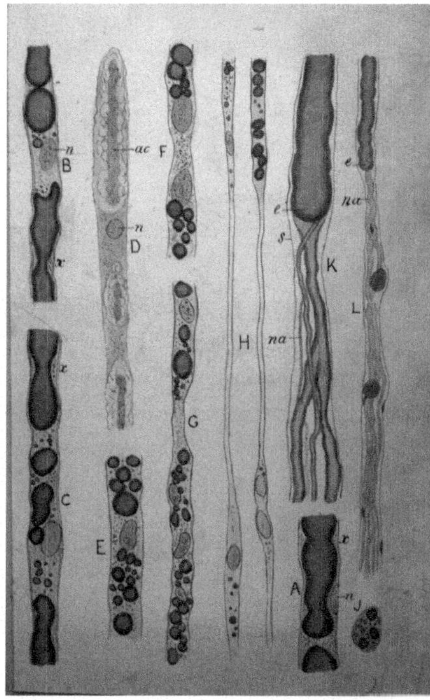

(b)

**Fig. 8.3** (a) Lesions of nerves. *Manual of Diseases of the Nervous System*, Vol 1, (1886), p.40. (b) Gowers' drawing. Image courtesy of the Queen Square Library, Archive and Museum.

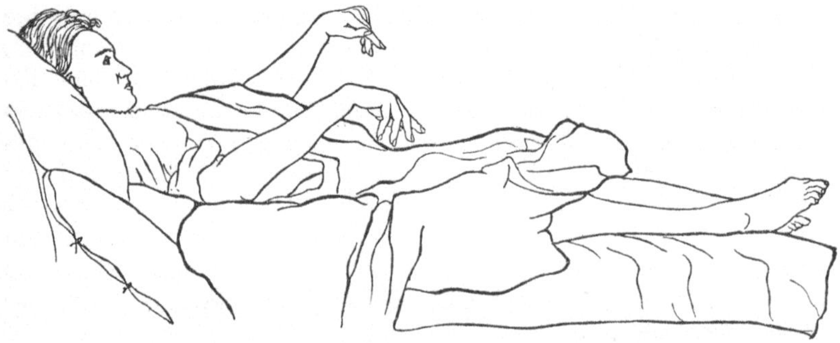

FIG. 53.—Multiple alcoholic neuritis; palsy of extensors of wrist and flexors of ankle. (From a photograph by Mr. Hyde Marriott, B.Sc.)

(a)

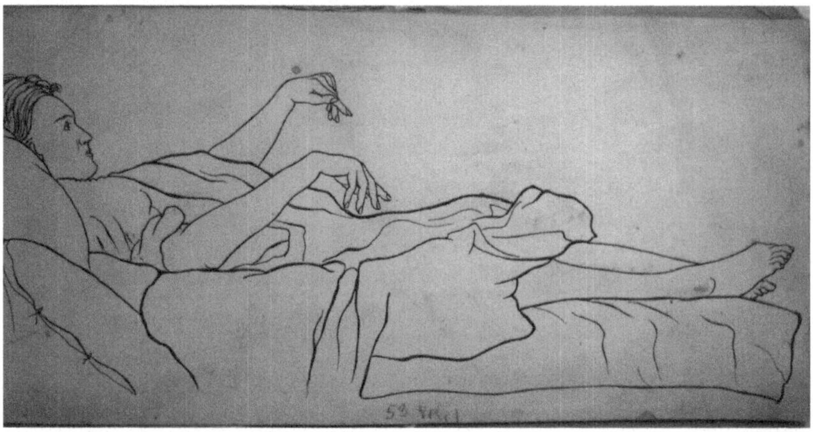

(b)

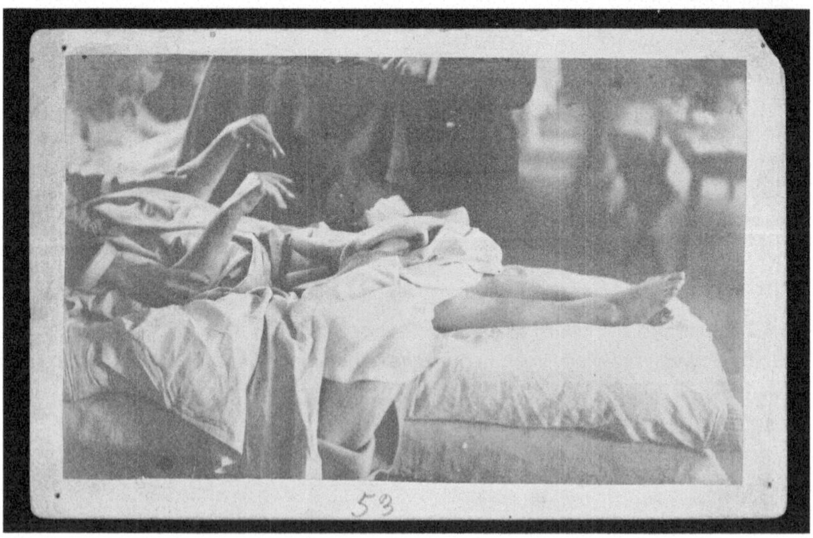


(c)

**Fig. 8.4** Multiple neuritis symptoms (a) Vol 1, (1886), p.97. (b) Gowers' drawing. Image courtesy of the Queen Square Library, Archive and Museum. (c) Photograph by Mr Hyde Marriott BSc, from which the figure was drawn.

FIG. 77.

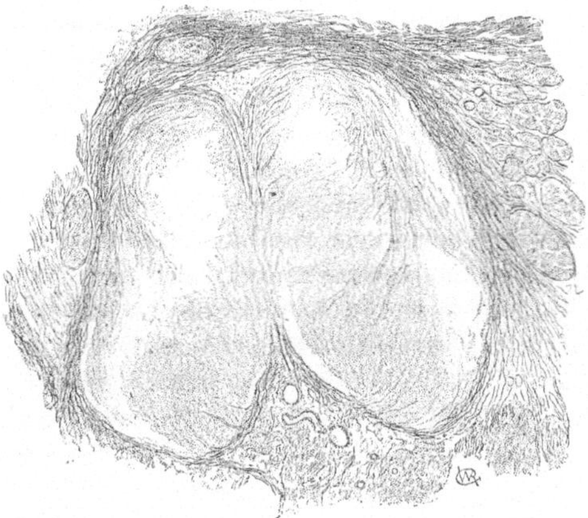

FIG. 78.

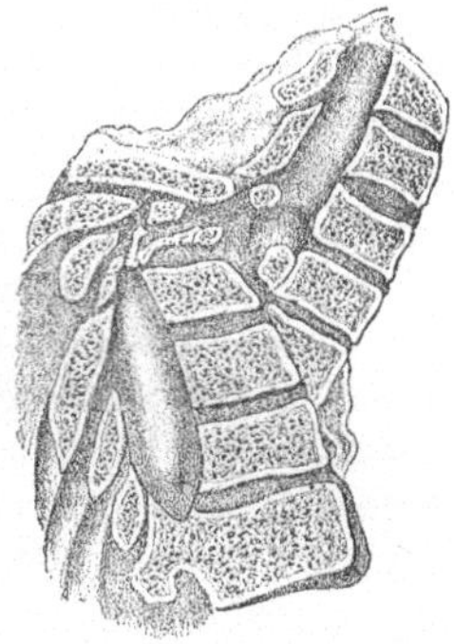

FIG. 77.—Spinal cord damaged by the fracture shown in Fig. 76. The elements of the cord itself are changed beyond the possibility of identification. The ascending degeneration is shown in Fig. 67.

FIG. 78.—Fracture of the body of the fifth dorsal vertebra and of its processes. (After Gurlt.)

(a)

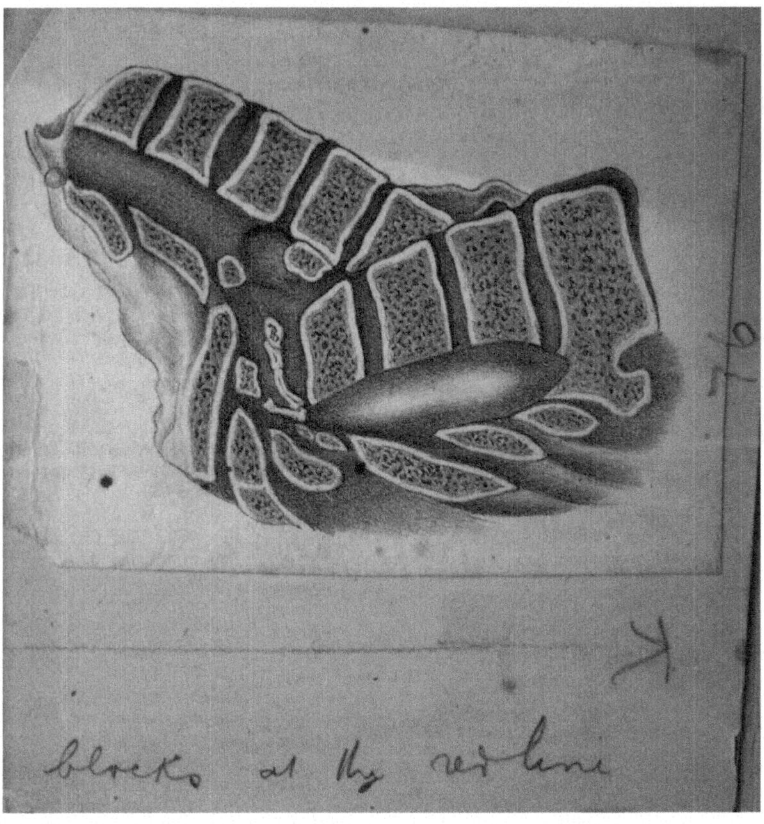


(b)

**Fig. 8.5** Fracture of the body of the fifth dorsal vertebra and of its processes. (a) Vol 1, (1886), p.166. (b) Gowers' drawing. Image courtesy of the Queen Square Library, Archive and Museum.

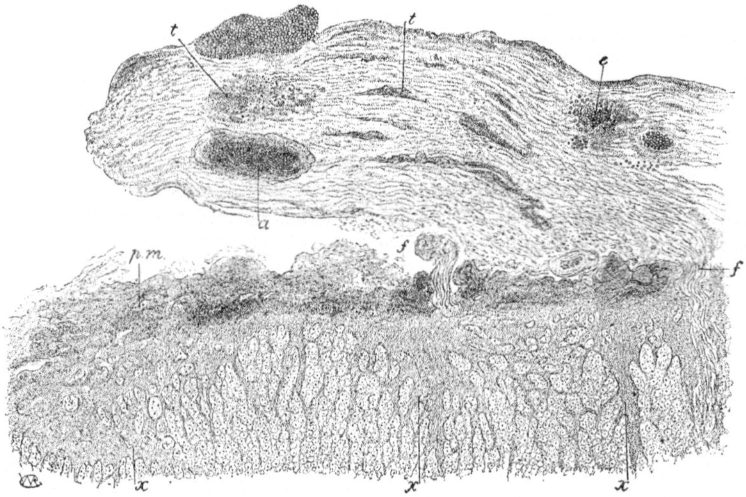


FIG. 83.—Chronic alcoholic meningitis. Section of edge of anterior column and of a large nerve-root; carmine preparation. *p. m.* Pia mater irregularly thickened and transformed into amorphous-looking tissue, from which wedge-shaped branching tracts (*x x*) extend into the white substance; *f. f.*, fasciculi of nerve-fibres entering the cord; *a.*, an artery in the nerve-root, enlarged and with thickened walls; *t. t.*, tracts of amorphous connective tissue; *e.*, a small extravasation.

(a)

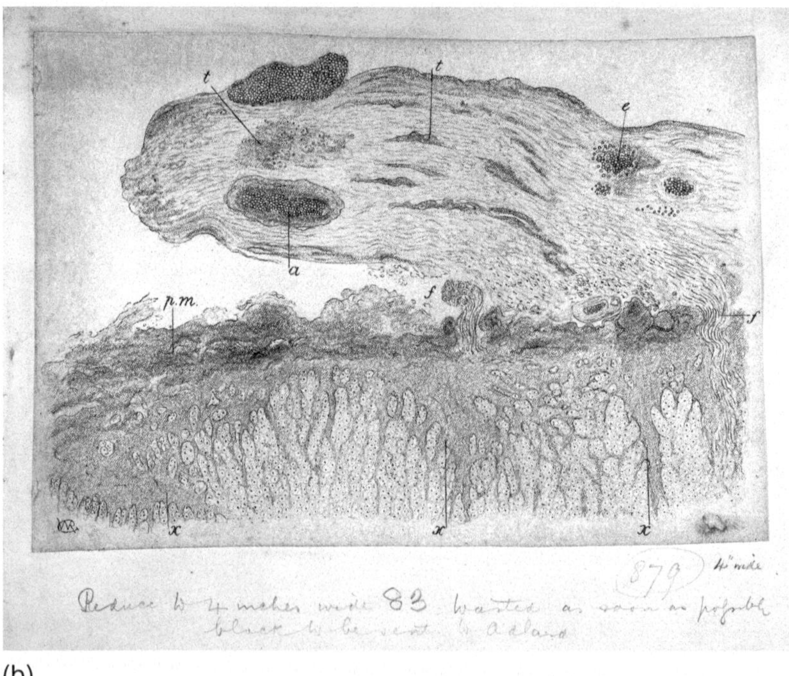


(b)

**Fig. 8.6** Chronic alcoholic meningitis. (a) Vol 1, (1886), p.197. (b) Gowers' drawing. Image courtesy of the Queen Square Library, Archive and Museum.

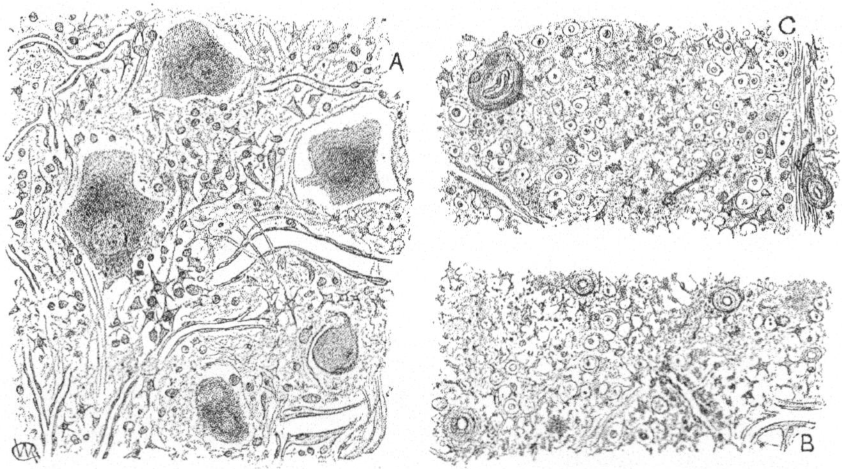


FIG. 86.—Portions of the section shown in the last figure, more highly magnified. A, from the left ant. cornu; distended capillaries with numerous nuclei; larger vessels with slight distension of perivascular sheaths; numerous round and stellate cells; ganglion cells, swollen, with shrivelled processes. C, from front of post. column; scattered nerve-fibres separated by amorphous material in which small cells can be seen, round and irregular, some distinct, others indistinct, vessels with thickened walls. B, from near the posterior surface, shows similar changes but with more open spaces from which nerve-fibres have perished. (From sections prepared by Dr. Money.)

(a)

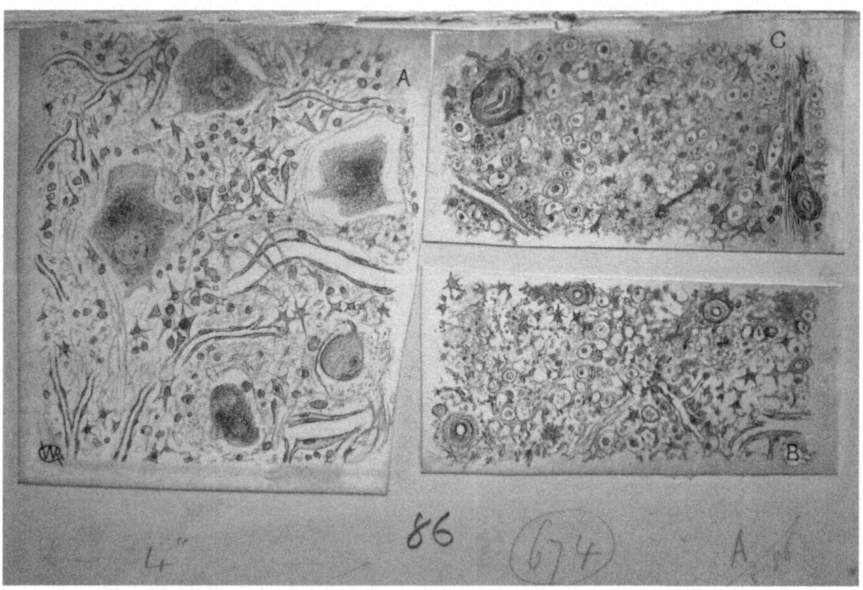


(b)

**Fig. 8.7** Subacute myelitis, lumbar region (from sections). (a) Vol 1, (1886), p.216. (b) Gowers' drawing. Image courtesy of the Queen Square Library, Archive and Museum.

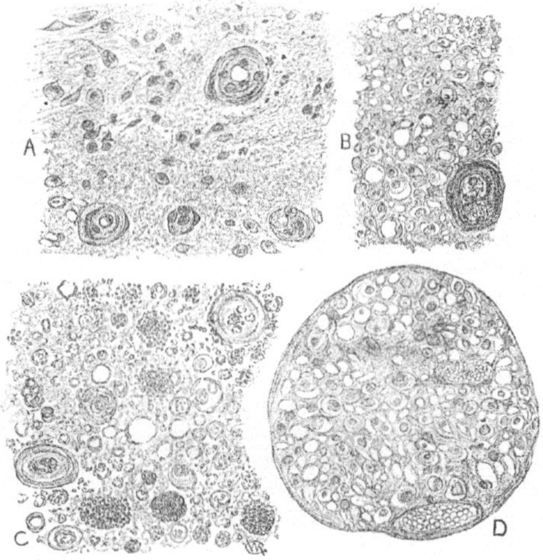


FIG. 99.—Pressure-myelitis: portions of the section D in Fig. 98 more highly magnified. A, from the grey matter, numerous angular and fusiform cells; vessels with walls thickened by a growth of cells, narrowing the cavity, which in some is obliterated. B, from the white column; thickening of the interstitial tissue, nerve-fibres in part destroyed, in part narrowed; a vessel with thickened walls. C, glycerine preparation from white substance, abundant products of degeneration of the nerve-fibres, in part aggregated into granule-masses. D, section of a nerve-root passing by compressed area; increase of interstitial tissue, many nerve-fibres narrowed, some with swollen axis-cylinders.

(a)

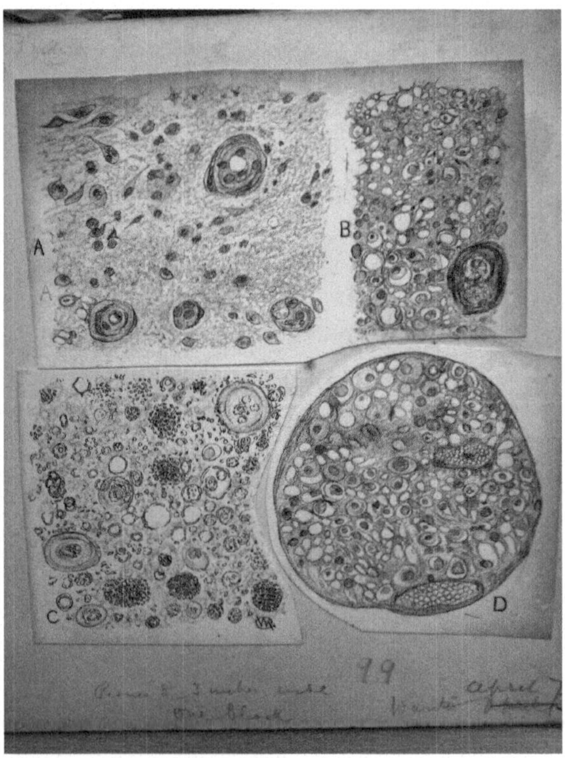


(b)

**Fig. 8.8** Pressure-myelitis. (a) Vol 1, (1886), p.248. (b) Gowers' drawing. Image courtesy of the Queen Square Library, Archive and Museum.

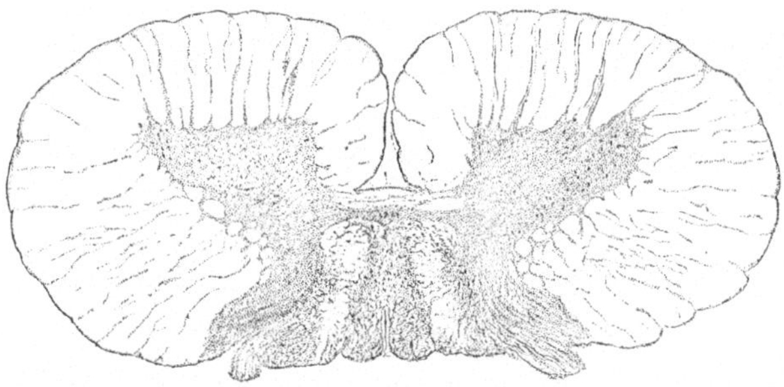

FIG. 112.—Tabes with ataxy of the arms as well as the legs. Section of cord in cervical region, showing sclerosis of the post.-med. column and root-zone of post.-ext. col. Degeneration of left ant. cornu.

(a)

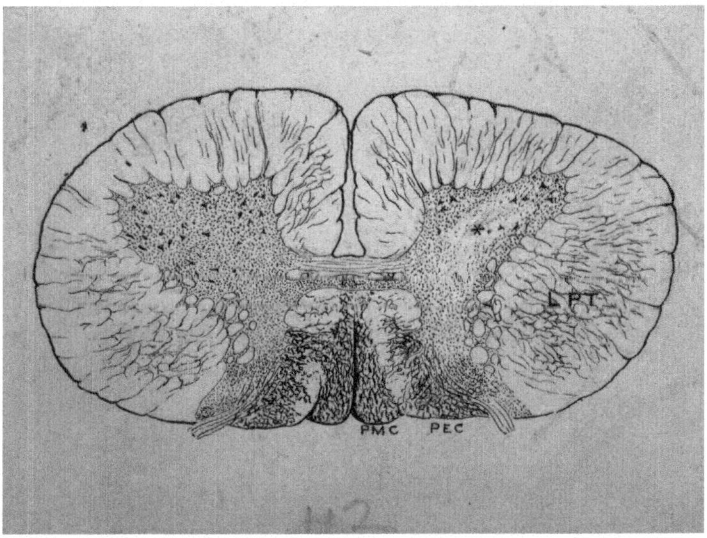


(b)

**Fig. 8.9** Tabes with ataxy of the arms as well as the legs. (a) Vol 1, (1886), p.308. (b) Gowers' drawing identified as Fig. 112, but which appears to be the substitution of an adjacent transverse section of the same spinal cord. Image courtesy of the Queen Square Library, Archive and Museum.

TUMOURS. 419

FIG. 156. FIG. 157. FIG. 158.

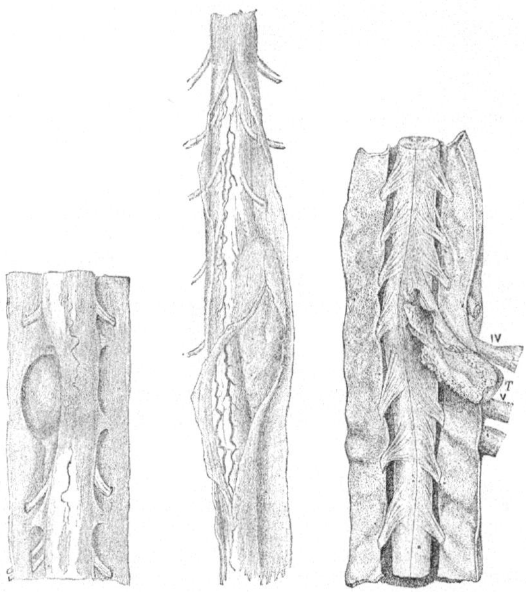


FIG. 156.—Tumour growing from the inner surface of the dura mater, and compressing the spinal cord in the mid-dorsal region. The tumour, 3 cm. long, was a sarcoma in which the cells were arranged in concentric groups, the centres of which had undergone calcification. The spinal cord was softened and dark in tint at the compressed part.* (After Lancereaux.)

FIG. 157.—Sarcoma growing between the arachnoid and pia mater in the mid-dorsal region of the cord. The tumour had sprung from the meshes of the arachnoid, and was only slightly adherent to the pia mater. The spinal cord was compressed and softened. In the figure the dura-matral sheath has been laid open, except at the top, and the arachnoid has been opened over the lower half of the tumour which, 5 cm. long, lies on the posterior and (right) lateral aspect of the cord.† (After Lancereaux.)

FIG. 158.—A tumour (T) growing from the dura mater, and compressing the right side of the spinal cord at the origin of the 4th, 5th, and 6th cervical nerves. The tumour was a spindle-celled sarcoma springing from the arachnoid.‡ (After Leyden.)

(a)

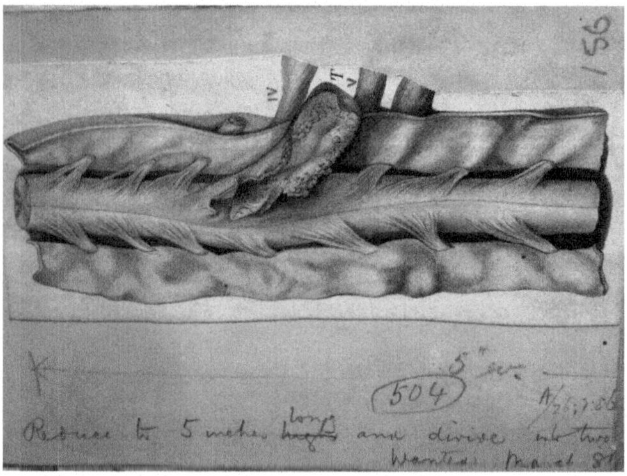


(b)

**Fig. 8.10** Tumours. (a) Vol 1, (1886), p.419. (b) Gowers' drawing for fig. 158. Image courtesy of the Queen Square Library, Archive and Museum.

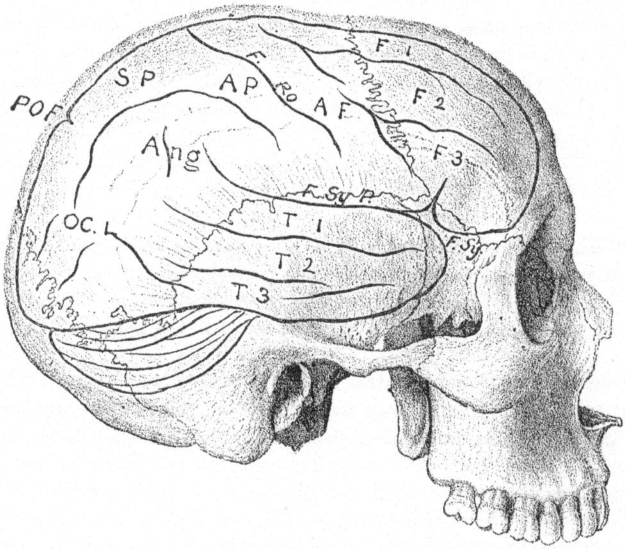


FIG. 4.—Diagram of the relation of the convolutions to the skull. F 1, 2, and 3, upper middle and lower frontal convolutions; A F, A P, ascending frontal and parietal; S. P, sup. parietal lobule; Ang, angular gyrus; Oc L, occipital lobe; T 1, 2, 3, the temporal convolutions; P O F, parieto-occipital fissure; F Sy and F Sy P, fissure of Sylvius and its posterior limb.

(a)

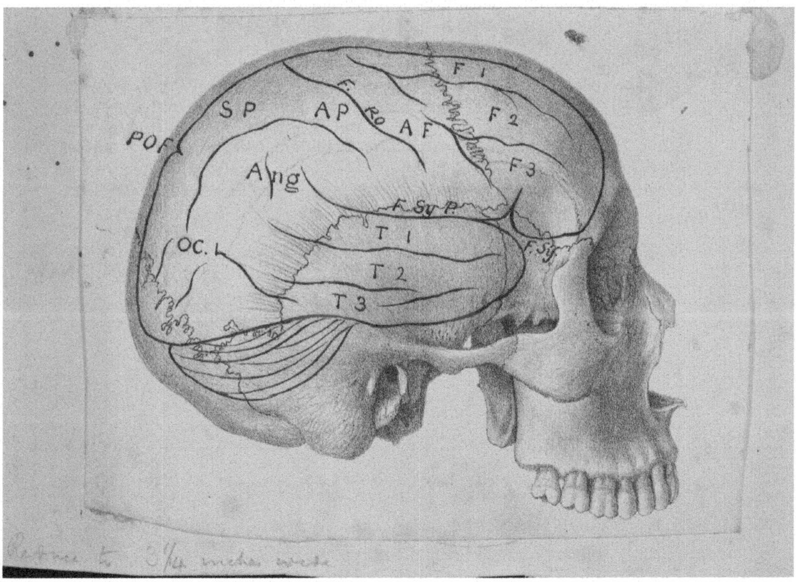


(b)

**Fig. 8.11** General relation of the brain to the bones of the skull. (a) Vol 2, (1888), p.7. (b) Gowers' drawing. Image courtesy of the Queen Square Library, Archive and Museum.

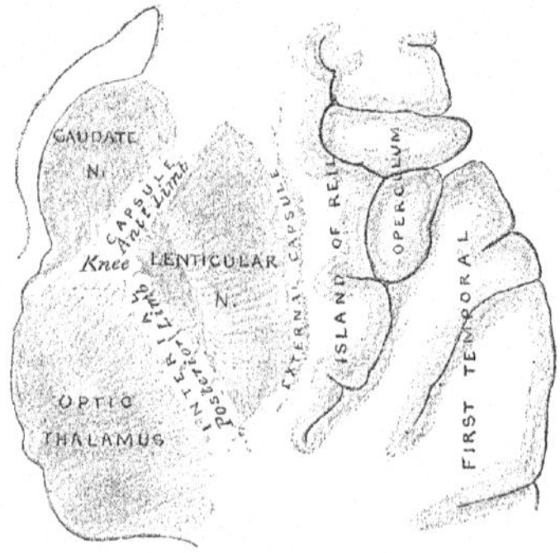


FIG. 19.—Diagram of horizontal section through the central ganglia and internal capsule.

(a)

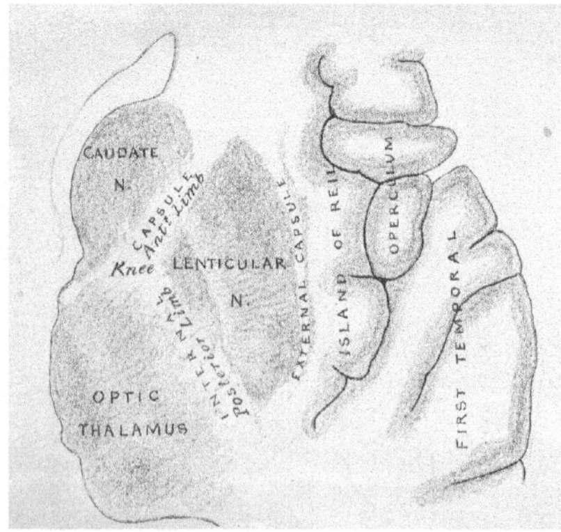


(b)

**Fig. 8.12** Diagram of horizontal section through the central ganglia and internal capsule. (a) Vol 2, (1888), p.23. (b) Gowers' drawing. Image courtesy of the Queen Square Library, Archive and Museum.

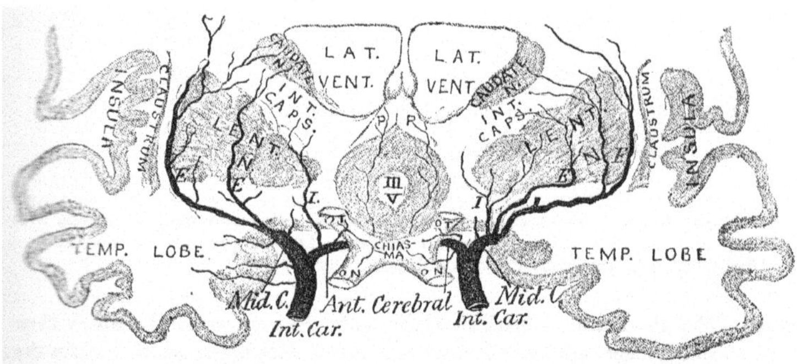


FIG. 43.—Diagram of the blood supply to the central ganglia by the lenticulo-striate arteries, external (*E*) and internal (*I*). III V, third ventricle; P P, pillars of the fornix; *Mid C*, middle cerebral artery. (After Duret.)

(a)

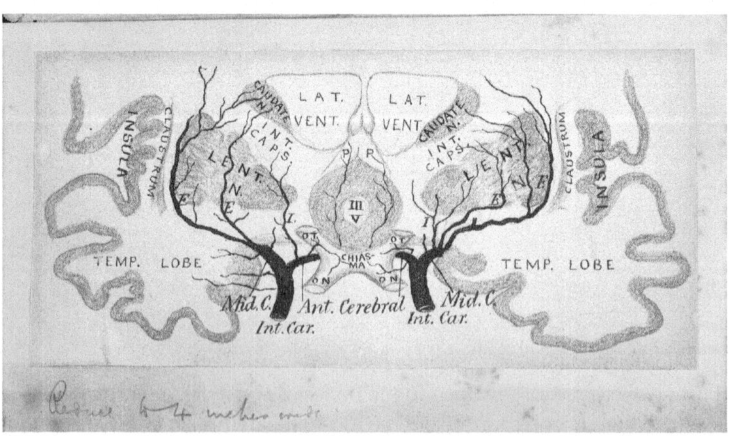


(b)

**Fig. 8.13** Diagram of the blood-supply to the central ganglia by the lenticulo-striate arteries. (a) Vol 2, (1888), p.55. (b) Gowers' drawing. Image courtesy of the Queen Square Library, Archive and Museum.

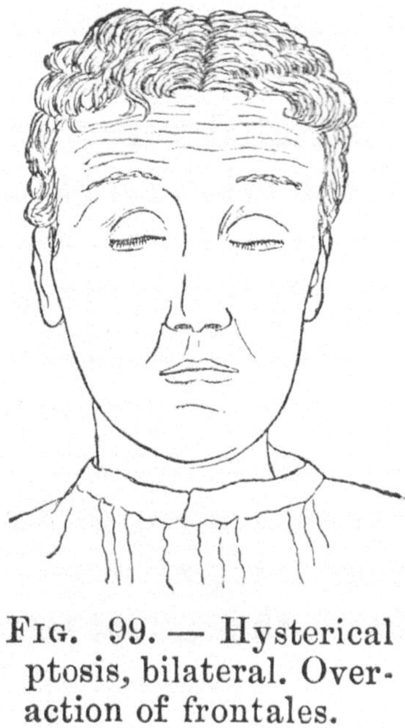


(a)

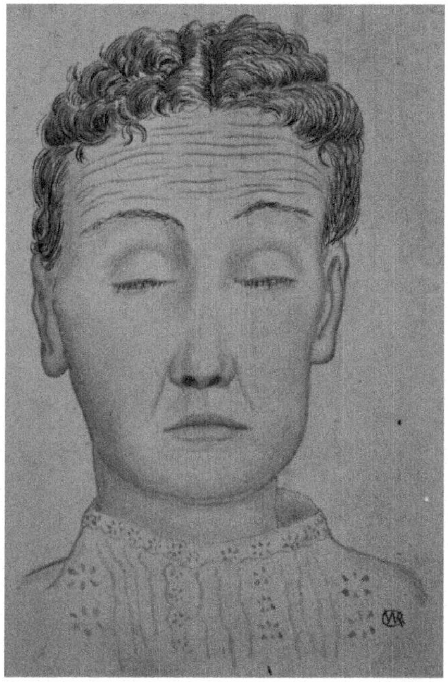

(b)

**Fig. 8.14** Hysterical ptosis. (a) Vol 2, (1888), p.188. (b) Gowers' drawing. Image courtesy of the Queen Square Library, Archive and Museum.

Gowers *Manual* was by no means the first textbook of clinical neurology. In the seventeenth century Thomas Willis had written two works, *Pathologia Cerebri* and *De Anima Brutorum* (both translated into English by Samuel Pordage). Together, these covered the neurological knowledge of the time, though after the passage of two centuries much of that knowledge had been superseded. Apart from books on special aspects of neurology, Romberg's *Manual of the Nervous Diseases of Man* had appeared in two editions in the nineteenth century (the second edition was translated into English, in two volumes, by Sieveking).[29] This work has often been regarded as the first modern textbook of neurology. However, it was in itself incomplete. Romberg promised there would be a further volume, but this never appeared.

Between 1870 and 1880, three medium-sized neurological textbooks were published, each written by a single author. In 1871 Hammond published *A Treatise of the Nervous System*,[30] and Rosenthal published *A Clinical Treatise in the Diseases of the Nervous System* (translated into English by Putzel in 1879);[31] nine years later, Samuel Wilks' attractively written *Lectures on the Diseases of the Nervous System* appeared.[32] There were also multi-authored accounts of neurology in von Zeimmsen's *Cyclopaedia* (1878)[33] and in Russell Reynolds' *System of Medicine* which first appeared in 1868.[34]

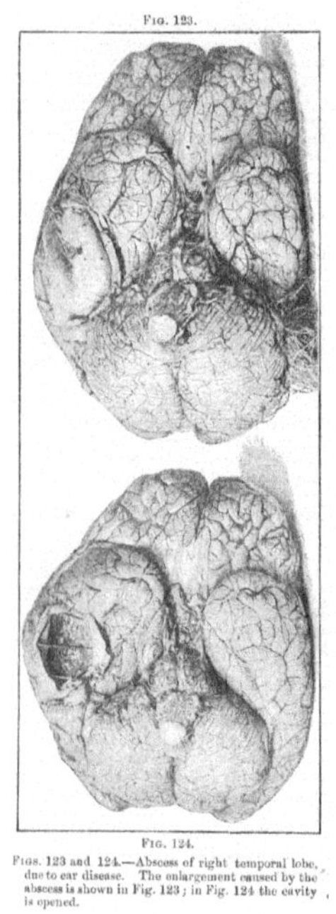


(a)

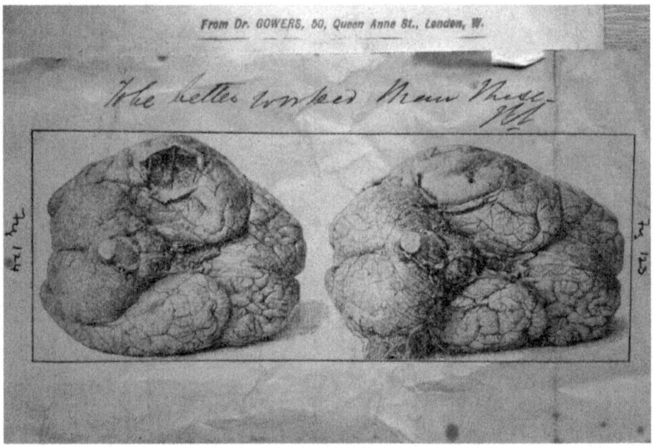


(b)

**Fig. 8.15** Abscess of right temporal lobe. (a) Vol 2, (1888), p.440. (b) Gowers' drawing. Image courtesy of the Queen Square Library, Archive and Museum.

In 1881, five years before Gowers' *Manual* was published, J. & A. Churchill had published the exhaustive two-volume textbook, *A Treatise on the Diseases of the Nervous System*, written by the Manchester physician James Ross (1837–92), followed by a substantially expanded and extensively referenced second edition in 1883.[35] Both the contents of the first edition, and its author's erudition and industry, were very favourably reviewed in several journals, receiving particularly laudatory comments from John Hughlings Jackson.

It is interesting to speculate why Gowers should have chosen to compete against such a contemporary work, and why the London publishers J. & A. Churchill published both the *Treatise* and the *Manual*. But Gowers did compete, and so effectively that Ross's textbook is now almost completely forgotten while Gowers' *Manual* is revered.

How did Gowers achieve this with his *Manual*? The simple answer would be that his *Manual* was both better written and better organized than its competitor. It was also a little smaller and cheaper and included a wider range of neurological disorders. There were probably other reasons too. Ross had spent a number of years working in general practice in the north of England before becoming pathologist and later physician to the Manchester Royal Infirmary and joint professor of medicine at Owens College,

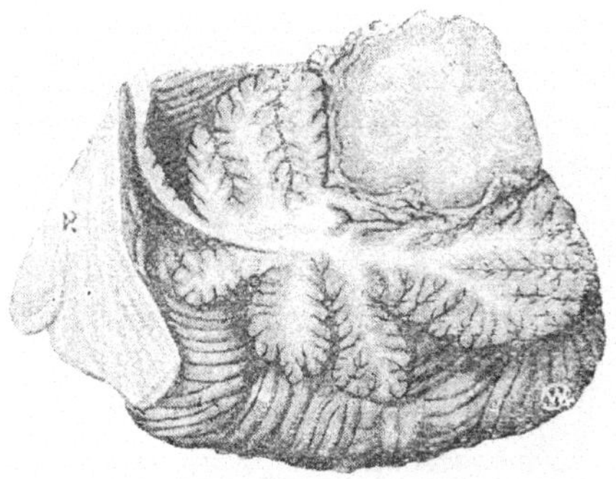

FIG. 127.—Tubercular tumour of the middle lobe of the cerebellum. The patient, a young child, was admitted into University College Hospital dying from general tuberculosis. P. Pons.

(a)

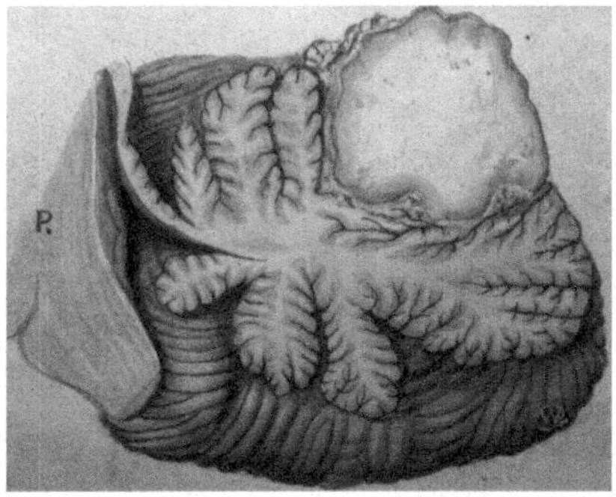

(b)

**Fig. 8.16** Tubercular tumour. (a) Vol 2, (1888), p.457. (b) Gowers' drawing. Image courtesy of the Queen Square Library, Archive and Museum.

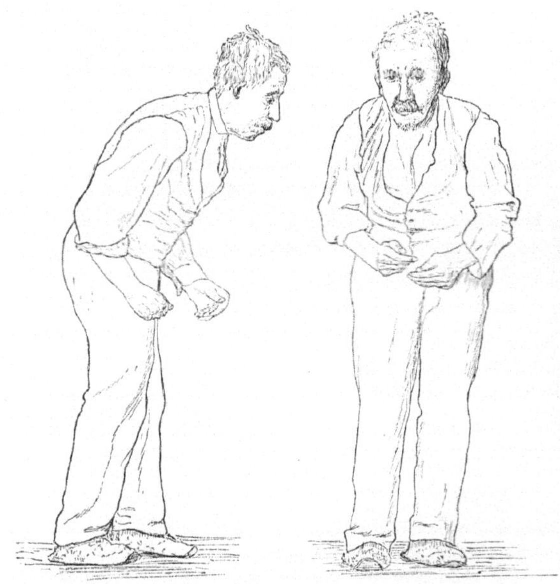

FIG. 145.—Paralysis agitans. (After St. Leger.)

(a)

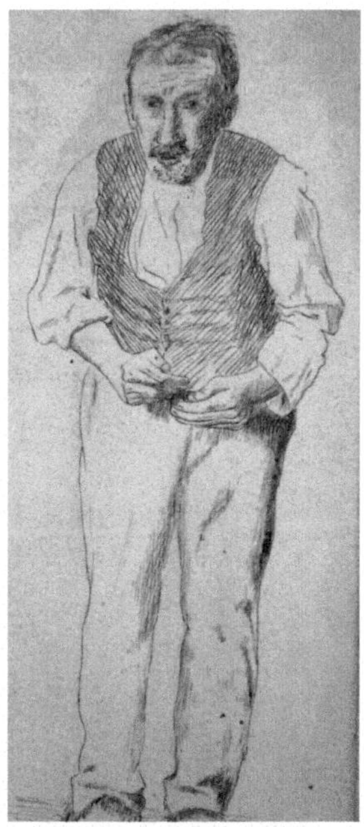

(b)

**Fig. 8.17** Paralysis agitans. (a) Vol 2, (1888), p.591. (b) Gowers' drawing. Image courtesy of the Queen Square Library, Archive and Museum.

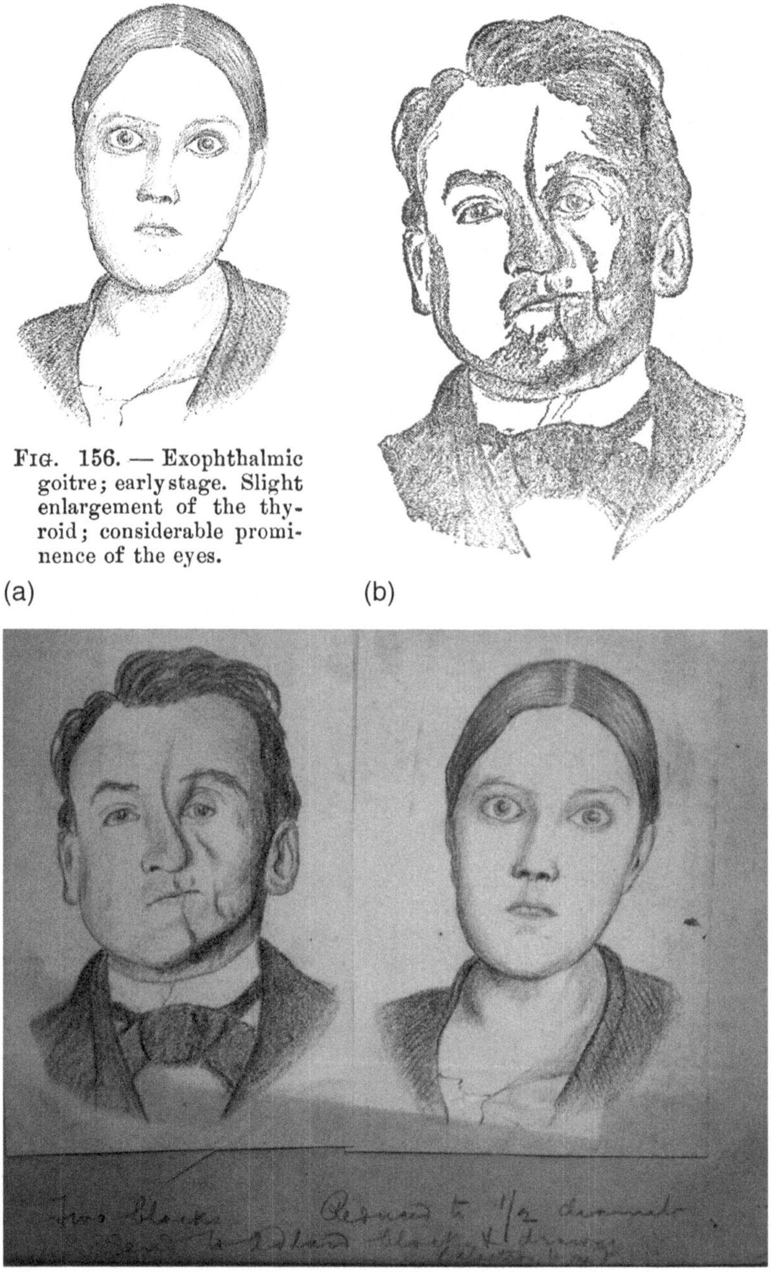


**Fig. 8.18** Facial hemiatrophy. (a) Vol 2, (1888), p.810. (b) Vol 2, (1888), p.805. Image courtesy of the Queen Square Library, Archive and Museum. (c) Gowers' drawings.

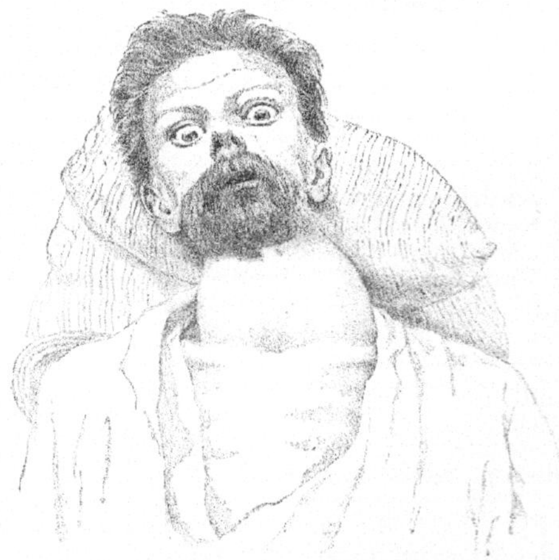

FIG. 157.—Exophthalmic goitre. Defective descent of the upper lid on looking down. (After Wilks.)

(a)

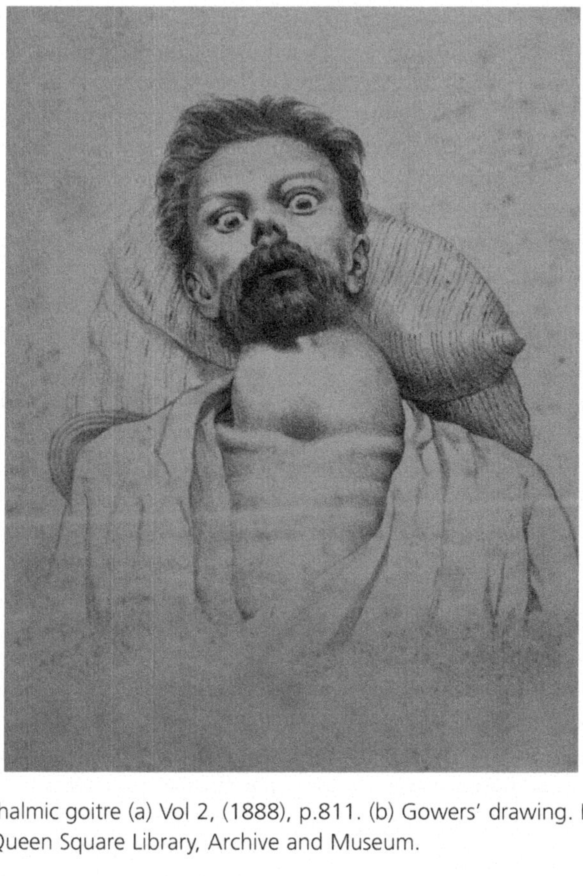

(b)

**Fig. 8.19** Exophthalmic goitre (a) Vol 2, (1888), p.811. (b) Gowers' drawing. Image courtesy of the Queen Square Library, Archive and Museum.

Manchester. When he wrote the *Treatise* he had not had the exposure to first-hand clinical neurology that Gowers possessed. Gowers drew on his own experience whereas Ross drew on the experience of others. As a result, Ross's *Treatise* reads as if he was trying to teach himself neurology, whereas Gowers' *Manual* gives the impression that he wanted to teach others what he already knew well. Ross's *Treatise* contained more neuroanatomy than was probably necessary, though this was particularly well illustrated, but had proportionately less physiological interpretation of neurological dysfunction than was in Gowers' *Manual.*

Ross was also at a disadvantage working alone in a provincial city without the daily contact with other neurologists available to Gowers. Nonetheless he was a man of formidable intellect and an exceedingly hard worker. If he had been able to bring out a third edition it would have been interesting to see whether his *Treatise* or Gowers' *Manual* would have dominated the market. After the publication of the second edition of his *Treatise,* Ross was preoccupied in producing a condensed version (still some 700 pages long) for the American market. He then wrote the first English-language monograph on aphasia, while his health deteriorated, before he struggled to complete a co-authored monograph on peripheral neuritis. He died at the age of 52.

Given the state of knowledge in the 1880s, there are really no areas of weakness in Gowers' *Manual.* The modern reader will note that certain modern disorders are missing and others might have been categorized differently. Thus, for instance, mention of Huntington's disease was relegated to a footnote in the first edition, whereas there was a good deal of material on chorea in general. Myotonia congenita was described, but not myotonic dystrophy (which was not delineated until early in the twentieth century). Some disorders considered at length in the *Manual* have now become unimportant or virtually non-existent, such as neurosyphilis and diphtheritic paralysis, while the cause of others is understood differently.

The true nature of certain disorders that Gowers described, such as saltatoric spasm and ataxic paraplegia, are uncertain. Ataxic paraplegia is not an identifiable neurological disease today, though Gowers devoted a separate nine-page section to it in his *Manual.* The disorder tended to develop in middle-aged males, and often no cause could be traced, though it could follow a period of sexual excess. Its course was slow but relentlessly progressive, the gait resembled that of tabes but the knee-jerks were increased rather than lost, and ankle clonus was often present. There was impairment of sexual and sphincter function. Pathologically, sclerosis of the posterior and lateral columns of the spinal cord was present. Gowers allocated it a place in the spectrum of neurological disease between the hereditary ataxias and idiopathic spastic paraplegia, but could not take matters beyond that stage. The various suggestions as to its nature made subsequently, e.g. that at least some instances of it may have been cases of subacute combined degeneration (vitamin $B_{12}$ axonopathy),[36] do not accord particularly well with Gowers' description of the pathological appearances.

Some sections of the *Manual* have attracted particularly favourable comment: the sections on locomotor ataxia, Parkinson's disease, writer's cramp, epilepsy, and migraine. When he wrote on migraine, Gowers may have benefited from having as a neighbour Edward Liveing, author of the classical book on migraine published in

1873. Gowers' *Manual* contained a very good account of aphasia, though from a survey of all Gowers' publications one gains the impression that he was not particularly interested in higher cerebral function. However, Critchley points out that Gowers had played an 'interesting though minor role' in collaboration with Hughlings Jackson, carrying out pathological examinations of a number of brain tumour fatalities. In particular, the case of Eliza Joad who had died of 'a large glioma of the hinder part of the right temporo-sphenoidal lobe, with other smaller growths near and in the right hippocampus major':

> This patient during life had shown a peculiar mental confusion with an inability to recognize persons, objects and places. Jackson called this symptom 'imperception' … 'a defect as special as aphasia' … and herein we find the first recorded instance of what Finkelnburg later termed 'asymboly' and what—following Freud—we now speak of as 'agnosia'.[37]

In the *Manual*, Gowers employed an important concept that he had mentioned in his *Diagnosis of Diseases of the Spinal Cord* and which has stood the test of time. This was that the motor pathway comprised two elements, an upper and a lower motor neuron. This idea is so much part of current neurological thinking that it seems as if it has always been known. In interpreting the mechanisms producing various neurological disorders Gowers often invoked the existence of functional centres in the nervous system. These hypothetical centres were responsible for the initiation and coordination of various bodily activities. He tended to give the impression that these centres were structural realities whose locations had usually not yet been finally established, although he made shrewd guesses as to where they would prove to be situated. Gowers' approach in this matter was probably stimulated by contemporary mapping of cerebral cortical function, much of it carried out by his Queen Square colleague David Ferrier.

The work of producing both the text and the illustrations for the *Manual* caused Gowers' health to start to deteriorate. He had undertaken a massive task in an era when manuscripts were handwritten, often at night under gaslight, but at least Gowers could lessen the physical impact by creating his initial drafts in his impeccable shorthand.

Second editions of the volumes appeared in 1891 and 1893, in a run of 1500 copies, for which Gowers received a profit of just over £312. In January 1899 a third edition of Volume 1 was published. Gowers, by now becoming frail, had the help of a co-editor, his assistant, friend, and colleague, James Taylor. Critchley suggests that the sales of the third edition were reduced because of the appearance on the market of Allbutt's *A System of Medicine by Many Writers*,[38] published by Macmillan in 1899, and perhaps this is why the third edition of Volume 2 on which Gowers and Taylor had been working, was never completed.

Critchley's biography contains an overview of textbooks that, in his view, stood close to the *Manual*. It is interesting to note that he did not include Ross's *Treatise*. It appears he was not aware of its existence. He did comment that Gowers brought a cohesion, a consistency of style, and technique that gave the *Manual* its rare individuality and interest.

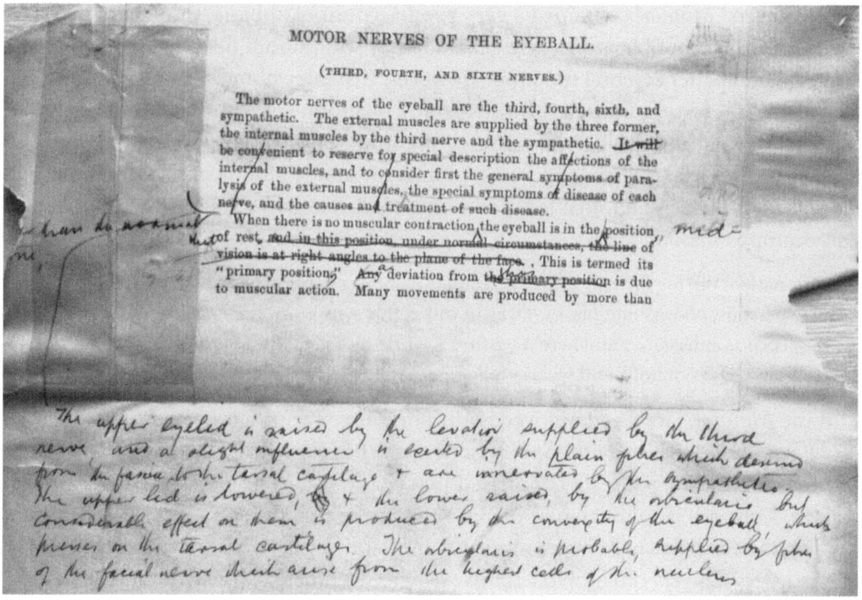

MOTOR NERVES OF THE EYEBALL.

(THIRD, FOURTH, AND SIXTH NERVES.)

The motor nerves of the eyeball are the third, fourth, sixth, and sympathetic. The external muscles are supplied by the three former, the internal muscles by the third nerve and the sympathetic. It will be convenient to reserve for special description the affections of the internal muscles, and to consider first the general symptoms of paralysis of the external muscles, the special symptoms of disease of each nerve, and the causes and treatment of such disease.

When there is no muscular contraction the eyeball is in the position of rest, and in this position, under normal circumstances, the line of vision is at right angles to the plane of the face. This is termed its "primary position." Any deviation from the primary position is due to muscular action. Many movements are produced by more than

**Fig. 8.20** Handwritten amendments to p. 168 of Vol. 2, 2nd edn (1898) intended for a third edition of Volume 2 that was never published.

## Reviews of the *Manual of Diseases of the Nervous System*

Reviewers in both the *BMJ* and *The Lancet* responded enthusiastically to the first volume in October 1886. It must have been an anxious month for Gowers. The review in *The Lancet* appeared first, opening with the words: 'In the space at our disposal it is impossible to do justice to works like the one that lies before us. … In the presence of such ability, learning, and originality, criticism can only take a favourable direction. The style and manner are accurate, studied, and adequate—never diffuse'. The *BMJ* referred to the fact that neurology had been classed as one of the 'doubtful specialities' but that 'compared with other isolated branches of medical practice' its position could scarcely be questioned. It concluded:

> The work, therefore, while serving to initiate the general reader in the elements of that science, ranks higher than a mere text-book on the subject. The author's object has been, in our opinion, skilfully and successfully carried out, and a perusal and study of this book will place the student and practitioner in possession of all the leading and essential facts necessary to investigate and treat diseases of the nervous system, according to the most recent improvements of our knowledge at the present day.[39]

The *Manual* received an unqualified review in the *American Journal of the Medical Sciences*:

> It may be said, without reserve, that this work is the most clear, concise, and complete text-book upon diseases of the nervous system in any language. And when the large number of such works which has appeared in Germany, France, and England, within the past ten years is considered, this implies high praise.

But, using the 'time-honoured dictum' of reviewers, it follows its praise for the quality of the print and the illustrations, with the mildest criticism:

> The subject of neurasthenia deserves a more careful study than is accorded to it by the author, but the English specialists fortunately see less of this disease than do Americans, and hence know less about it.[40]

Two other issues of the American journal carry reviews of different editions of the *Manual*. The first, a review of Volume 1 of the second edition, suggests the book is a little too 'diffuse'. It takes issue with Gowers for being too sympathetic to litigants complaining of injuries such as 'railway spine' and does not mention 'malingering', an interesting criticism because Gowers was used as an insurance assessor. The reviewer complains that Gowers sheds no light on the 'neurotic' victim 'whose suffering is assuaged with a verdict'.[41] However, this is mild criticism of such a comprehensive work. In 1887, the journal also carried a composite review of works by Ferrier, Bastian, and Gowers.[42]

Bearing in mind that the *Treatise* by Ross was still in print at the time, that neurologists should have been aware of it, and that it had been very well reviewed in the medical press, it is interesting to note that *The Lancet* review of the first edition of Volume 1 of Gowers' *Manual* stated:

> Space exigencies forbid, or we should have liked to point out further excellences in Dr Gowers' work. Whether we contemplate the erudition, meditate on the suggestiveness of the original matter, admire the illustrations, or think of the care that has been bestowed in apportioning the space to each subject according to its importance—from whatever point of view we regard the book we must express the opinion that, judged by its first volume, no better manual of nervous diseases has been presented to the medical profession.[43]

Nearly a century later, McHenry wrote of the skill exhibited in Gowers' drawings:

> The illustrations were nearly all his own work, and by means of suppressing unnecessary graphic detail, he was able to emphasize his presentation in a manner which even modern photography can not achieve.[44]

Critchley refers to Gowers' pique when Armand de Watteville, after warmly praising the *Manual*, concluded his review in *Brain* by saying that 'in order not to derogate to the time-honoured tradition of reviewers always to find some fault with the work under notice, we shall attract Dr Gowers' attention to some verbal mistakes in the course of the book'. He gave several examples, including questioning Gowers' application of Latin rules: 'We find that Gowers adopts the absurd "pontine" for "pontal"'.[45] Critchley commented:

> Nothing could have piqued Gowers more. Already a stylist and a purist, he might have borne with adverse comment upon his neurological doctrines, but his prose was sacrosanct. It is probable that de Watteville's inappropriate sneers were never forgotten.[46]

Gowers had published two articles in the earliest issues of the Neurological Society's journal *Brain* in 1878 and 1880. There have been rumours that despite the fact that Ferrier and Hughlings Jackson were on the editorial board and de Watteville ceased to be editor in 1901, Gowers refused to have anything further to do with *Brain* until 1910, when the journal published his Hughlings Jackson lecture.[47] This does not explain the twenty-year gap in his contributions to *Brain*, nor the fact that Gowers was one of the 'distinguished individuals' who helped select papers from 1908 to 1914. It has been alleged that Gowers refused to join the Neurological Society because of his dislike of de Watteville, and remarked that the society was founded by a charlatan (de Watteville) to keep out a quack (Julius Althaus).[48] Gowers instead regularly published in the *Medico-Chirurgical Transactions.* The Medical and Chirurgical Society of London had been formed just after the beginning of the nineteenth century by a splinter-group from the Society of Medicine who protested at the high-handed tactics of the president at the time. In 1907, together with a number of other societies, including the Neurological Society, it amalgamated with the Royal Society of Medicine. The more likely explanation seems to lie in the history of the numerous learned medical societies at the time. It is interesting to note that the *BMJ* wrote in 1915 that reputations were at the time largely made in certain of the societies—the Pathological, the Clinical and the Medico-Chirurgical.[49]

In 1893 the Royal Medico-Chirurgical Society awarded Gowers the quinquennial Marshall Hall Prize for the *Manual of Diseases of the Nervous System* as the best original work in the English tongue dealing with the anatomy, physiology, or pathology of the nervous system.

At Queen Square the *Manual* was later referred to as 'the Bible of Neurology' and it is still regarded by many neurologists as the greatest comprehensive account of clinical neurology ever to be written by a single author.

## Professor of clinical medicine, University College Hospital

In 1887 Gowers was appointed professor of clinical medicine at UCH. For sixteen years, from 1872 to 1888, he had held simultaneous staff positions at Queen Square and at UCH, where he was appointed assistant physician in 1872, and promoted to physician in 1883. Most of Gowers UCH undergraduate lectures after 1883 were published in *The Lancet*, the last appearing in 1909.

Gowers was a loyal supporter of his *alma mater*, as his opening address to the 1884 intake of medical students demonstrates:

> Of your choice of place of study I need say little. For more than half a century University College has shown other schools how medicine should be taught. Almost every important step in medical education has first been taken by her. Thanks to her example she now has many rivals, but remains surpassed by none and equalled by few, whether the test of comparison be that of method or quality of result.[50]

He gave the first clinical lecture of the UCH winter season at in 1905. This lecture, entitled 'A metastatic mystery', had the characteristic rhetorical introduction that exemplified all his talks:

> Gentlemen, I have been asked to give you the first clinical lecture of this winter session. Many of those present, I doubt not, have just effected the transition to the Hospital, which constitutes the mid-point of the student's career. Others see, not far away, the gate of exit, beyond which lies an unknown future. To those who are beginning their clinical work and to those who are near its end, the case I have chosen as my subject presents much that should instruct and also much that can hardly fail to interest. It presents pathological features of great rarity and yet sufficiently related to that which is common to be useful. It constitutes moreover, a good example of diagnostic method and of this you cannot have too much. It also shows how important and direct is the relation to the sciences some of you have just mastered to the work on which you are now entered.[51]

In his clinical lectures, his advice was always pragmatic, based on experience and experiment rather than concepts and notions:

> When I say you cannot have too much of diagnostic method I mean that the power you will hereafter need, the power of discerning the nature of disease, can only be gained by constant exercise. You should systematically follow the process of diagnosis in every case observing its elements and their relative weight. Avoid the easy habit of taking in the diagnosis as a whole and being satisfied with the recognition of the disease. It is only by thoughtful perception of the reasoning, which varies in detail in every case, that you can gain the ability to deal in like manner with cases that are unfamiliar. The power will come unconsciously. …
>
> We must always remember it is the balance of evidence that determines diagnosis. The sciences concerned with disease deal largely with probabilities, almost wholly so in internal medicine. The probability varies in degree but usually falls far short of certainty. We must learn to take probability as our guide. We have to act. To act we must decide, and to decide we must weigh the evidence, and deal with the probable as if it were certain. Sometimes we shall be wrong, but generally we shall be right; if we hesitate between two opinions we shall be powerless. Remember that also in practical life, in dealing with patients, the habit of discerning the probability and acting decisively is all-important. Nothing is so necessary to every practitioner as the confidence of his patients. To gain that he must manifest some measure of confidence in himself. If you wait before forming even a probable opinion, at any rate be decided in delay. Remember, decisive hesitation is far wiser than hesitating decision.[52]

One past student described his clinical lectures as 'profoundly interesting and original, and not only in the physiology of the nervous system, in which he was pre-eminent. Brown wrote that Gowers had 'a pungent humour, which was greatly appreciated by his audience'.[53] His obituary in the *BMJ* commented that, at a time when neurology was beginning to emerge from a stage in which pathology was confused and diagnosis summary:

> Gowers insisted on tracing symptoms to their origin and an accurate regional diagnosis being made. The students gave him the nickname of 'primary lesion', and respected what they did not always fully understand. [54]

Gowers' teaching was not well adapted to the ordinary run of young students, and he did not welcome female students. In common with many (but not all) of his peers, Gowers was uncomfortable about women training for medicine. When his career began there were only eight female doctors in Britain. Embroiled in what was a heated debate over decades, it appears he was particularly averse to the London School of Medicine for Women, founded by Sophia Jex-Blake in 1874. By 1876, under new legislation, British medical examining bodies were allowed to include women students. But the fight to gain qualification was the source of major political and social controversy. By 1902, there were still only 212 female doctors.

Gowers remained opposed to the London School of Medicine for Women throughout his career, and also against UCH admitting female students. In January 1896 he wrote a note to one of his house physicians, which appears to differentiate this political debate with what was happening on the other side of the Atlantic:

> I thought all those ladies were Americans, and if so I thought I might have invited them to come round with me on Saturday. If they are from the School of Medicine for Women, it is a different matter and of course, I shall take no notice of them. The whole question however rather inclines me to feel more strongly than I did the undesirability of having the lady students in the Hospital. I think every one of the Physicians of the Hospital beyond myself is strongly opposed to it but I think some of the Assistant Physicians may be in favour of it. I don't think there is the slightest chance of their being admitted at present. I don't suppose there would be objections to a lady pursuing research in the laboratory but that is another thing. I would teach them and examine them separately. But yesterday shows the practical inconvenience of the presence of ladies.[55]

He was quite prepared to give a warm tribute to the American Neurological Association's Dr Sarah McNutt's work on diplegia 'whose investigations constitute, I think, by far the most valuable contribution to medical science that the profession has yet received from its members of her sex'.[56]

He was also prepared to demonstrate how deeply he felt over other issues close to his heart. He was profoundly affected by the terrible suffering and destruction he had seen syphilis wreak on its victims. In his 1889 Lettsomian lectures, given six years before the organism that caused the disease was identified, he passionately advocated what he saw as the only effective prevention: celibacy outside marriage:

> With all the force that any knowledge I possess can give, and with any authority I may have, I assert—as a result of long observation and consideration of facts of every kind—that no man was ever yet the slightest degree better for incontinence; that for it every man must be the worse morally, and that most are worse physically; and in no small number the result is, and ever will be, utter physical shipwreck on one of the many rocks, sharp, jagged-edged, or on one of the many banks of festering slime that are about his course, and which no care can possibly avoid.[57]

The report of his lecture earned him praise in the *New York Medical Record* and a leader in *The Lancet*, which wrote 'There is much in our profession to make us sad, but there are few sights more pitiable than to see a youth committed to all the horrors of syphilis ... a disease which is rivalled by no other in its total capacity for wrecking happiness, and health, and life'.[58]

When Critchley asked Ernest Gowers to provide some background material for his 1949 biography, Ernest chose to include the following extracts from a lecture Gowers gave in 1884, at the age of 39. It was the introductory lecture on the opening of the medical session at UCH. Ernest chose the extracts because they would 'serve to illustrate both his literary style and his outlook on his profession':

> The mode in which the various studies should be pursued will be sufficiently explained to you by those whose task it is to teach them. I would only impress on you one general principle, which should ever be kept in conscious view. It is a trite observation, often repeated, familiar enough in the abstract but never enough familiar in daily effort, that the object of study is two-fold.
>
> You are here for education as well as for instruction. You are here to acquire the knowledge of fact and rule and theory that you are to apply hereafter in the daily work of your lives, but you are here also to obtain the mental training needful for that application, needful to enable you to use that knowledge under conditions that are ever new and ever changing, to distinguish fact from fancy when they present themselves in unfamiliar aspect and often in borrowed garb—to trace new facts, new laws, among the manifold combinations of phenomena that will be around you in every day's work. …
>
> The extent to which you obtain this training rests largely on yourselves. It is at once an important, perhaps the most important part of your work, and it is that in which your teachers can do least for you. They can put before you fact and reason, but they cannot, or can only in a small degree, compel you to observe, to realise for yourselves the value of evidence, to distinguish fact from theory, and to be on guard against the fallacies that lurk on all sides. They can test your knowledge: they or others can 'coach' you or 'grind' you, but the process of the instillation of facts, represented by these somewhat inapt metaphors, may leave you wholly untrained for subsequent work. Your 'coach' may carry you through the lofty portals of Lincoln's Inn and Pall Mall, or the lower archway of Blackfriars, and leave you altogether unfitted for independent progress. Your 'grinder' may pass you through his mill with such success that you emerge - a flabby mass of factitious atoms kept in the semblance of form by the sack of a diploma; but it is only by your own continuous effort that you can gain cohesion and the power of organic growth. And this effort must be made from the commencement of your studies. …
>
> If we look around us, and read much of the medical literature of the day, it is difficult to avoid the conclusion that there is, to put it mildly, room for improvement. To put it more exactly, there is no department of science in which there is so much imperfect observation, hasty generalisation and fallacious reasoning as there is in medicine. I was going to say 'there is no department of intellectual work', but as that would include politics, the statement might be open to question; so I will leave you one comforting comparison. But in medicine, almost every day, fancies are formulated as if they were facts, theories are elaborated on data absurdly inadequate, and almost every conceivable error in reasoning is gravely perpetrated, and what is more, these things are welcomed with acclamation, when in any other department of science they would be put by with a smile. …
>
> There is another and very different province in which self-training is desirable. When you come to the practical study of disease, strive to acquire the habit of entering into the feelings of the sick and into their modes of thought, to such a degree as to ensure a considerate tenderness in dealing with them. Never forget that a patient means one who suffers and that you come into contact with the tenderest parts of human nature. Remember that those in whom pain, disease and death are stern and trying realities of the

> present or the nearer future, the mental tone is altogether changed; and do not judge the sick by the standard of the sound. Invest suffering with the reverence that is due to its sad mystery. ...
>
> It is true that to enter fully and deeply into suffering, with the sympathy that is not only intelligent but 'with-suffering' is impossible. A doctor's work would then be simply beyond endurance. To him, as to no other, the darkest side of human nature is ever open; in his ears the deep undertone of sadness rings through every chord and melody of life, now in the wail of pure distress, now in the discord of passion, now rising into the sweet still sad music of patient resignation and self-sacrificing love. Well is it for the world that it is impossible to understand without enduring, or the helpers would be few. As it is, our lives are often saddened by the suffering that we cannot but share. No statement more untrue was ever uttered than that familiarity with the sight of suffering destroys the capacity for sympathy in medical men. ...
>
> To relieve suffering, to cure disease, and above all to preserve health—these are the objects of your life. It is to achieve these that your energies are tasked, your drudgery bestowed, your days and your nights devoted. Each hour's work sees, or should see, these ends in some measure achieved. Failures must come, and, baffled in many a struggle, you may at times despond; but remember that the good you do is always far more than you can see. Our failures are obtrusive; our greatest triumphs imperceptible.[59]

However, as Liddell wrote in Gowers' entry in the *Dictionary of National Biography*, by the 1880s the strain of overwork was beginning to show in his lectures:

> He was a fluent and lucid lecturer and a bold and incisive clinical teacher. But, often strained and tired by overwork, he sometimes seemed dogmatic and impatient of criticism, and was even given to occasional sardonic if humorous invective. The immense labour of writing the *Manual* permanently impaired his enthusiasm and energy.[60]

When pressure of work forced him to resign from the staff of University College Hospital in 1888, *The Lancet* reported his resignation, commenting: 'It may surprise some to hear that Dr Gowers' resignation comes comparatively early in life, for his work has been so extensive and has become so familiar to all that he seems to have accomplished more than many men of advanced age'.[61]

At the end of 1892 he decided that for reasons, which he 'could not explain by letter' he should cease attending the Queen Square outpatients room.[62] He wrote formally to the board:

> I have now worked in the outpatient room, as a member of the permanent staff, for nearly, if not quite, twenty years, seeing outpatients, for about half that time, twice a week. Previously, for about four years when Medical Registrar, I saw about three quarters of the patients on all four days of the week. I think that the time has come when it is reasonable, and also right, that I should ask to be relieved of attendance in the outpatient room the more so since it has been impossible for me, of late, to give the proper amount of time to the work. There exist also other reasons, not of a personal nature, which make the step desirable, but I think it is not necessary for me to enter into these. Should the Board see fit to permit me to retain the small number of beds allotted to me, I shall be glad to do so and shall be content with them until such time as a re-arrangement takes place. I should hope, by this means, to continue some of the teaching, which seems, in the past, to have been found useful to many.[63]

No explanation of the reasons 'not of a personal nature' that caused him to take this step has come to light, though it may have been the success of his private practice as a consultant. After the end of the Christmas holidays he received a reply from Queen Square conferring on him the title of 'extra physician'. From then on he spent less time demonstrating cases in outpatients but concentrated on his private practice and inpatient care.

His teaching involved preparing two or three keynote lectures each term. In addition, he explained to students that 'the changed conditions' of his work at Queen Square prevented him from continuing his outpatient teaching, and that he would try to show students a case each week as a substitute.[64]

Critchley reminds us that by 1880 Gowers had already established a reputation not only in British medicine but also in international circles:

> His writings proclaimed his brilliance and energy. His practice was growing. Already known to a comparatively small circle as a great lecturer, his superlative gifts as a clinical demonstrator were not yet common knowledge.
>
> We may remind ourselves of Gowers' relationship to the outstanding figures in British, Continental and American neurology. In 1880 he was 35 years of age. At Queen Square, Jackson was 45 and Bastian 43. Horsley was as yet a newly-qualified young man of 23. In France, Charcot was 55, Raymond 36, Pierre Marie 27, while Babinski was the same age as Horsley. Oldest of the French was Duchenne, then in his 74th year. Closest to him among the French was Déjérine, then 31 years of age, whose career was to run on parallel lines to his own. The great figures in German neurology included Erb aged 40 years; Friedreich 55, Westphal 47, Quincke 38, Strümpell 27, Wernicke 32, Meynert 47, while Möbius was 26 and Oppenheim only 22. In Philadelphia lived Weir Mitchell, the outstanding American neurologist, then aged 51.[65]

Critchley added that by 1886, only six years later, 'no British medical man was better known and appreciated in America, France and Germany'.[66]

Gowers' obituary in the *BMJ* noted that he achieved great success in practice, and for a good many years was one of the busiest consultants in London. He may have destroyed his consultancy records when he retired and moved house. If not they were destroyed by his family after his death, when they also sold most of his library.

> Far from being spoilt by success, he was very much the better for it; without any diminution in the earnestness and confidence with which he expressed his conclusions and settled opinions, he grew more tolerant and ready to listen, and the attention with which he received a doubter's question was sometimes even embarrassing'.[67]

## Chapter 9

# Life outside work

Gowers devoted himself so wholeheartedly to his work that he had little time for friendships, although he always made time for his family. Between 1870 and 1900 he combined his work as a physician with research, teaching, and publishing books and articles. He became increasingly in demand as a consultant, and enlisted help in running his practice, first from Dr Walter Coleman and later Dr James Taylor. The practice expanded into two of the rooms at 50 Queen Anne Street. But few records have survived about his consultancy such as what other staff he employed or whether his self-effacing, shorthand-writing wife helped him run the practice. He appears to have done all his writing at home. The only hint about his fees comes from a letter to Rudyard Kipling's brother-in-law, which is impossible to interpret as he does not cite an hourly rate, and there is an almost undecipherable letter from J. M. Barrie apparently asking to be excused from some treatment. There are few other hints as to who his patients were. He acted as an insurance assessor for the Guardian Assurance Company (and wrote several articles about this work in the *Phonographic Journal*).

He continued to have intermittent bouts of ill-health. Throughout the 1870s he had suffered from a grumbling appendix, and applied his diagnostic skills to himself:

> Between 26 and 34 I had five or six definite attacks of perityphlitis, the last of great severity. In none was there any spot of greater tenderness to suggest that the affection started in the appendix. My personal observation generated a strong conviction of the origin of the form from which I suffered. In his teaching Sir William Jenner used to insist on the variation in the amount of peritoneum over the caecum in connection with intussusception, which he held to occur chiefly when the covering is so complete as to give rise to a mesocaecum and consequent mobility.

He went on to describe his most recent attack:

> I suppose that there was no indication of suppuration, for Sir William Jenner, who kindly looked after me, did not think a surgeon's opinion necessary. In the course of a few weeks the whole gradually disappeared, in spite of an incidental attack of catarrhal jaundice. It was before the days of 'appendicitis'. I wonder whether, with such extensive induration I should have escaped operation at the present day. I do not think my prospects of recovery would have been increased thereby. … I have met with several illustrations … that a severe attack of peritonitis, whether operated upon or not, is usually the last. I think the explanation is that the connective tissue is left in an altered cicatricial condition which becomes less and less prone to inflammation as the cicatricial change is more and more complete.[1]

Doctors were not immune from the outbreak of typhoid fever in Marylebone in 1873. *The Times* reported that a number of prominent medical households, including that of Gowers, were affected:

> The outbreak of typhoid fever to which attention has been this week drawn in Mayfair and Marylebone is one of the most remarkable and severe with which we are acquainted. A great number of families have been attacked, and eminent medical men have largely suffered. We are acquainted thus far with about 165 cases occurring in 47 families inhabiting [the area around] Harley Street. ... Among households attacked are those of ... Dr Murchison, Dr Gowers and Dr Liveing ...
>
> We have said that circumstances point very strongly to the milk-supply being the source of the poison; and so much is this the case that Sir William Jenner and Dr Murchison, who have been called to see a number of the patients, have thought it their duty to represent the urgent nature of the emergency to the vendors of the milk, and to advise them to suspend their sale of milk.[2]

However there is no evidence that Gowers or his mother had contracted typhoid. It is most likely to have been a child of one of their domestic staff.

Gowers' health started to break down seriously in the 1890s, and he became crippled by severe and constant back pain. He was clearly becoming daunting to many students and colleagues by this stage. His obituary in *Nature* commented that the early struggles and difficulties he experienced sometimes made him seem 'a little austere', but that as time went on his kindness asserted itself more and more, and that his death would be deeply mourned, not only by those who benefited from his professional skill and knowledge, but by many who had experienced generous kindness at his hands.[3]

This kinder side of Gowers is clearly seen from Ernest's descriptions of him as a father. The humour and generous kindness is revealed both in his 'children's diaries', and from his correspondence with close friends. Ernest described his father's personality in his later years:

> Small talk bored him; he hated to be bored and was sometimes shatteringly outspoken. But his real nature was sensitive and affectionate and generous to a fault, and in those who got to know him well and understood him, when as pupils or patients, he was apt to inspire a devotion amounting almost to idolatry.
>
> He had few intimate friends, and those he had were mostly outside his own profession. He liked people who could tell him things he did not know. His longest and closest friendships were with Thomas Bonney, the eminent geologist, and Augustus Jessopp, a Norfolk Rector, antiquarian and essayist. He enjoyed the society of people who had unusual experiences; notable among these were Mr Morrison, the well-known Peking correspondent of *The Times* and Dr Jameson.

We have discovered more about the nature of Gowers' friendships with the two younger men, Morrison and Jameson (discussed below), from correspondence that has come to light. It is easy to understand why Gowers formed friendships with the other two men, Bonney and Jessopp. Bonney, twelve years Gowers' senior, was a fellow of St John's College, Cambridge, and emeritus professor of geology at UCL. Jessopp, twenty years older than Gowers, was a specialist in the history of East Anglia, and had been a close friend of Meredith, Tennyson, and Browning (he lived to the age of 90, becoming 'chaplain in ordinary' to Edward VII). Another of Gowers' friends was the Reverend Page-Roberts, whose church in Vere Street was attended by the Gowers family. Page-Roberts probably also consulted Gowers professionally, as all three of his sons suffered from muscular dystrophy.

Ernest explained why some people found his father daunting:

> He was of medium height and of spare build, with thick hair and a square-cut beard, both of which whitened at an unusually early age. His way of speaking was loud and oddly deliberate. His pale blue eyes had a penetrating quality disconcerting to anyone who had a mind to be anything but frank with him. Patients and students sometimes found him alarming. He could not tolerate sloppy thinking or circumlocution, and was at no great pains to conceal the fact.

## Paterfamilias

Family was far more important to Gowers than his friendships. He had married Mary Baines in her home town, Leeds, on 6 April 1875. Their elder son William Frederick (nicknamed Willie) was born on 31 December 1875. He was followed by Edith, born in 1877, Ernest in 1880, and Evelyn in 1884. According to Ernest, Mary Gowers lived for her husband and four children 'a life of self-effacement'. But in his father's 'friendships of the heart there was one person who had no rival, his elder daughter Edith. She laid herself out to interest herself in the things that interested him, and was his constant companion throughout his life'. She became a competent shorthand writer, and when she grew up and her father had become ill and frail she helped him by sometimes transcribing his lecture notes from his shorthand drafts.

Queen Anne Street crosses Wimpole and Harley streets, and lies between Wigmore and New Cavendish streets. William and Mary Gowers raised their four children in number 50, two rooms of which were used for his consultancy. There was a night nursery and a day nursery, and by 1881 there were five living-in staff: a cook, nurse, nursemaid, housemaid, and butler.[4] Weymouth Street was behind the house 'on to the back of whose houses my night-nursery used to look along the length of the mews from which the noises of stamping horses, jingling harness and cursing coachmen used to give me company in bed', wrote Ernest to a friend, years afterwards.

William's mother Ann Gowers lived with the family until she died in 1882, aged 75, having suffered from chronic gastritis; her son recorded her death after suffering 'exhaustion, three days'. She had been the only close family presence in his life until the time of his marriage. He expressed his sense of loss to Thomas Barlow: 'A mother's death is as you say, a severe trial and it is the more so to me since for twenty years, from the death of my father to the time of my marriage, my mother and I had been each other's only companion, she having no other [surviving] child'.[5]

Gowers went out of his way to provide his own children with the kind of rich family life he had never experienced in his own isolated youth:

> He did allow himself one non-intellectual relaxation. His love of chess remained, but he had little time for games, and he found that if he played it in the evening its stimulating effect interfered with his sleep. But after dinner he would play billiards or table tennis with his children. At both his zest was greater than his skill, and I fancy the real reason for this exception to his usual habits was not that he enjoyed the game but that he enjoyed above all things giving pleasure or instruction to his children.

No subject could be raised in conversation without his 'wanting to know anything about it that he did not know already', and family meals were punctuated by visits to the shelves of reference books. Gowers always made time for his children:

> It is astonishing to me that at the busiest time of his professional life he should have been able to find the time that he gave to them. It was not only that whenever he had free time in the afternoon he would take them out in the carriage with him, perhaps to some historic building, perhaps to some exhibition or amusement, perhaps to Lords or the Oval, perhaps for a country walk on Putney Heath or at Finchley. He wrote animal stories for them in prose and verse; they were of high merit and have delighted three generations of his descendants. For more than ten years he wrote for every day that had anything out of the ordinary in it what he called the 'children's diary', a whimsical and witty account of the day's doings as seen through the eyes of the children, recorded with all his great gifts of imagination, selectivity and literary skill and charmingly illustrated by his pen.[6]

In fact, when Gowers began these diaries in 1884 he wrote them by hand, as well as illustrating them with his own sketches. But in 1885, always fascinated by new inventions, he bought himself two new gadgets: a typewriter and a camera. Both were primarily for use in his consultancy, but that year he took a photograph of each member of the family on their birthday, which he glued into the diary, as well as taking photographs of some of the places they visited. He used the typewriter to make the diaries easier for the children to read, and some of the spelling mistakes suggest that Gowers did not always transcribe the shorthand notes he made during the holiday himself.

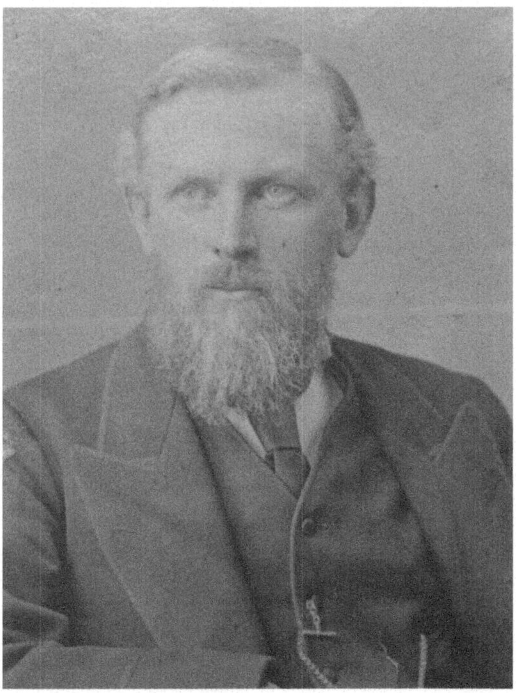

**Fig. 9.1** 'Papa' aged 40, from the 1885 'children's diary'.

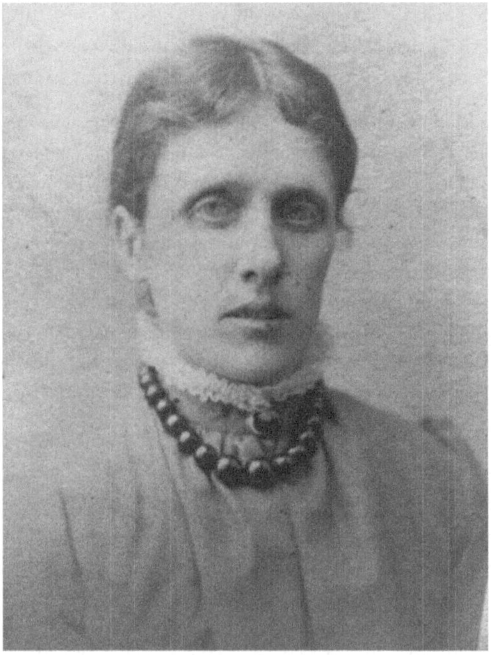

**Fig. 9.2** 'Mama' Mary Gowers.

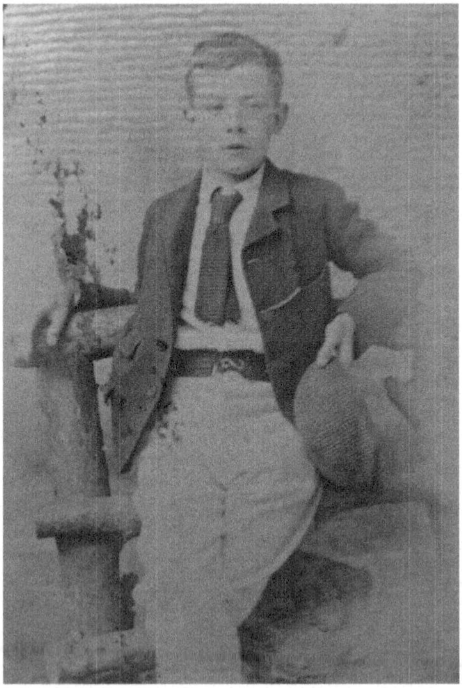

**Fig. 9.3** 'Willie' [William Frederick] on his tenth birthday.

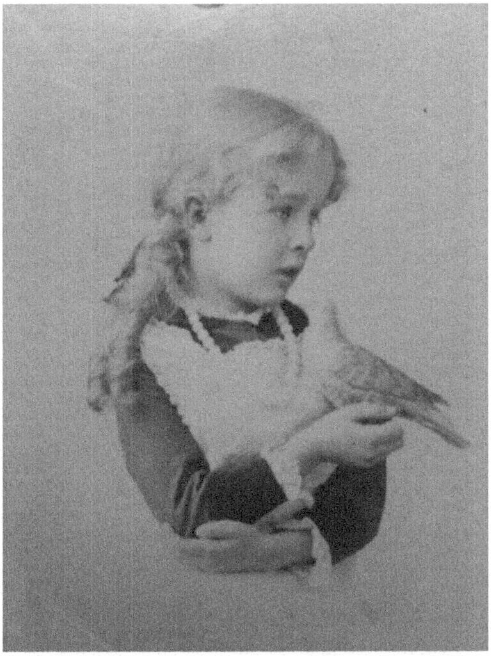

**Fig. 9.4** Edith on her eighth birthday.

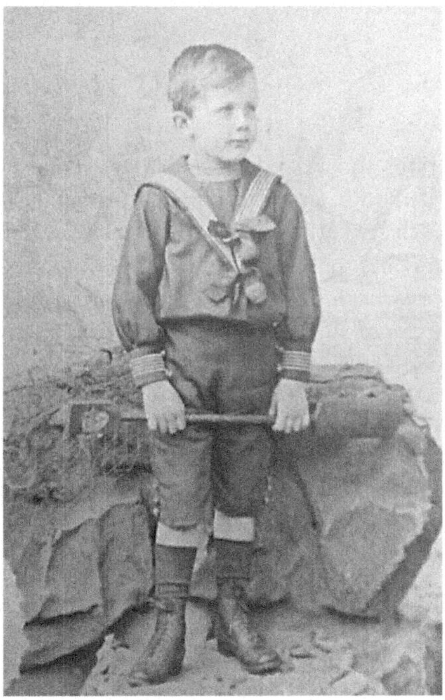

**Fig. 9.5** Ernest on his fifth birthday.

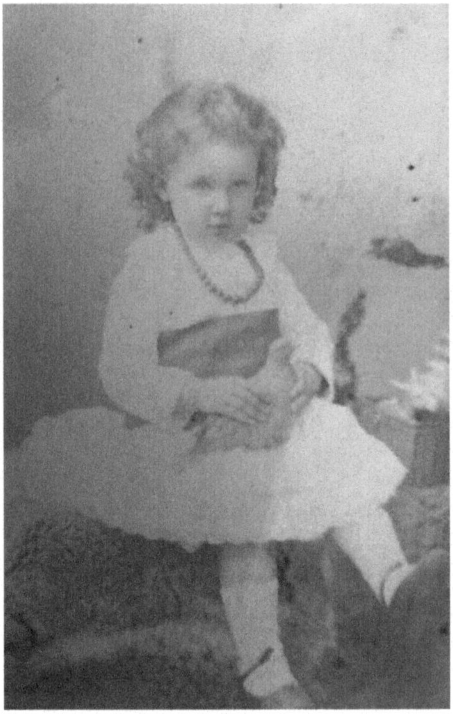

**Fig. 9.6** Evelyn on her third birthday.

Many of the descriptions are of day-to-day holiday events, including four separate holidays spent in Bournemouth, and several in Southwold. By 1884 he records taking the elder children to watch cricket at Lords, to the Health Exhibition, to the Zoological Gardens at Regents Park, and to the Natural History Museum in Kensington (which had opened three years earlier). In July 1885 the family visited the city that Gowers described as the 'grimy gloom' of Leeds to see their Baines relatives, staying with their grandfather at Weetwood Lodge.

They played cricket and croquet and went for country walks. One day Gowers took the children to collect Grandpapa (Frederick Baines) from the '*Mercury* office', and on another travelled alone to pay a nostalgic visit to the farm at Bentley where he had spent a year working with Joseph Hurst. He drew a sketch of the farm in the 'children's diary'.

Then, when the holiday came to an end, he drew a picture of the family queuing to board their train from Doncaster station, showing an advertisement for the *Leeds Mercury* in the background.

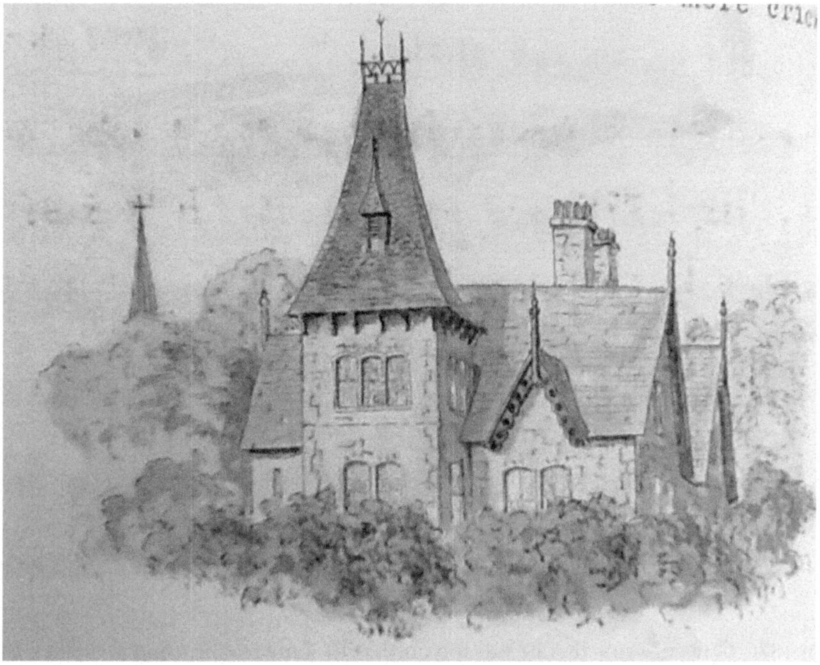

**Fig. 9.7** Weetwood Lodge, Leeds, Frederick Baines' family home.

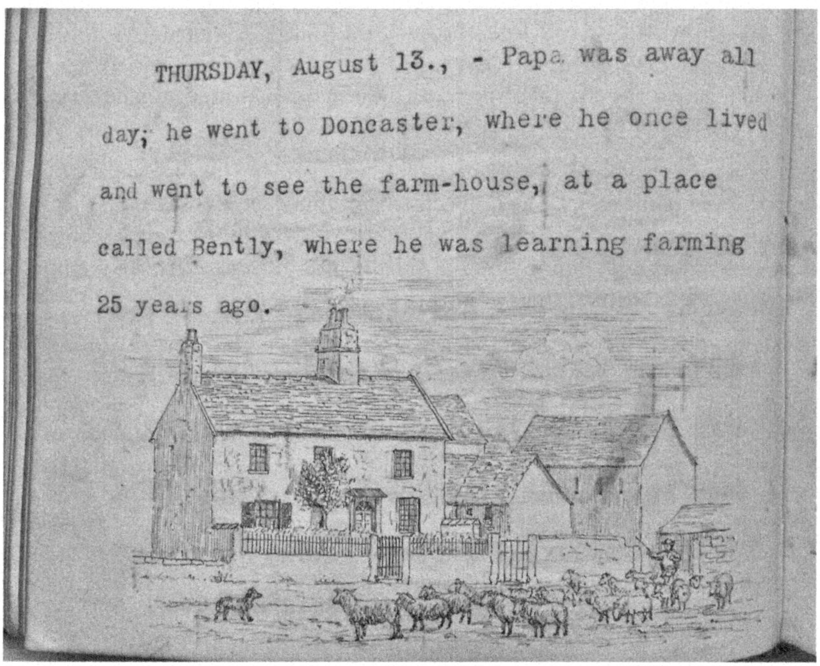

THURSDAY, August 13., - Papa was away all day; he went to Doncaster, where he once lived and went to see the farm-house, at a place called Bently, where he was learning farming 25 years ago.

**Fig. 9.8** Joseph Hurst's farm.

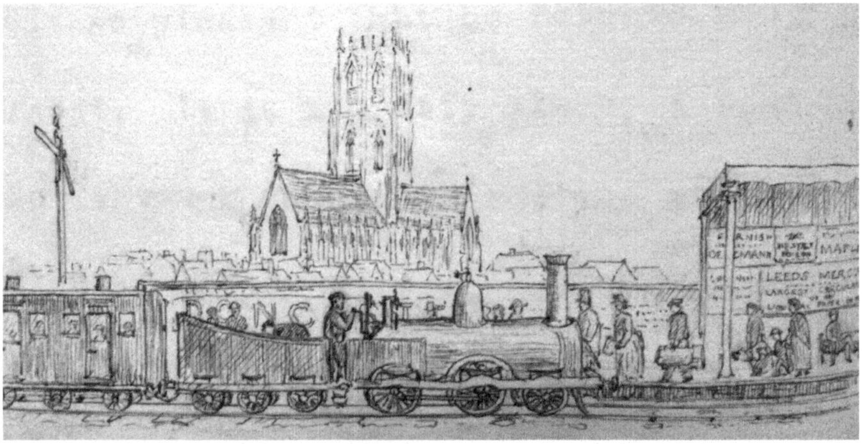


**Fig. 9.9** The end of the 1885 Leeds holiday. The family boarding the train at Doncaster station (advertisement for the *Leeds Mercury* in the background).

In 1886, Gowers wrote that he was too busy 'with some real printing' to make diary entries. He was half-way through the huge work of compiling his *Manual*, and he records how the elder two children had helped him make copies:

> The months of January and February passed with very little to note, and that little Papa was not able to write down, as he was very busy, beginning to print his large book, the *Manual*, as it is called. Willie and Edith helped him, sometimes by copying what he had written in the copying press, and a little with the pen. Papa has given them each a stenographic pen because they both have learned to write so nicely. …

Copying machines involved an original, written with copying ink, being placed against a damp sheet of tissue paper. The iron copying machine pressed them together, making a copy appear (in reverse) on the tissue. In March Gowers took his elder son, 10-year-old Willie, with him to the J. & A. Churchill printing office 'to see how the printer is getting on with the big book':

> Our business in Bartholomew Close took us to a close within a close, for we went down a narrow passage in a corner, an old-fashioned sort of place, at the bottom of which stood a strange old building, with narrow passages and break-neck stairs—the printing office from which Papa's book is some day to come out into the world. We saw a sheet of the book being printed off, the clean white paper go in and come out covered with Papa's ideas and drawings. One of the figures in the sheet was a drawing that Willie had seen Papa make. Then we went into another room and saw a press in which the sheets are pressed smooth after being printed. It was a hydraulic press, and can give a pressure of more than a hundred tons, equal, say, to fifty wagons full of coal one on the top of another. And as Papa's ideas will have to undergo that pressure before they go out to the world; they are likely to be rather flat, not to say thin, when they have passed through the ordeal. Then we went up the cranky stair-case to the large room in which the compositors were at work, with nimble fingers, moving so quickly putting up the type.

They had an April holiday in Bournemouth, and August was spent at Southwold. At the end of September 1886 Willie started his formal schooling at University College School, and received an excellent report at the end of the term. Then came a festive Christmas:

> During the still hours of the night, when young eye-lids had fallen over tired but anticipating eyes, SANTA CLAUS paid his mysterious visit, and found the customary receptacles suspended in the customary places, and he did not leave them empty. When morning broke, and wondering hands felt their way into the stockings in the dim December light, the soft recesses were found to contain various small but useful articles.

Gowers described the children enjoying their Christmas lunch:

> At mid-day, the time-honoured and welcome bird made its appearance on the table, and four small but ardent ornithologists proceeded to take part in the minute dissection of portions of its pectoral muscles. The study of anatomy usually occupies only the fingers and the eyes, but the scientific zeal today was so great that it led to the employment of every available sense, including even the sense of taste, in the investigation of the minute characteristics of the tissues of the bird. Nor was this the only object that excited their interest. Elongated bodies, of curious aspect, smooth externally and mottled internally, lay around the carcase. These objects were also investigated in the same minute manner, and a singular harmony was discovered between the impressions made on the sense of taste of the investigators by the inside of these elongated bodies and by the flesh of the turkey. A vast quantity of greenish material was found inside the bird, but there was some difference of opinion as to its qualities. When this examination had proceeded for some time, and most of the fragments operated on had disappeared in a mysterious manner in the course of the examination, the instruments of dissection were laid side by side and removed, and so also were the remains of the carcase.

Then came the traditional Christmas pudding, brought to the table covered with a flame of lighted brandy:

> A remarkable phenomenon then occurred. Prior brought into the room a large soft-looking mass, and from this mass twigs, with leaves on them, appeared to be growing, while all about it played a lurid lambent flame, and the leaves crackled in the tongues of fire which seized them. Alarming as was the appearance, this did not deter the brave and zealous students of nature from subjecting this to the same process of examination that had yielded such interesting results in the case of the bird, and the conclusion ultimately reached was that it was composed of the dried seed-vessels of a foreign shrub, the fat which lies behind the peritoneum of the sheep, the ground seed of a kind of grass, and of some other substances. It excited great interest. The last part of the proceedings consisted in the examination, in like manner, of some very singular objects which turned out to be the enlarged seed-vessels of certain trees encrusted with crystals obtained by evaporating the juice of a gigantic kind of rush, or grass.

Gowers took the older children to the Botanical Gardens to work off their lunch, then returned home for a game of billiards on the table he had bought the family as a Christmas present.

The following Christmas was far less joyful, because Edith had been struck down by typhoid fever six weeks earlier.

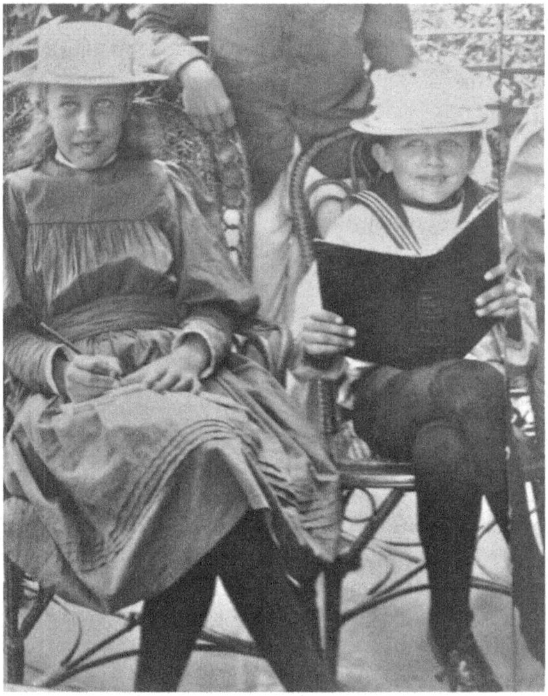

**Fig. 9.10** Edith and Ernest.

In December, after describing an accident in which Willie had suffered severe cuts after putting his arm through a window, Gowers described in detail how Edith had been afflicted:

> On the evening of this accident, Edith did not seem very well, but she never likes accidents or the sight of blood, and we thought that she had been upset by hearing of the cut. But the day before, she had not seemed very well, and had not been to Church. On the day after the accident she seemed to be better, and went out, but in the evening she was found to be feverish, and the next morning was so unwell that she did not get up.
>
> The day after that, Dr Barlow came to see her, and thought that she would soon be well. However, day after day passed, and she did not mend, but rather got worse than better, and at last, on the Sunday following it was found that she was suffering from typhoid fever. She had been moved each day on to the sofa in the day-nursery, but now she had to be kept in bed, and the others were not allowed to go near her. It was very sad for her, but, although she did not know what was the matter with her, she was very good, and submitted to all the arrangements without complaint. A nurse was obtained from University College Hospital.

Edith became increasingly ill over the next few days, and had to be sponged frequently with cold water:

> She liked this at first, but afterwards she got so weak and weary, that it tired her, and she was very glad when it had not to be done quite so often. Her lips got parched, and she was very thirsty.

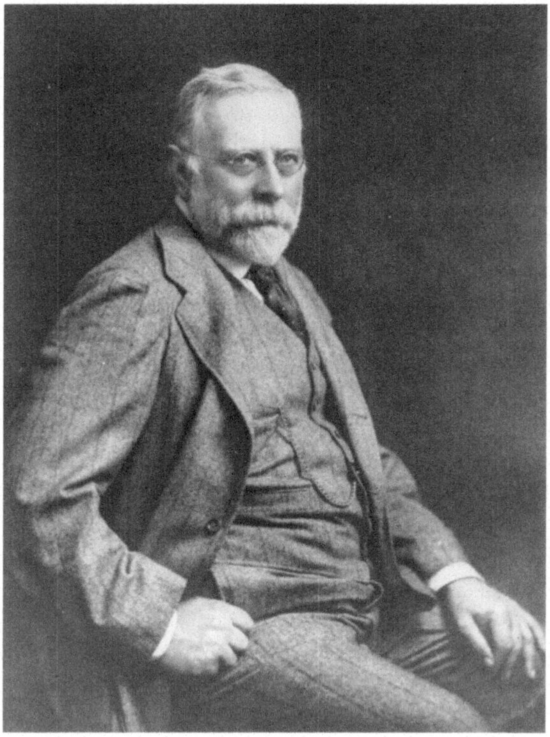

**Fig. 9.11** Sir Thomas Barlow, 1845–1945. In 1870 Barlow succeeded Gowers as assistant physician to William Jenner at UCH. Reproduced with permission from Museum & Archives Service, Great Ormond Street Hospital for Children NHS Trust.

> So the weary days went on. Dr Barlow came to see her two or three times every day, and was very very kind. He liked to see his little patient, and would stroke her face and hair, and see if any more 'spots' had come out. Then Sir William Jenner came to see her, and came again. He is the greatest living doctor, and is the doctor to the Queen.
>
> After a while, a very curious thing happened to her, and an unpleasant thing too. She left off speaking. Try all she could, she couldn't utter a word or even whisper one. Before this, however, she had become deaf, and now she could not hear what was said to her or say anything to us. This state of things lasted for more than a week. Then she began to hear a little better each day until she could hear very well, but still she was not able to speak. She tried so hard, we could see how hard she tried but she could not speak.

The illness continued throughout December, but by Christmas Day Edith was beginning to improve slightly:

> A very quiet Christmas Day, partly because it is Sunday, partly on account of dear Edith's illness. She is still so ill that she has to be kept free from any excitement, and we are not able to tell her that it is Christmas.

Willie turned 12 years old on 31 December, but they celebrated two birthdays that day. Edith's fever was coming down and the family decided she was well enough to hear how ill she had been, and for how long. At last, after six weeks, she was released from her isolation and a birthday was held for her, in place of the one she had missed.

In 1888 another phase began, when Willie was sent to Rugby. Gowers chose to send both Willie and Ernest to Rugby. The underlying principles of Thomas Arnold's reforms as headmaster of Rugby had been: adherence to religious and moral principle, 'gentlemanly conduct', and academic ability. One of Arnold's successors, headmaster from 1858 to 1869, was Frederick Temple, later to be Archbishop of Canterbury, who also was a 'liberal Anglican', 'open-minded, and in favour of open-mindedness'.[7] Temple, who supported Darwin's theories of evolution, wrote one of the articles in the controversial *Essays and Reviews*, thus becoming embroiled in a four-year dispute. The choice of Rugby, therefore, suggests that Gowers was comfortable with the liberalizing church, and with sending his sons to a 'Broad Church' Anglican school. Mary Gowers' father Frederick Baines, despite his Nonconformist background and beliefs, had already sent his son to Rugby. Amongst Ernest's contemporaries were Frederick Temple's second son William who, like his father, became Archbishop of Canterbury, and Richard Tawney. William Temple defended the working-class movement and supported economic and social reforms; Richard Tawney became famous as an economic historian, social critic, and Christian socialist. The Rugby ethic was evident in both men.

On Ernest's eighth birthday Gowers recorded that he had 'gone through much suffering' (Ernest was not a robust child), but 'all are now fairly well, and able fully to enjoy the day'. The family frequently visited Gowers' beloved Southwold. Ernest wrote that the churches of Suffolk gave ample scope for his father's antiquarianism, and both they and the Southwold fishing industry 'gave him just the right material for his pencil'. When the children were older Gowers decided that they should broaden their horizons, so in the 1890s they went further afield, including a holiday at Shanklin, Isle of Wight, in 1891. In 1895 they went to Wales, and also visited their Yorkshire relatives.

Gowers always took his sketchbook with him. Sketching was a common pastime in the nineteenth century, before the first cheap cameras appeared in the 1880s, so this was not an unusual hobby. But, as with his shorthand, he approached his drawing as a dedicated perfectionist. He once asked Foster Kennedy, his last house physician: 'What are you going to do for your holiday this year? I am going to do clouds'. One year he would 'do' clouds, another he would 'do' ferns, another he would 'do' mosses. He may, like Ruskin, also have wanted to draw in order to teach himself the laws of nature. But the sketchbook was always there, whatever type of knowledge he was pursuing. He sketched pastoral or seaside scenes such as boats, houses, barns, bridges, or local characters.

Just after Christmas in 1891 Gowers took Willie abroad to celebrate his sixteenth birthday in Cannes. Cannes had been developed largely by the efforts of Henry (Lord) Brougham, and had become the 'sanatorium of Europe'. It was a fashionable health resort where Willie's grandfather Frederick Baines was living because of his frail health. This appears to be the first trip Gowers took outside the United Kingdom. He kept a diary on this holiday, with descriptions of their surroundings echoing the close visual observations of his apprenticeship days. He refers to himself as 'Papa' and Frederick Baines as 'Grandpapa':

> Our abode is a very sumptuous one, the best rooms in the hotel [the Prince of Wales], a sitting room on the first floor in the middle of the hotel, with a bedroom on each side of it. The sitting room is the only one that has a balcony. It contains six tables, two sofas and eight easy chairs besides other chairs, so that we have an abundant choice of comfortable positions. The rooms are those always occupied by the Duke of Cambridge when he comes to Cannes, and he is coming to these rooms on the 11th of January, the day we leave. …
>
> Willie has had many drives with Grandpapa. This morning he had some presents from Grandpapa and the Aunts, which he chose in the town, whither he walked with Auntie Edith, especially a very pretty scarf pin. Papa gave him a wonderful little lamp to burn colza oil for his study at Rugby, and a box of pencils and sketchbook. We lunched with Grandpapa, who is staying at the Hotel Paradis, not far away.

Gowers spent most of the holiday confined to the hotel with a heavy cold. On New Year's Day 1892 he wrote:

> We have thought much of the dear ones at home today. Papa had to keep to the garden on account of a cold, except for a drive into the town in the afternoon in Grandpapa's carriage, when Willie accompanied him, to go to the chief booksellers and stationers and change a book at the library there, and get an inkstand and some ink.

Despite being confined to his room, he was fully occupied:

> Papa's cold still makes him a prisoner, but Willie had a pleasant drive in the morning with Uncle Talbot and the Aunts Edith and Agnes. In the afternoon he walked down into the town and obtained a small paint-box for Papa, making an excellent choice, which was quickly utilised over a lovely, but too short sunset.

He still enjoyed a glass or two of wine, and he encouraged Willie to do so. There are several references to splendid hocks or clarets enjoyed over dinner. Gowers was as struck by the beauty of the Esterel Mountains, as Monet had been four years earlier:

> Tonight's sunset was again beautiful, rosy streaks of clouds above the Esterel Mountains, but more dark clouds, and the fiery hues soon vanished, while the sky beyond had not the deep red tint near the horizon which sometimes adds such beauty to the scene. But the sharp-edged Esterel Mountains never fail to give peculiar grandeur to the contrast with the nearer and lower hills of Cannes dotted with houses, and of the pale sea which lies at the base of the mountains, and beyond them extends far off to the horizon beyond which, one thinks with strangeness, lies Africa itself.

There was a severe influenza epidemic during the winter of 1891–2. On 11 January 1892, Gowers and his son crossed the English Channel on their return to London from Cannes:

> It was a very little misty, but the whistle went on until some lights appeared in front of us. These, we afterwards found, were the lights of the South Foreland towards which the Captain was taking us! It turned out that the regular captain was ill with influenza with some 49 others of the people employed on the boats, and our Captain was making his first passage across the Channel.

> After the return of the travellers from Cannes there were but few incidents to record. The influenza had possession of London and England. Indeed, it may be said to have seized upon the whole world for it was left behind at Cannes and passed at Paris, as well as found at London and heard of in distant America and various parts of the globe. Two days after the return, the Duke of Clarence died, the eldest son of the Prince of Wales, who was shortly to be married to the Princess Mary, the daughter of the Duke of Teck.

Willie was about to return to Rugby, where he was moving into the sixth form. Before he went, he and Edith had lunch with Mr Page Roberts, then Willie was taken to see the pantomime, Humpty Dumpty, by Dr James Taylor. Ernest returned to his preparatory school. The end of the girls' holiday was marked by the return of their governess, Miss Pearce. Gowers added a postscript to the diary, commenting on the influenza epidemic:

> The influenza has made death busy killing the old people of the country, and some of the deaths deserve record that the children may, in future years, remember that they were alive when some of the old or great ones of the former time passed away. Thus Professor Adams of Cambridge is just dead, who made out from the irregularities of the planet Neptune that there must be another outside it, and said this in the year Papa [Gowers himself] was born, 1845. Owing to an accidental delay, however, the planet was actually first seen by a Frenchman, Levrier. He and Adams are regarded as entitled to joint honour as discoverers of the planet.
>
> The Duke of Devonshire has also died, who was the Chancellor of the University of Cambridge and owned the greater part of Eastbourne. The oldest chorister in the country is dead also, a man named Mitchell who was a chorister in St George's Chapel at Windsor Castle for 77 years. He was 83 when he died, and began to sing in that chapel when only six years old.
>
> Cardinal Manning is also dead. He was the greatest English Roman Catholic since the death of Cardinal Newman about a year ago. He was first a clergyman in the Church of England like Cardinal Newman, but did not leave the Church of England for the Church of Rome for many years after Cardinal Newman 'went over', as it is said.

At the end of February 1892 'Grandpapa' Frederick Baines also died:

> This has been a very, very sad day, for a telegram came to tell us of the death of dear Grandpapa this morning at Cannes. He loved his London grandchildren dearly, partly for their mother's sake and chiefly for their own, and was always delighted to have them with him. ... He is the last of the children's grandparents, and the one whom they will always remember best, and whose look and words and love should never fade from their memory.

True to his Congregational upbringing, Gowers noted that in 1892 Christmas fell on a Sunday so was spent in 'a quiet manner befitting the occasion, but unlike the ordinary Christmas style'. It was a cold winter and the children spent much of the holiday on their ice-skates. Willie turned 17 on the last day of the year:

> Willie's eighteenth year takes him quite out of the proper range of notice in the journal, but it is difficult to drop him from its pages, in which his doings have figured so largely. He has shot up in height until he can certainly look at his father on a level, if indeed he cannot almost look down on him.

Gowers noted in the 'children's diary' that they now preferred to refer to their parents as 'Father' and 'Mother' rather than the 'Papa' and 'Mama' that he had always used in his diaries. Willie, in another act of rebellion, wrote from Rugby and reprimanded his sister for writing to him in shorthand, asking her never to do so again. In 1894 Willie, who had excelled as a sportsman, particularly cricket, was awarded a classics scholarship to Trinity College, Cambridge. Ernest won a scholarship to Clare College, Cambridge in 1900.

## Hobbies

By the 1890s the pressure of Gowers' work was easing, his children were growing up, and he had more time in which to indulge the two recreational interests 'that never failed, whatever by-paths of knowledge he might follow from time to time': drawing (and etching) and that of the antiquarian, 'and especially the student of church architecture and ornament'.[8]

### Archaeology

Augustus Jessopp and Gowers shared a love of East Anglia, its countryside, and its history.[9] Gowers' interest in the history of East Anglia started in his apprenticeship days, when Bryan Dale asked him to report on details about the churches he passed on his walks around Coggeshall. In 1894 and 1903 Gowers published articles in the *Proceedings of the Suffolk Institute of Archaeology and Natural History*: the first on the flint-work inscription on Blythburgh Church, and the second on the ruined chapel of Mells, near Wenhaston.[10]

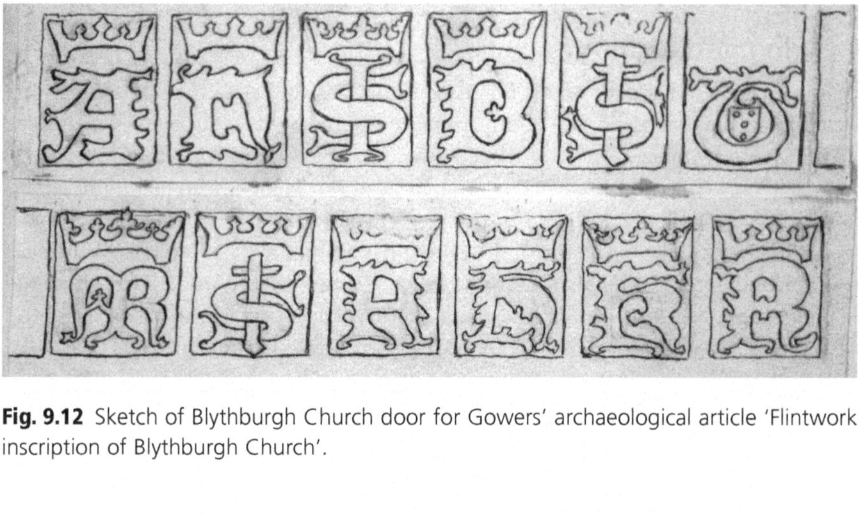

**Fig. 9.12** Sketch of Blythburgh Church door for Gowers' archaeological article 'Flintwork inscription of Blythburgh Church'.

In September 1889, the 75-year-old Sir James Paget had visited Lowestoft, and Gowers spent a day showing him around nearby Southwold, giving him an etching as a memento. After the visit Paget put Gowers in touch with the Suffolk Archaeological Society:

> Dr Raven, Vicar of Fressingfield, not far from Halesworth—I am sure he will give you any information that he can, either personally or by letter, and he is one of the most active members of the Suffolk Archaeological Society. It was a singular pleasure to meet you today and to have your guidance in Southwold. I do thank you for it and again for the beautiful etching which will often remind me of the day.[11]

The Reverend Canon John James Raven was also a Fellow of the Society of Antiquaries. He became a friend and correspondent of Gowers, who also, formally or informally, gave him medical advice. In 1895 the Gowers family had a holiday at the coastal town of Barmouth, in north Wales, during which Gowers wrote to Raven, who had recently been ill:

> I am delighted to hear that you are able to persevere with work. You have had a narrow escape and suffer quite enough to induce you to have your church well warmed next winter. If you don't you deserve—I won't say what beyond a very poor congregation. We have been spending our holiday here & seeing something of the scenery of this part—the younger ones much. There does not seem much of Roman interest around here.
>
> I am glad you enjoy the *Spectator*. It is to Edith that you are indebted for its dispatch—she makes it a point of conscience & is only sorry that it so often is kept on the waiting room table until too late to reach you in time for your Sunday afternoon. Unfortunately the newspaper post goes out before the letter post to which we send—otherwise you would have it a day earlier. But we are glad to know that it interests you & also your father. I often think that this or that in it would appeal to you. This number raises the question which I dare say you have long settled. Do you at the Creed turn towards Jerusalem or towards the place where the sun rises? In either case you must rest on enough symbolism to avoid floundering.[12]

## Drawing and etching

Gowers never lost his enthusiasm for recreational drawing and etching. Many of his sketchbooks have survived. An album containing some of his best sketches, examples of which appear on page 193, was recently discovered at Queen Square.

In 1880 Gowers was approached by Francis Seymour Haden, who had founded the Society of Painter-Etchers. Haden, a surgeon, had attended art school in Paris, believing in the importance of the use of drawing for training the hand and eye of the surgeon. Haden became a highly accomplished etcher and an important spokesman for etching during its revival in the nineteenth century. He was also brother-in-law of the artist James McNeill Whistler.[13] He made his approach to Gowers in 1891:

> I understand that among your many other claims to distinction you are an Etcher, and that you have by you some unfinished plates that you had it in your mind to let our council [the Society of Painter-Etchers] see. Might I suggest your doing so whether they are finished or not? My idea being if I may venture to say so, that one who has done so many things well is not likely to do anything badly.[14]

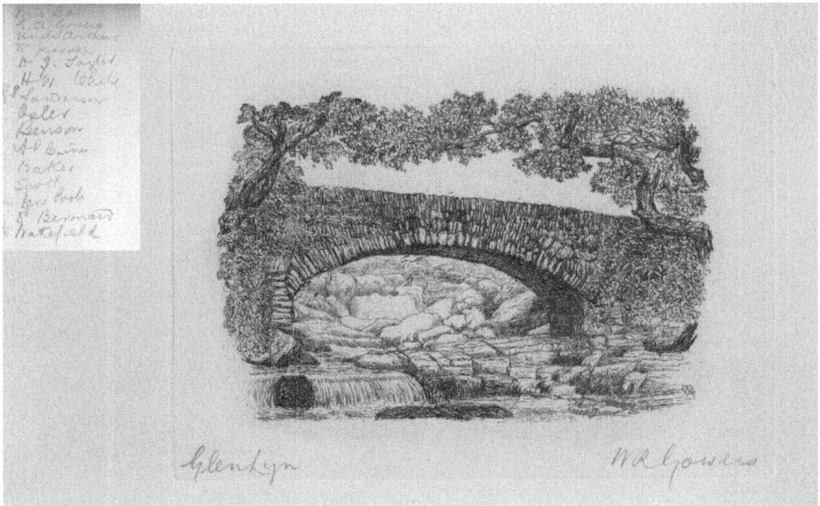


**Fig. 9.13** Gowers' sketch 'Glen Lyn'. Recipients listed: Mrs Best, E. A. Gowers, Uncle Arthur, Dr Jessopp, Dr J. Taylor, H. W. White, R. S. Sanderson, Osler, Benson, A. P. Baines, Baker, Scott, Lane Pool, Dr Beronard, Wakefield.

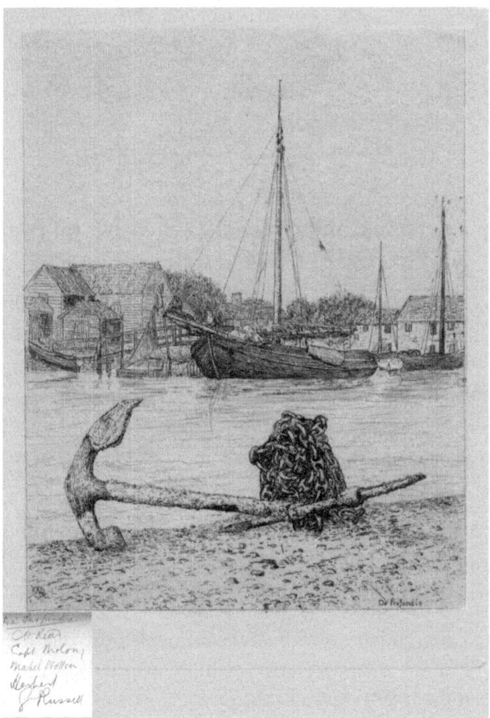


**Fig. 9.14** Gowers' sketch 'De Profundis'. Recipients listed: C. H. Read, Capt Molony, Mabel Wotton [novelist], Herbert, G. Russell.

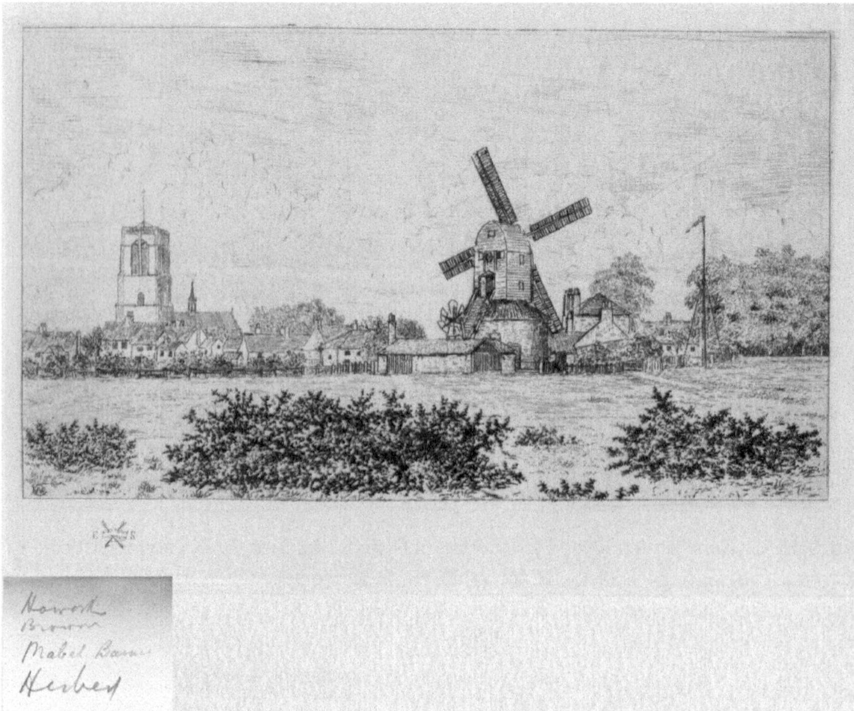

**Fig. 9.15** Gowers' sketch 'Windmill'. Recipients: Howorth, Brown, Mabel Baines, Herbert.

Gowers sent Haden an etching, and received a somewhat lukewarm response a few days later:

> I am greatly obliged by your kind present of your Blyth trawler and will bring it before the Council on the 27th, though being only one specimen of your art it will not conduce to your election. It is, however, full of quality and fine and delicate feeling, with a charming distance and an unusual sense of atmosphere. May I recommend you to get, if you can—I fear it is out of print—some early notes of mine 'About Etching'[15] since they will show you what I call the mental side of the art, and why you, of all people, surgeons and physicians should cultivate it.[16]

Gowers was not admitted into the society's exclusive membership.[17] However, when Haden was knighted in 1894 for his work as president of the Society of Painter-Etchers, Gowers wrote to congratulate him. Haden replied:

> I receive your kind congratulations with all the more pleasure that they are founded, if I may venture to say so, on an appreciation (wholly unusual) of the connection which really exists between the intellectual and the physical part of us, each part receiving—as you suggest it does—an exaltation from the other. For my own part I have always seen, or thought I have seen, a close connection between the two, and have preached that

connection continually, and have even gone farther in suggesting that by relying as much as possible on the natural way of the hand and as little as possible on the adventitious aid invented for its guidance we were setting up a habit of self reliance which we should find the greatest use to us as practitioners and, this being so, I should have been an arrant coward if I had not, in the face of a vast amount of prejudice, practised what I had preached.[18]

In 1894, Gowers sent Seymour Haden a copy of his short book exploring how the energy in an epileptic seizure was generated: the *Dynamics of Life*[19] (see Chapter 10), and received a further lukewarm and convoluted response:

I must not delay to thank you for the 'Dynamics of Life' because, after two attempts to make myself master of your views, I have failed to do so. That chemical action may be set up by vital energy—by the degradation of [?] which is the result of that energy I can understand; what I fear I shall never be able to take on is that chemical action or any other physical expression of force can take the place, or any part of the place, of the vital impulse which has its seat in the brain and which alone, I imagine, is capable of generating and evolving vital energy. Or, perhaps I have misunderstood you in supposing you think differently. Anyhow, I have been greatly interested in your paper and think it very ingenious if not very convincing, and am much more ready to attribute my non-acceptance of your views to my own stupidity than to any failure on your part to make them clear.

By the way—to descend to the dynamics of the etching impulse—have you anything to submit to me in that line? If you have, I am sure we shall see nothing mere chemical about it.[20]

Gowers had more success with the Royal Academy than with the Society of Etchers. In 1888 one of his drawings, 'Anchor boat at Walberswick', was exhibited at Burlington House and in 1896 reproduced in *The Artist*. Ernest wrote that it was one of the proudest days of his father's life when it was accepted by the hanging committee of the Royal Academy.

Gowers was unsuccessful with watercolours and never tried oils. Later in the 1890s he corresponded with another artist Charles Napier-Hemy about the use of colour in etchings. Hemy, said to be the finest marine artist of his generation, lived in Falmouth in a boat fitted out as a studio. He was probably one of Gowers' patients. When he was ill, Hemy wrote to say how drawing took his mind off his pain.

In 1887, the College of Physicians asked Gowers to commission a memorial painting of one of his old lecturers, Dr Wilson Fox, who had been professor of pathological anatomy at UCL, physician to UCH, and physician-in-ordinary to Queen Victoria. He approached Valentine Prinsep, writer and Pre-Raphaelite artist. The painting was exhibited by the Royal Academy in 1889. Prinsep added a postscript to one of his letters to Gowers:

But I wished to write to you a few words of admiration of your lecture at the reopening, or opening your Hospital, or rather of your instructive themes in print in full in the *Lancet*. I hope this is not a liberty, but it strikes me at once a philosophic exposition and a practical teaching concerning the deep mysteries of our organism as more and more fully revealed in our days. How amazing the subject, so expounded as you expound, is. It fills one with a sort of awe, such as David felt when he said 'I will praise thee; for I am fearfully and wonderfully made: marvellous are thy works; and that my soul knoweth right well'.[21]

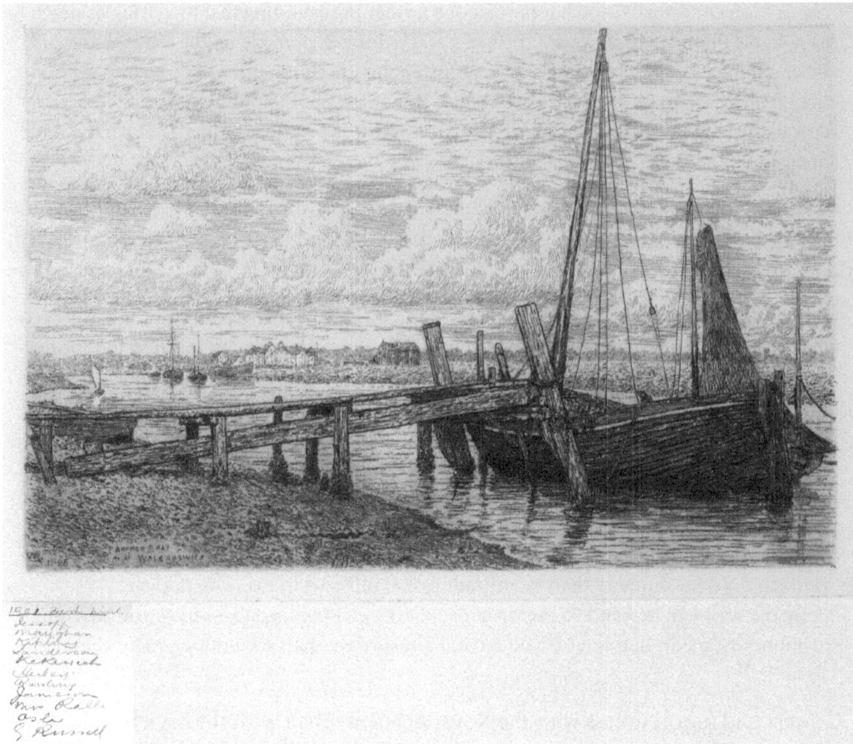

**Fig. 9.16** Gowers' 1886 sketch 'Anchor boat at Walberswick', hung in the Royal Academy in 1897. Recipients of '1901 fresh prints': Jessopp, Maugham, Kipling, Sanderson, Kekewich; Herbert, Rawlings, Jameson, Mrs Rolls, Osler, G. Russell.

## A 'clubbable' man?

Ernest wrote that Gowers was not a 'clubbable' man, but it seems that he was not quite as antisocial as his son recalled, especially in his later life. Duty compelled him to attend some obligatory social events, particularly the frequent fundraising dinners for the National Hospital, which may have seemed arduous. But he was also a member of a number of clubs or societies devoted to subjects that interested him, such as the Zoological Society of London (to which he was elected a fellow in 1895) and the Botanical Society. He used the Zoological Gardens for his research. In 1902 he sent his assistant to make dissections of the facial muscles of monkeys, which demonstrated that zygomatic muscles were present in animals though in a different form from those of humans, referring to what he called the 'myasthenic snarl' in his paper on 'Myasthenia and ophthlamoplegia'.[22]

Botany was also an enduring interest. Throughout his life Gowers maintained a keen interest in clinical pharmacology. He must have felt well-qualified in the field, because as early as 1878 he applied, though was unsuccessful in a close-run contest, for the chair in materia medica at UCL. Undeterred, he wrote several papers on medical therapeutics, and used bromides, arsenic, belladonna, eserine, chloroform, opium, chloral, cocaine, strychnine, and paraldehyde in his everyday practice. He was also a strong advocate of Indian hemp for several nervous disorders, as was his mentor Russell Reynolds. He continued his close interest in botany after he arrived in London, and was elected a fellow of the Royal Botanical Society in 1885.[23] He had an 'intimate knowledge' of mosses.[24] A paper he wrote on them has not survived.

But there were other clubs he joined which offered interesting and influential company, and while he may have joined them in order to help his career, to judge from his correspondence with friends, it does not sound as though he tried to avoid spending evenings there. In 1872, while still a bachelor, he joined the relaxed Savile Club, from which he resigned in 1881. The Savile was said to have been 'a little place for those aspiring to the dignity of membership of a certain club [the Athenaeum], reputed to be duller and more austere, to wait in'. The club was formed in 1868 to bring together men of different professions and opinions under 'a careful process of election'. Amongst its founders were Sir Norman Lockyer, pioneer of astrophysics, who also founded the journal *Nature* and London's Science Museum; the neurologist Charlton Bastian and the physiologist Michael Foster. Robert Louis Stevenson, Rudyard Kipling, and Charles Darwin were all members of the Savile.[25] Gowers was seldom seen there, preferring to stay at home with his young family when he was not concentrating on his career. However, when he was older, and his family was growing up, he was elected a member of London's exclusive Athenaeum Club. He was added to its waiting list in 1874 by Dr Sharpey, his old lecturer, and Leslie Stephen. Leslie Stephen, author, literary critic, editor of the *Cornhill Magazine*, and first editor of the *Dictionary of National Biography* was also an 'uncassocked clergyman who had lost his faith as a result of the *Origin* [*of Species*] and 'now admired Darwin as a god'.[26] His role in nominating Gowers comes as rather a surprise as there is no other evidence of them knowing one another, though they both lived in Bloomsbury. Gowers was seconded by Dr John Marshall, the man who beat Lister to the surgery chair at UCH in 1866 and in 1873 had become professor of anatomy at the Royal Academy.

When Gowers eventually became a member, in February 1890, 179 members voted for him, with two of the infamous 'black-balls' against him. Each 'black-ball' reduces the count by ten votes (men could wreak revenge over old feuds, as happened when Charles Darwin black-balled St George Mivart). The Athenaeum drew its members from men of achievement in science, literature, and the fine arts. It was here that Herbert Spencer and Francis Galton discussed their ideas on genetics in the smoking room after lunch. Spencer wrote that his election 'was an incident of moment to me, affecting greatly my daily life throughout the future', and he remained a member for 37 years. Spencer probably discussed biology with Gowers. He certainly wrote to him at one stage bemoaning the narrowness of scientists: 'the immense majority of writers in the special divisions of science have a horror of wide views, and prefer to limit themselves to their details and technicalities'.[27] Gowers left no record of his evenings at the Athenaeum, although it is clear that he used the club regularly and Critchley recorded that he enjoyed visiting the club and meeting men 'whose conversation was stimulating'. In 1894 he proposed his friend, William Osler, as an honorary member, a limited-term privilege for distinguished overseas visitors, having first met Osler when the Canadian physician visited Queen Square in 1878, and he also offered to nominate Rudyard Kiping as a member.

## Empire and adventure: Morrison, Jameson, and Kipling

Letters from Gowers to his young Australian friend George Morrison, and those he received from Rudyard Kipling, shed light on the generosity Gowers showed towards his friends. These friendships grew out of his innate curiosity. 'If I were to pick out my father's most outstanding characteristic' wrote Ernest, 'I think it would be his insatiable thirst for knowledge of every sort. Apart from drawing, the only form of recreation he really cared for was learning something fresh'.

Critchley wrote that Gowers played no active part in politics, and that it was doubtful whether public affairs or even medical politics interested him.[28] However, Gowers was enthralled by what he read and heard from contemporary explorers, scientists, and archaeologists. As Ernest recalled, he particularly enjoyed the society of 'people who had had unusual experiences' men such as George Ernest Morrison, Leander Starr Jameson, and Rudyard Kipling. These friendships drew him into imperial politics, even if only on the margin or behind the scenes.

### G. E. Morrison ('Morrison of Peking')

Gowers initiated his friendship with Morrison in 1895. Morrison, who later became famous as a journalist, traveller, and political adviser to the Chinese government, was nearly 20 years younger than Gowers. He epitomized the sense of adventure Gowers admired. By the age of 18 he had walked along the coast from Adelaide to Melbourne and taken a 1500 mile canoe trip alone up the Murray River. He started a medical degree at Melbourne University, but in 1882 his studies were 'rudely interrupted—because he recommended an excessive dose of medicament as a cure for syphilis at the intermediate examination'.[29] In 1883, at the age of 21, he was speared in New Guinea when he led one of Australia's earliest expeditions from Cape York across the Torres Strait. Nine months later he went to Edinburgh to have the tapering spearhead removed from his side, and in 1887 completed his medical degree in Edinburgh. He returned to China and travelled 3000 miles from Shanghai to Rangoon; spent the next two years as the resident surgeon in Australia, in a Ballarat hospital; and made another trek between China and Burma.

After returning to Britain, he completed his MD thesis on 'the hereditary transmission of malformations and abnormalities' in August 1895. He also published an account of his travels: *An Australian in China*.[30] Gowers read the book, which included observations of medical interest, a discussion of Chinese doctors, the prevalence of goitre, the medicinal use of narcotic drugs, and what Morrison concluded was the Chinese 'blunted sensory nervous system': 'No people are more cruel in their punishments than the Chinese, and obviously the reason is that the sensory nervous system of a Chinaman is either blunted or of arrested development'.[31] This type of speculation about inherent racial differences was not unusual at the time. In the eighteenth

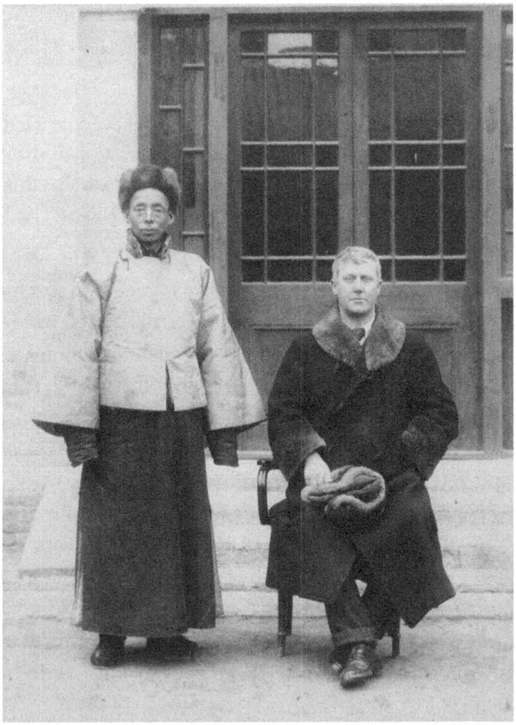

**Fig. 9.17** George Ernest Morrison with Sun Tienlu. Taken by S. Yamamoto in Peking, China, c. 1910. Reproduced with permission from Collection: Powerhouse Museum, Sydney.

century nervous diseases had been viewed in class terms, restricted to the upper classes. In his discussion on hysteria in the *Manual of Diseases of the Nervous System*, Gowers himself linked susceptibility to nationality or race, and the process of civilization:

> Both race and civilisation have probably more influence on the occurrence of hysteria than has been recognised or studied. It is almost unknown among barbarous races, and seems to be a product of the cerebral development that accompanies the process of civilisation. In certain stages of civilisation, peculiar forms of the disease have attained great development, as in Europe during the Middle Ages. Among races that have attained, apparently, an equal civilisation, hysteria reaches a higher degree in some than in others, in the French, for instance, than in the English; no doubt in consequence of the underlying differences in nervous constitution that are recognised in the expression 'national temperament'.[32]

Gowers was also interested in what Morrison had written about the use of opiates by the Chinese. He wrote to the young man suggesting they meet, and it proved a fruitful meeting for Morrison. He had always been interested in becoming a journalist, and when he arrived in England he had approached various newspapers offering himself as foreign correspondent, without success. At the time, Gowers was physician to the editor of *The Times*, George E. Buckle. Morrison had not approached *The Times* and Gowers offered a helping hand. Many years later, in a letter to Moberly Bell, manager of *The Times*, Morrison described what happened next:

> Who spoke of me to you I never heard for certain, but I believe that a letter written by Sir William Gower[s], the physician to Mr Buckle, or a conversation at the Athenaeum Club between Sir William and Mr Buckle, introduced my name which was then communicated to you. Then you wrote to me. You asked me to call upon you at *The Times* . . . [I] was astonished beyond measure to receive such a request.[33]

Gowers' intervention ensured Morrison's future career as a foreign correspondent. Buckle held a private dinner at which Morrison was introduced to Moberly Bell, a self-confessed 'radical with imperialist leanings' as well as Flora Shaw, his assistant manager. Shaw was a friend of Cecil Rhodes, and a highly influential writer for *The Times* promoting British imperial interests.[34] As a result of the meeting, Morrison was appointed as a special correspondent in Asia.[35]

Morrison's offhand reference to Gowers understates the efforts Gowers exerted on his behalf and the warm friendship he offered. The Gowers family welcomed Morrison into their home in 1895, and he often dined with them. Gowers urged him to learn shorthand before he set out again, and Edith took shorthand dictation from Morrison to help him submit articles to a publisher. They approached Henry Cockayne Cust, editor of the *Pall Mall Gazette* and were told that Morrison ought to go on his knees 'and pray for a political earthquake somewhere', because it would be pretty sure that he would be sent there.[36]

Not only did Gowers negotiate Morrison's meeting with Buckle and Moberly Bell, but he was also instrumental in setting up a 'secret' aspect of the arrangement through Sir Charles Wilson, director-general of military education at the War Office (who Gowers had probably met through the Royal Society).

> Sir Charles Wilson has offered to give you a note of introduction to the head of the Intelligence Department of the War Office. He thinks it is important that they should know of your journey and should tell you, without giving you any commission or putting you in any kind of relation to them—what information they need that should you choose you might give it to them on your return.[37]

The tone of the letters is covert: 'It has occurred to me that if you would prefer to have no direct communication with them it might be managed easily. Though I don't see that it matters if you are quite free and any information on return is quite voluntary'.[38] Just before Morrison left, at the end of November 1895, Gowers sent him notes, almost daily, with advice or requests. On the 19th he asked Morrison to go and see Sir Thomas McIlwraith, ex-premier of Queensland, who had gone to London for health reasons in 1893, and so probably was Gowers' patient. After Morrison had left London Gowers wrote, chiding him for not saying he was going via Paris: 'I would have got you to call on a man who resembles a baboon more closely than any human being I have seen in the flesh re the figure. But he is a very interesting man and much interested in you. He is and has been for long Blowitz' lieutenant in Paris' (Henri Blowitz was Paris correspondent for *The Times*; Gowers was probably referring to Blowitz' deputy, Wallace, who eventually succeeded him). Gowers urged Morrison to send articles for the journals of 'small societies'. However, it was not long before Morrison became a celebrity and needed no further help from Gowers.

The time delays were frustrating when the men corresponded. An exchange of letters could take nearly a year. In May 1896 Morrison wrote to Gowers; the letter arrived in London in September. Gowers met Buckle at the Athenaeum who told him Morrison was 'somewhere on the frontiers of China', so Gowers wrote again:

> Of course we spotted your letters to *The Times*. Edith at once recognised the story of your Algerian fellow traveller. I wonder so much what you are doing this Sunday evening Nov 15th! It seems so strange. Here is the back drawing room you know so well—there is the chair you used to sit in—there are the mother, Edith, Evie, just as of old, only I should say—just as, but older—actually by a year! ... Edith keeping up her shorthand, Evie keener than ever on her stamps but finding it harder to get those she hasn't got as her collection grows, and Edith keener than ever on her autographs. And myself? I jog along much the same. We had a good holiday at Falmouth and Cornwall, but a very sharp attack of influenza in October has taken the good away—followed, as it was by true gout, and convalescence hindered by a lecture at the College of Physicians. ...

Gowers speculated about Morrison's capacity for getting out of scrapes:

> You have a sort of charmed life. The only reasonable conclusion is that you have an eel-like integument when difficulty and peril tries to grasp you—chiefly due I think to your belief that it is so and to the effects of that belief. I shall have to extend my definition of the art of life. I have been accustomed to say that it is 'to anticipate the improbable' I ought to add 'to feel sure that the probable will not occur'.[39]

Although able to follow Morrison's articles in *The Times*, Gowers missed more personal news: 'When you write to anyone else I wish you would direct the letters to be sent to me for perusal'.

## Leander Starr Jameson

One of the men Gowers wrote to Morrison about was Leander Starr Jameson. The historian C. P. Fitzgerald wrote 'All men belong to the age of their lifetimes, and few if any escape the prevailing climate of opinion, prejudices, and assumptions'. Fitzgerald describes the age in which Morrison wrote as 'the heyday of the late phase of the British Empire' when 'to be an imperialist was no badge of shame; on the contrary it was a privilege conferred by the good fortune of being born a subject of the Queen':

> It carried duties also; Britain had a worldwide responsibility not only to the subjects of the Queen abroad, or in the colonies and overseas Empire, but to mankind, as a just guardian of the best interests of civilization, which were almost to be identified with those of the Empire itself.[40]

Gowers' friendships with Morrison, Jameson, and Kipling, show him caught up in this mood. Gowers had been one of Jameson's lecturers at UCH. Jameson had been an outstanding student who received a gold medal in materia medica. He was appointed resident medical officer after graduating with an MD in 1877, and became friendly with other medical men such as Jenner, Erichsen, and Russell Reynolds. However, in 1878 his health broke down from overwork, and hoping that a change of climate

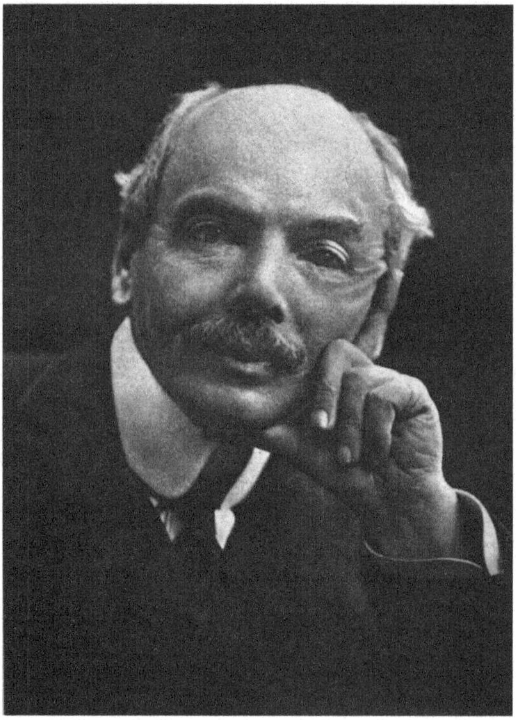

**Fig. 9.18** Leander Starr Jameson.

might help, he answered an advertisement to become the partner of a doctor with a large practice in South Africa. He made a great deal of money in the practice, much of which he lost through gambling. Not long after arriving in South Africa he fell under Cecil Rhodes' influence, becoming both 'the energetic instrument of Rhodes' vision' and also more interested in politics than medicine.

Rhodes had established the British South Africa Company in 1889, ruling under charter on behalf of the British crown. The company had powers that included the right to annexe and administer land. Jameson abandoned his medical practice in 1890 and accompanied the Pioneer Column, the army raised by Rhodes through the company, when it occupied Mashonaland. Afterwards he was appointed the company's administrator of both Mashonaland and Matabeleland. But administration bored him. One of his most harmful acts was land alienation, lavishly granting vast areas to men such as Sir John Willoughby, his military adviser.[41]

On 29 December 1895, he launched the short, abortive 'Jameson raid' into the mineral-rich Transvaal, ostensibly to protect the Uitlanders (primarily British migrant workers) from acts of aggression by the Boers. Hopelessly outnumbered, he surrendered to the Boers on 2 January 1896. His liberation army was captured and imprisoned in Pretoria. Rhodes is said to have complained that 'Old Jameson has upset my apple cart. Twenty years we have been friends and now he goes and ruins me'.[42] Whether this act was one of protection or part of a scheme of the British government or Cecil Rhodes (or both) to foment an uprising of the Uitlanders against the Boers was immediately and hotly debated.

The day after the raid *The Times* published a letter from Gowers defending Jameson as a cautious man who had never risked the lives of others rashly. Gowers argued that Jameson would have gone to protect lives, though ostensibly asked to help with the raid, and wrote that 'This will be found true unless all his past is untrue'.[43] However, later that year Jameson was tried and convicted at the Old Bailey for violating the legislation regulating mercenary activities by British citizens.

Before the trial started Jameson had time to write to Gowers about Russell Reynolds, who was dying. Jameson wrote that he had tried to see Reynolds some time earlier 'but even then he was too ill to see anyone ... Certainly now I should not think of intruding on him'. Reynolds died in May 1896.

Jameson was sentenced to fifteen months in jail, but was released early on the grounds of ill-health. His military commander, Colonel Willoughby, was sentenced to ten months. Jameson lived in the Burlington Hotel after his release, where Gowers tried to visit him without success, leaving an invitation to dinner, which was refused because Jameson felt that he could not go to any functions, public or private, until Willoughby had been released. Cecil Rhodes also stayed firmly out of the public eye in the Burlington. After the trial, Gowers again came to Jameson's defence through a letter to *The Times*:

> When the Jameson disaster was first announced you permitted me to call attention to the evidence his past career afforded regarding his probable motives. It may not be inopportune to mention now a fact which strikingly confirms the statement of his counsel that his object was to prevent the fighting which he believed to be inevitable. A few days after his arrival in this country Dr Jameson said to me, 'When I started it was with the feeling that, if a single shot was fired, I should have failed'.[44]

Gowers wrote an account to Morrison:

> You left, I think, before the Jameson raid. Just after his return, I got him to dine here with someone through whom the highest personage in the realm would at once hear his account. I heard the whole story, including some things that have never come out. Poor fellow. He has got through a third of his time at Holloway prison. It was the wildest of actions from the purest of motives—one of the mistakes that are catastrophic in their disaster. I taught him the beginnings of medicine.[45]

## Rudyard Kipling

As he had with Morrison, Gowers initiated his friendship with Kipling. He described how this happened in a letter to Morrison:

> I have made a new friend—made last April. Friends are very few in this world, and I think the word is right in the case of a man who wrote the other day to me before anyone after his relations to say 'It is a boy, a blockheaded boy' [on the birth of Kipling's son John]. You will understand my estimate of it when I tell you it is Rudyard Kipling for you will agree that an intimate friendship with him must be a precious thing. But what you cannot

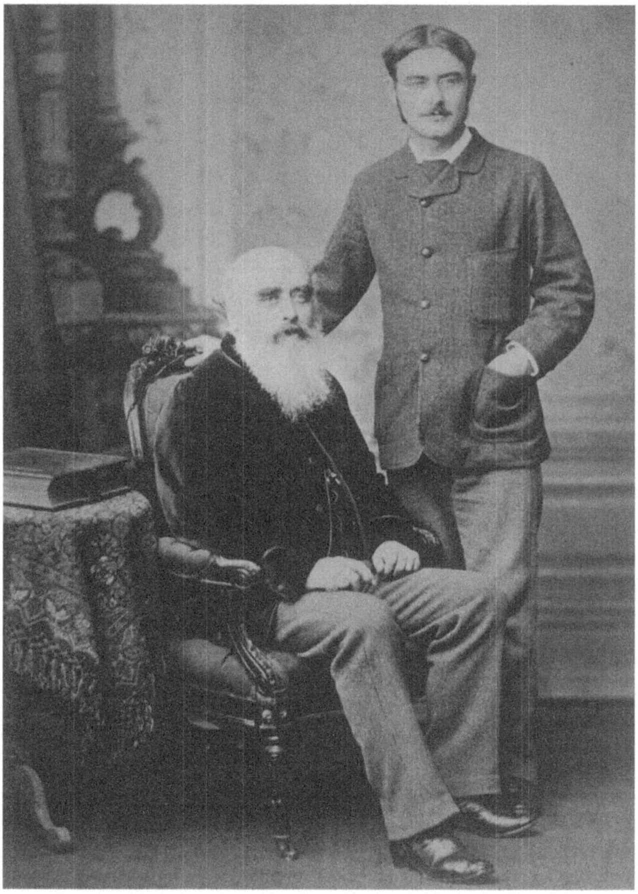

**Fig. 9.19** Rudyard Kipling with his father John Lockwood Kipling. Reproduced with permission from the National Trust and archive at the University of Sussex.

guess until you meet him, when he is 'free' as he always is with us. For he 'struck home' with all of us just as you did. Personally, he is everything that is brightest and finest and best in his writings only much more. Earnest, as his 'Recessional' in *The Times*, but ever bursting out in some flash, such a personality as I have never met the like of—revealing to me for the first time the full meaning of the word 'genius'.

It came about like this. A year or two ago I wrote to him in America to thank him for the rest his tales gave me and the letter pleased him. Last year he came to England to live near Torquay. One or two small services, very small, came into my head—a suggestion about the Athenaeum Club which was new and resulted in his special election last spring—advice as to local doctors which turned out to be most useful. So when I spent an Easter fortnight at Torquay we met and quickly became warm friends and he looks to me for guidance on matters medical and has stayed one night with us. I think I know him perhaps more thoroughly, partly through personal medical help, than anyone else except his father—you know how I talk frankly, and he responds as frankly. Think—he is only 33. 'Plain Tales from the Hills' was out before he was 19. You must know him when you come back.[46]

In January 1893, Kipling published his story 'Love-o'-women'. In it he describes locomotor ataxia, suffered by the central character Tighe. In their article on 'The medical Kipling' Vora and Lyons suggest that Kipling consulted Gowers when writing this:

> Kipling identifies the social stigma and shame attached to certain neurologic diseases and sexually transmitted diseases. He also shows the private suffering, guilt, and depression prevalent in patients with chronic, disabling, painful disorders. ... The diagnosis 'Locomotus attacks us' seemed well known, even to Tighe, who whispered it to the doctor. ... Kipling seems aware of the association between sexual promiscuity, syphilis, and loçomotor ataxia.[47]

Kipling, the authors suggest, would have become aware of this association either through Gowers or Sir William Osler. The fact that some time after the story was published Kipling sent Gowers a copy of his book of short stories, *Many Inventions*, in which 'Love o' women' was published, seems to confirm that it was Gowers.

In a discussion on differentiating between simulated or genuine epileptic fits, Critchley tells the story of a man falling into an attack of some sort in front of Russell Reynolds and Gowers who were walking down a street together. They did not know whether it was genuine or feigned. Gowers felt that the latter was likely 'though the choice of spectators may have been unintentional'.[48] It seems Critchley was right in suggesting that Gowers may have advised Kipling about the simulation of epileptic fits for the (undated) poem 'The post that fitted', about a man who wanted to extract himself from his engagement to a Miss Minnie Boffkin. The poem also ends with an allusion to one of the issues of the day, whether epilepsy is hereditary, discussed by Gowers in 1897 in a letter to *The Lancet*: 'Should epileptics marry?'[49]:

> Ere the steamer bore him Eastward, Sleary was engaged to marry
> An attractive girl at Tunbridge, whom he called 'my little Carrie.'
> Sleary's pay was very modest; Sleary was the other way.
> Who can cook a two-plate dinner on eight poor rupees a day?
> Long he pondered o'er the question in his scantly furnished quarters —
> Then proposed to Minnie Boffkin, eldest of Judge Boffkin's daughters.
> Certainly an impecunious Subaltern was not a catch,
> But the Boffkins knew that Minnie mightn't make another match.
> So they recognised the business and, to feed and clothe the bride,
> Got him made a Something Something somewhere on the Bombay side.
> Anyhow, the billet carried pay enough for him to marry —
> As the artless Sleary put it: — 'Just the thing for me and Carrie.'
> Did he, therefore, jilt Miss Boffkin—impulse of a baser mind?
> No! He started epileptic fits of an appalling kind.
> [Of his modus operandi only this much I could gather: —
> "Pears' shaving sticks will give you little taste and lots of lather."]
> Frequently in public places his affliction used to smite
> Sleary with distressing vigour—always in the Boffkins' sight.
> 'Ere a week was over Minnie weepingly returned his ring,
> Told him his 'unhappy weakness' stopped all thought of marrying.
> Sleary bore the information with a chastened holy joy,—

Epileptic fits don't matter in Political employ,—
Wired three short words to Carrie—took his ticket, packed his kit—
Bade farewell to Minnie Boffkin in one last, long, lingering fit.
Four weeks later, Carrie Sleary read—and laughed until she wept—
Mrs. Boffkin's warning letter on the 'wretched epilept'. . . .
Year by year, in pious patience, vengeful Mrs. Boffkin sits
Waiting for the Sleary babies to develop Sleary's fits.

In September 1896 Kipling had left the United States to resettle his American wife and two young daughters, Josephine and Elsie, in England. Initially they lived in Rock House, Maidencombe, near Torquay. However, they found themselves depressed and ill-at-ease in the house, and wondered whether the problem lay within themselves or with the house, concerned that it might not be built according to the oriental principles of feng shui. Kipling's biographer writes that it was at this time that he started 'the long chart of his clinical history' and went up to London to see a doctor.[50]

When Gowers suggested that Kipling might like to become a member of the Athenaeum Club, they corresponded about who might propose him for membership. Gowers was worried about whether he himself carried enough 'weight' with the members, to which Kipling replied:

> Very many thanks for the June A Committee list. I do not think that either Sidney Colvin or Walter Besant are at all unfriendly to me: and I fancy Lord Kelvin might assist but of this latter I am not at all sure. If Grant Duff has any kind of a memory he will not love me. It will be curious to see what the outcome of it may be. Personally, of course, I would sooner come up under your name than any other because it is to your kindliness I owe the suggestion: but you know best. My father John Lockwood Kipling, CIE is I think known by about every other man on the list. I don't know whether that would help at all.
>
> PS: It occurs to me with an awful distinctness that I have occasionally made light, in print, of His Excellency Lord Wolseley our present Commander-in-Chief and that in the ordinary course of things it may be necessary to do it again. Now the question is? ? ?[51]

Sir Sidney Colvin was an art and literary scholar, and museum administrator; Sir Walter Besant, a writer and campaigner for authors' rights; Lord Kelvin, a mathematical physicist and engineer. Grant-Duff, a politician, had been appointed by Gladstone as under-secretary for the colonies in 1880, and in 1881 governor of Madras. Viscount Wolseley had been appointed governor and high commissioner in South Africa with the rank of local general in June 1879: 'He attempted to intimidate the Boers of the Transvaal into an acceptance of annexation, and is therefore seen to have contributed to future difficulties in southern Africa'.[52] The issue of who should propose Kipling was resolved. In April 1897 he was elected, proposed by his uncle-in-law, Edward Burne-Jones and seconded by Henry James.

The Kiplings left Rock House in 1897 and moved to Rottingdean, in Sussex, to live with Rudyard's aunt 'Georgie' Burne-Jones and her husband. Kipling searched for suitable houses around Sussex and Kent in which to make a more permanent home as his wife was expecting another baby. Eventually they settled on The Elms, a house near the Burne-Jones's. Kipling appears to have consulted Gowers about the effect of the environment on his health.

> You are indeed a kind man. The note gives us just the sort of information we want to arrive at. We shall go out on a small tour of inspection in a few days but we shall be back here again before you come down. Houses—of sorts—are offered to us in scores but I have a reasoned horror of clay and India has taught me to sniff over any drains. There is a place (we are going to look at it) in the Isle of Thanet—near Minster St Nicholas at Wade they call it which has taken our fancy—but I am by no means sure of the wisdom of living on flat ground.

Gowers may have commented about a lack of trees in the Thanet area. Kipling wrote:

> You are indeed the kindest and most thoughtful of men, though what you say of 'St Niklus' makes me cold at my heart. I will not live without trees and I do not intend to go four miles every time I wish to see one cast a shadow. As to London, as things are at present the wife and I go up to town this morn; and straight to Ramsgate the same day to make a preliminary survey. We shall then find out what we don't need and after that shall settle down to the laborious work of finding what we do need. We shall only be in town on our return for a later afternoon and a night, this time. Will you please let me know where you stay when you come to Torquay and I will call as soon as you are at liberty. With many thanks for Dr Thornton's letter.

John Walker Gregory was another of Gowers' close friends. He had matriculated in 1886 having taken night classes at Birkbeck College, and was appointed assistant in the geological department of the Natural History Museum in 1887. In 1893 he was awarded a DSc for studies primarily in palaeontology. He had a passion for travel combined with scientific observation, writing *The Great Rift Valley* in 1896, and *The Dead Heart of Australia* in 1906. Gowers was anxious to influence an appointment to the British Museum, and they exchange letters on the politics involved. On 3 February 1897 Gregory ended one of his letters:

> In regard to the dinner you mention, it is too good to come off. I have an immense admiration for Kipling. I have a paper on him in hand. His 'Seven Seas' has entitled him to a grave in the Abbey as the poet of the Empire. The pathos of pioneer work, is the fate of the men, who spend their lives in a hard, unnoticed fight, and die quite unknown; while report-writing humbugs get all the credit of their labours. I do not know anyone else who has so fully realized, or at least who has proclaimed the fact, that the British Empire has been built up by the privates of the 'Legion never enlisted'. I tried to express it at the end of my preface, backed up quotations from Carlyle. I wish Kipling's 'Song of the Dead' had been published then. And then the accuracy of Kipling's geographical allusions is marvellous. The only things I can compare with them are Tennyson's botanical allusions which are all perfect. So to meet Kipling, Jameson and Hansen together would be a never-to-be-forgotten treat. I did not know you had been over Hansen's nerves. I hope they have held better than his Myxostoma conclusions. He seemed to work with marvellous patience and care, and yet his conclusions have not quite held.[53]

He was probably referring to the Norwegian physician, G. H. A. Hansen, who had described the leprosy bacillus (*Mycobacterium leprae*) for the first time on 28 February 1873.

From the letters it appears that Gowers acted as informal broker between Kipling, Walford Davies, and the music publishers Novello. According to his son, Gowers certainly 'knew nothing of music':

> The only music he cared to listen to was that made by his children, to whom he allotted instruments and teachers of them at an early age. But it was not because he enjoyed the music that he liked listening to them; the noises they made often, I fear, hardly deserved to be so called. It was because he took an almost childlike (and sometimes to them embarrassing) pride and delight in all his children's accomplishments, especially when they were outside the range of his own.

Walford Davies served as organist to a number of London churches, and later became Master of the King's Music. He was only 11 years older than Ernest, and may have taught him to play the organ, because Ernest himself became an accomplished organist. Gowers helped Kipling find a publisher for a musical setting by Walford Davies of 'Our lady of the snows' (1897), a poem written after the Canadian government had decided to favour imports from Britain. Kipling wrote:

> Yr letter and mine to hand: overleaf I send the authorization for Novello who, I see is a business man. As to Laurier—Prime Ministers come and go but Canada we hope will last: and moreover I've never dedicated anything outside my own family. All the dedications will do is to make people who don't like Laurier (there are many of' em) dislike the song. Don't let's import any side issues into this job. It's too important. I'm awfully glad Novello have jumped at Davies; and hope he'll do lots of good work for' em. Tell him to go ahead with a free mind; & vary and transpose as he pleases—so far as I'm concerned. I'm no musician. I'd sooner have Ernest represent my interests at a key board than myself; but make an appointment just now I simply can't!

Walford Davies reminded Gowers of this incident several years later, after Gowers' wife died.

> It is very long since we met. But our communications over Kipling's 'Lady of the Snows' (do you remember?) remain a most pleasant memory to me. I scarcely ever pass the Athenaeum without thinking of the evening (which you may easily have forgotten) when we drove with Kipling down to that august Club after dinner. Kipling had just been made a member. As we passed through the streets K exclaimed—'this is the grandest sight in the world'.[54]

Kipling and Gowers continued to exchange letters through the 1890s:

> I've been away for awhile and the result is a pile of letters as high as a hat-box. But before I tackle them I must make haste to thank you for the two little books. I think Dr Jessopp could do as big work as 'he had a mind to', to use an Americanism if he'd turn his mind in that direction[55], and your little volume[56] has given me a heap to think upon. You see, I use nerves largely in my business, and I think what you say about them is right. ...
>
> Dr Jessopp's opinion would be very horrifying if there was not always the blessed consolation that we are all, who live, much too close to people and things to take them at their proper values. Tisn't what I've done that is of any special use: it's what I've started a whole heap of other men to do that will in ten or twenty years begin to show itself. Wait till the young Canadian and Australian émigrés begin to turn up and then we shall see what we see! But, after all, the whole world is so bound together that it's futile and illogical for any one man to say that he did this that or t'other. We combine chemically.

Kipling had just sent Gowers *Many Inventions*:

> Your note must have crossed the copy of *Many Inventions*. I write in the stark bare end of chaos—we've packed up all our belongings and go to town tomorrow—consequently I may be a little confused. As to the 19th, I fear I can't accept your kind offer for the night: me being bound to return to my roost but chaperone me to the show you must or they'll cast me out: for in the turmoil of packing I've lost the R. S. Soiree ticket! What am I to do about it? Please advise me at the Savile, 107 Piccadilly. YES! This represents the joy with which we (I speak for Josephine and myself) will take Sunday rides to the Zoo! It's just what we want. Please send me some (tickets) soon as the children say.
>
> PS The darkness has rolled away like a cloud—only a few draggled edges left which I believe is the results of today's wintry weather. I'm a new man as to the lining of my head. Not so sure as to the lining of my guts which still complain.[57]

Kipling may not have enjoyed the soiree; he had a character in *Kim* (1901) say that 'Nine men out of ten would flee from a Royal Society Soiree in extremity of boredom'! Gowers took advantage of his membership of the Zoological Society of London to offer Kipling tickets to Regent's Park Zoo as an outing for his five-year-old daughter Josephine, the little girl to whom Kipling told animal stories at bed-time, stories which he published as the *Jungle Book* and were recently discovered to have been dedicated to her.[58]

## South African rest cure, and losing touch

By 1897 Gowers was so ill that he was ordered to take a complete rest. He had suffered severe back pain for a number of years, culminating in a breakdown at the beginning of the year.[59] On Kipling's advice, he chose to take a round trip to South Africa, sailing from Southampton on the Union Castle Line's ship *The Gaul* in July 1898.

Kipling had made the first of his annual pilgrimages to escape the British winter in South Africa at the end of January 1898, a time when tensions were rising between the Boers and the British, and his love affair with South Africa was just beginning. He had met Cecil Rhodes on a brief visit to South Africa in 1891 on his way to Australia. Like Jameson and Flora Shaw before him, he fell under the spell of Rhodes, and had dined with Rhodes and Milner when elected to the Athenaeum in April 1897. The Kiplings lunched with Rhodes almost as soon as they reached the Cape in January 1898, and Kipling was 'mesmerized'.[60] He wrote to Gowers afterwards:

> One doesn't (and you won't either) feel quite so earnest about WEG after a visit to South Africa. I wonder what I will think of Dr Jim [Jameson]. I've never met him; but I suppose we'll hear of him again. We saw a bit of Rhodes in Cape Town.[61]

'WEG', was the British prime minister, William Ewart Gladstone, who was opposed to military imperialism and was a strong supporter of minority rights. His government passed anti-slavery legislation which made life harder for the settlers. But he recognized the missionary potential of imperialism, supporting conversion rather than oppression.

At the time of Queen Victoria's diamond jubilee celebrations in 1897, Kipling was surrounded by his extended family, including the Burne-Jones's and Stanley Baldwin, his cousin, at Rottingdean. Rudyard Kipling later claimed that he wrote his famous poem 'If' ('If you can trust yourself when all men doubt you . . .') in 1895, in response to the news of the Jameson raid, although it was not published until 1910 (in *Rewards and Fairies*). However, his biographer, Lord Birkenhead, records that by 1897 Kipling had become worried about what he had heard about the Jameson raid.[62] But he had recovered enough from his Torquay depression to write his hymn, *Recessional*, to celebrate the diamond jubilee, and a number of poems in support of the British efforts in the Boer War. The Kiplings moved to The Elms shortly before the birth of a third child, their son John, in August 1897.

Willie Gowers had graduated from Cambridge in June 1898, and had not yet chosen a career. Gowers suggested that his son join him on the trip to South Africa and they sailed from Southampton on 2 July. Kipling urged them to stay away for three months to allow time for sightseeing ashore. Gowers did not take this advice, and the pair returned to England after only one month. 'Tradition relates' wrote Critchley 'that though enjoined to a regime of the strictest rest, he returned from this cruise with the second edition of his *Manual* rewritten, corrected and ready for press'.[63] However, Critchley thought that the trip took place in 1894. There is now no doubt that it was 1898, and that Gowers was revising the first volume ready for its third edition (fragments of the second volume of the *Manual* marked with Gowers' revisions for a third, but unpublished, edition found in the archives at Queen Square confirm that it was Gowers' work on the third edition that Critchley heard about).

Kipling promised to try to get to Southampton to see Gowers and his son off: 'Do you know that cabins on the starboard side of the ship going down are the best and do you know that deck-cabins in the winter which may be windy as you near the Cape are not admirable? There is a heap to learn even in modern seafaring'.[64] The travellers had interesting company on the journey out: Leander Starr Jameson, Dr Rutherford Harris, and Sir Walter Hely-Hutchinson. A parliamentary select committee had been appointed to examine the Jameson raid and whether members of the government, particularly the imperialist colonial secretary Joseph Chamberlain, had secretly encouraged it. Flora Shaw had had to explain telegrams between herself and Rhodes, which implicated her in collusion between Rhodes and Chamberlain. A number of men came back from the Cape to appear before the committee, including Harris, a man Rhodes had appointed secretary of the British South Africa Company when it was formed in 1889. Harris, like Jameson, was a qualified doctor whose indifferent health led him to practice in the Kimberley region, where he became closely involved with Jameson and Rhodes. He had helped to organize the Jameson raid. Hely-Hutchinson was a colonial administrator who had been governor-general and command-in-chief of Natal and Zululand since 1893. The Jameson raid and its aftermath did not seriously impede Jameson's career. He entered the Cape parliament in 1900, becoming prime minister of the Cape Colony from 1904 to 1908. In 1911 he was made a baronet, in 1913 became chairman of the British South Africa Company, and when he died in 1917 he was buried next to Cecil Rhodes in Matabeleland. But he remains a highly controversial figure in imperial history.

Perhaps it was the experience of listening to these men (particularly the persuasive Jameson) or the sight of Africa itself that cast a fateful spell on Willie for, not long after getting home to London, he returned to Africa to begin a career that eventually led him to enter the colonial civil service. He joined the British South Africa Company in

January 1899 and, with Jameson's strong support, was appointed first assistant native commissioner in Matabeleland. Willie and his father had been close, and had enjoyed travelling together to Cannes, and then South Africa. His father wrote to Morrison of the sadness losing his son to Africa had caused him:

> In the spring I had fallen into ill health so I became bold and took a return ticket to Natal. The voyage was purely pleasant and did me a vast amount of good. My eldest boy went with me, who had just taken a first class at Cambridge. Alas, he was badly bitten by S. Africa & nothing would satisfy him but to go back. Through Jameson he got a nomination to a post in the Native Commission and sailed in November and is now in a district near the Zambezi—much to my grief for he was and is fit for better things. It has been a real sorrow to me, but he was not too steady a worker and I had had my misgivings. My younger boy [Ernest], who has just finished at Rugby, is all I could desire in goodness and diligence.[65]

On his return to England in August 1898, Gowers went to stay at Hythe, in Kent, while he readjusted to being home. He had time to write to Morrison describing the trip:

> I am down here for three days to get let down gradually from sea to land before resuming work. I came ashore last Friday after 15,000 miles at sea! … I went round the Cape and up the coast to Durban, only sleeping ashore there & at Port Elizabeth. It has done me infinite good. I had the run of the hurricane deck, to which passengers are not admitted, and used to sit there day after day in quiet. We had not one wet day but just a taste of some days of very big head seas going out, & a full gale the night we left Durban. Oh I was sorry to leave the ship. I had Jameson for a companion going out and Sir Walter Hely Hutchinson the Governor of Natal, a charming man, sat opposite me at the Captain's table. Coming back the company was too much mixed, too many Johannesburgers, men and women. I met Miss [Mary] Kingsley of West African fame not long ago—a quietish pleasant young woman, not masculine as you might think. [James] Taylor is very well. I have had to associate him with me in editing the *Manual*, too big a task for me alone.[66]

To his obvious regret, Gowers gradually lost the close contact he had enjoyed with Morrison and Kipling, but for different reasons: the first being fame, and the second grief. Gowers wrote two more letters to Morrison, in 1899 and 1900. They almost plead for the continuing friendship of the now famous young man. In September 1899, he wrote:

> Having once got a glimpse of your most interesting personality and being constantly reminded of it by this or that, in *The Times* or elsewhere, I am sorrowed to lose all immediate touch with you. A year ago I wrote you a long, long letter, to which no answer has reached me. …
>
> We have been for a holiday to Scotland. The mother and I have come home first; the young ones are pursuing supplementary visits and return in a few days. How often they speak of you and wonder about you and how pleased we should all be to hear more directly from the famous Peking Correspondent of *The Times*. We are just now reminded of you afresh, because a Glasgow *Phonographic Monthly* is publishing at my suggestion your Ways of a Wanderer from the defunct *Phonographic Quarterly*. They copied your portrait out of one of the illustrated weeklies, in which there was no concealment about you.

> I am writing in the same old back drawing room and in one of its empty chairs your form would seem so natural. Evelyn is now going to a school at Eastbourne to be 'educated'. Edith is our precious mainstay at home.
>
> Did I tell you of my friendship with Kipling, established in the same kind of impertinent way as my friendship with you? I have not seen him since his illness but expect to do so in a day or two.

Morrison had visited London in 1899, but not been to see Gowers. When he returned for a break from his posting in China, he was lionized, and relished the attention of the influential set in London, commenting in his 1899 diary that all his 'old associates' seemed boring. This seems to mark the end of the friendship with Gowers. At the end of 1899 Morrison found himself in the middle of the Boxer Rebellion, and an inaccurate report of his death led *The Times* to carry a long obituary, to which Gowers contributed. He wrote his last letter to Morrison in November 1900 after the obituary appeared:

> My wife & daughters have repeatedly been asking me, 'Why don't you write & congratulate Dr Morrison on his return to life?' Well, I do so, & have done, heartily. I hope he liked his obituary notice in *The Times*, surely the pleasantest ever man yet was allowed by the fates to read. Buckle sent up to me for any information I could give him. But it was not much & the whole was a thoroughly spontaneous outburst of appreciation. I feared then that I had your death to answer for. Yet on consideration I could not believe I had had anything to do with it. If I had, I reasoned, my long letter to you of August 1898 would not have remained unanswered, nor should we have had the more than surprise of not seeing you when you came to London, tho' our back room was expecting you in vain each evening. When you next come to London you will be carried to the xth degree—or nth degree. An evening paper has had a special paragraph on the extent to which you will be lionized. You have certainly achieved an absolutely unique position of any of the Foreign Correspondents of the world & seem to be admired in every European country as much as in England. …
>
> Of course we have read with avidity everything about you and Peking & all the books about China from Walton below to Scudmore in the middle. The last and Milford give the best idea of Peking life. But how much there must be to make you angry & desire to smash things in general & in particular. Evelyn is at school in Eastbourne. Ernest is at Cambridge. Willie looking after natives by the Zambezi. Edith our home mainstay. All send kind regards and forgiveness.

Morrison remained resident correspondent for *The Times* until 1912, when he became political adviser to the president of China from 1912–20, and represented China during the peace discussions in Versailles in 1919. However, he was already ailing, and died in England in 1920.

Kipling's illness, alluded to by Gowers in his letter to Morrison, was the pneumonia that nearly killed him, and did kill his adored six-year-old daughter Josephine. He and both his daughters had become ill while in New York. Elsie recovered, but Josephine died in March 1899. Grief at her death led Kipling to retreat from his friends. Kipling and Gowers had remained in touch and Kipling had sought Gowers' advice when his sister Trixie (Alice) had shown the first manifestations of a serious illness in 1898. Her 'brilliant mind had been temporarily disordered' and she came back from India, where she had been living with her husband, an army officer. Gowers arranged for her to come under the care of an experienced nurse. But Trixie Fleming wanted to be with her mother and the nurse felt that she could be of little service once Trixie had moved to her parents' house. Gowers sent a report to her husband giving a thorough overview of his assessment of the case. The letter ends with a request for a fee, providing the only hint of Gowers' consulting rates:

> When I saw your wife Mr Kipling paid me the fee of two guineas. I have had, since, a great amount of correspondence and anxiety about the case. I do not care to mention fees to Mr Kipling, since I undertook the case, in the first instance, at the request of Rudyard. I do not know whether you care to be under a moral obligation to him for my help. Otherwise the minimum fee I can say is fifteen guineas, which is leaving out of account a visit to Brighton to talk over matters with Rudyard which may go down to the service of friendship.[67]

Kipling's sister suffered a series of nervous breakdowns. Eventually, to the dismay of some of her relatives, she made her name as a psychic, under the pseudonym Holland, as a result of her experiences in 'automatic writing'.

Kipling and his wife had found their ideal house, 'The Elms' in East Sussex, and had been looking forward to moving in, but their joy was short lived. Josephine's death may not have been the end of the friendship, but Gowers was becoming increasingly ill himself, and Kipling may not have wanted reminders of the visits to the zoo that

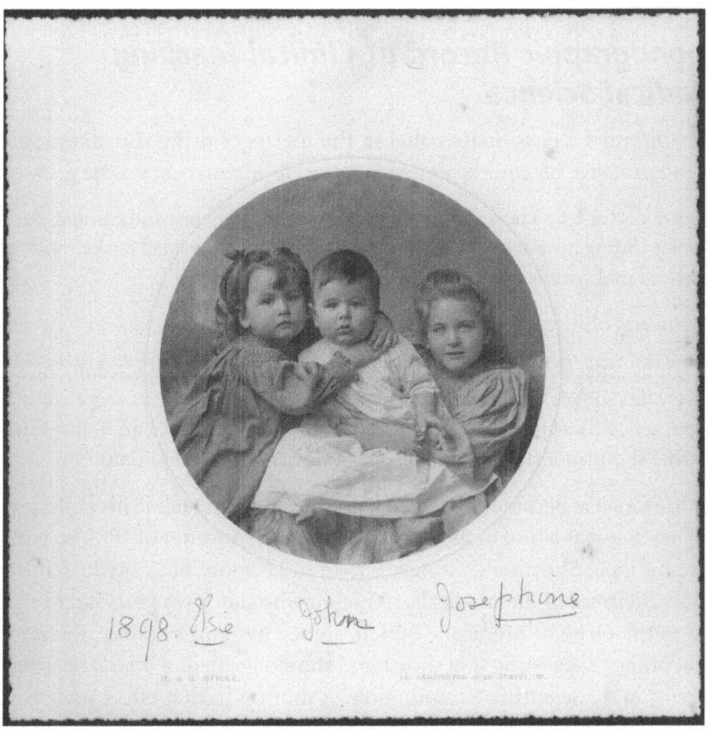


**Fig. 9.20** Kipling's children. Reproduced with permission from the National Trust and archive at the University of Sussex.

Gowers had arranged for Josephine. Kipling's cousin, Angela Thirkell, wrote that much of the 'Cousin Ruddy' she knew as a child died with Josephine. No one could talk to him about Josephine after her death.

The last surviving letter from Kipling to Gowers is dated 7 August 1902, just as Kipling and his wife were about to move into the house they would inhabit for the next 34 years, 'Bateman's', in the village of Burwash, East Sussex. It was a better retreat than Rottingdean:

> Yes, we migrate in a month or two: and for the reason that you suggest. But we are a few miles south of Tunbridge Wells in a heavily wooded land: and the Lord he knoweth when we can get in to our new diggings. The wife is being daily massaged for the pain in her arm (the other pain has altogether disappeared for the past two months) and I think that she is better. Certainly the detail of arranging about the other house amuses and interests her. That is good news about Ernest [just awarded a first in the Classics Tripos], and I hope your Zambezi boy didn't bring home too many fever microbes with him. Sometimes English air makes' em up most potently. Please give our best love to all your people and believe me. Yours affectionately, Rud.

Artist William Rothenstein commented that Kipling became stiff and unapproachable when they saw one another at the Athenaeum.[68] Perhaps Gowers felt this too. But by the mid-1890s Gowers' illness had also left 'indelible marks' on him, and he began to look older than his years. He, too, may have started to retreat.[69]

## The *Phonographic Record of Clinical Teaching and Medical Science*

Gowers maintained a passionate belief in the merits of using shorthand in medical research and practice, becoming almost fanatical in his advocacy as he grew older:

> Any young doctor who knew shorthand at once won his interest and commendation. At the bedside during his ward rounds he would often produce a small pocket-book and jot down a few rapid symbols recording an unusual point.[70]

In 1915, Gowers' obituary in the *BMJ* recorded that:

> In a previous generation, when neurology was more feared than studied in England, if a man knew this subject well, and especially if he carried an ophthalmoscope ready for use in his pockets, he was probably an old student at Queen Square, and if, in addition, he could write shorthand, almost certainly one of Gowers' house physicians.[71]

In later life Gowers became distracted by his desire to persuade his colleagues of the merits of shorthand as a tool in medical science. In the autumn of 1887 he participated in the International Shorthand Congress held in London, but noted ruefully that he was the only member of the medical profession who did. Two years later he prepared a petition to the General Medical Council, signed by Jenner, Lister, Richard Quain, and several others, suggesting that shorthand should be made a 'mark-bearing' subject for the Preliminary Scientific Examination. A motion to that effect was proposed to the council by Sir Dyce Duckworth, treasurer of the Royal College of Physicians, and seconded by Mr Wheelhouse of Leeds. However, as they were the only two council members who supported it, the motion failed.

In 1889, Gowers enlisted the help of Duckworth, Howard Marsh, and Dr Sidney Coupland in establishing a voluntary examination in shorthand for medical students, with prizes attached. Sir William Jenner and others helped to fund the project. Eight out of the 11 students who sat the exam in October 1889 passed. The £5 prize was awarded to Mr Caiger for an article submitted from South Africa. However, few students showed any interest, and the exam was not repeated.

In 1892 Gowers attended a special dinner to celebrate the 'phonographic jubilee' of Mr T. A. Reed, Sir Isaac Pitman's biographer, attended by 'ladies and gentlemen interested in phonography'. Reed had been stenographer to the Council of the British Medical Association for many years, and in 1895 would travel to India to record the proceedings of the controversial Royal Commission on Opium in India. Isaac Pitman presented Reed with an illuminated address and 'purse of 200 guineas' and praised Reed for his persistent advocacy of phonography over 50 years.[72]

Gowers was not prepared to give up his own persistent battle, and in 1894 he published two issues of a small shorthand periodical the *Phonographic Record of Clinical Teaching*. Contributors included Marcus Gunn, William Osler, and the dermatologist Dr H. Radcliffe Crocker. Gowers was so convinced of the significant role medical shorthand could play that he and his colleagues completed the 'arduous'[73] task of devising a list of 2500 specialized medical shorthand outlines, an undertaking he had originally suggested to Pitman while still an apprentice in Coggeshall. This list provided a standard 'outline' for each medical term to enable published shorthand medical articles to be written using consistent shorthand forms to help guarantee they would not be misread.

Gowers included a letter in the first issue of the *Phonographic Record* reminding readers of the noble history of shorthand schemes, such as that created by the 'great Roman orator Cicero', and Dr Timothe Bright's 'short, swift and secret' English shorthand system (for which Queen Elizabeth granted a form of royal copyright in 1588). Samuel Pepys, another early shorthand writer, used Sheldon's shorthand to record his notes on the Great Fire of London and the Great Plague.

After receiving expressions of interest from 150 medical men, the Society of Medical Phonographers was established later that year, by Gowers, a Dr Gray (of Oxford), and Dr Neil (of the Warneford Asylum, Oxford). Gowers became the first president. By April 1895 there were 139 members of the society, rising to 248 the following year. In January 1899 Gowers was succeeded as president by Sir William Thomson, the president of the Royal College of Surgeons of Ireland. Thomson was followed by David Ferrier, who held the position from 1903 until 1908. Gowers was then appointed for a second term, but dwindling membership forced the society to fold in 1912.

Gowers sold 120 copies of the first issue of his journal, which was soon renamed the *Phonographic Record of Clinical Teaching and Medical Science* in order to extend its range. It lasted for 17 issues, eventually ceasing publication in 1911.[74] The *Phonographic Record* contains lectures and articles by many of Gowers' contemporaries, as well as a miscellany of obituaries, clinical reports, reports from abroad, and jokes under the heading 'The humours of medicine'. Altogether just over 300 articles were published. The articles, such as university lectures, had often already been published in the standard journals. However, some were also written specifically for the *Record*, including a series called 'Problems of practical diagnosis' by Gowers himself. The impression one

Chapter 10

# 'Grand old man' of clinical neurology

## Queen Square in the 1890s

In 1893 the Queen Square board conferred on Gowers the title of 'extra physician'. In an undated letter to Burford Rawlings, Gowers had written to say that he was 'vexed' not to be able to get to the hospital that day, and had come to the conclusion that he should cease to attend in the outpatient room, 'light as the work is made by the consideration of my colleagues and yourself'.

He was still at Queen Square when the next generation of neurologists, including James Taylor, James Collier, Risien Russell and Kinnier Wilson, joined the staff.

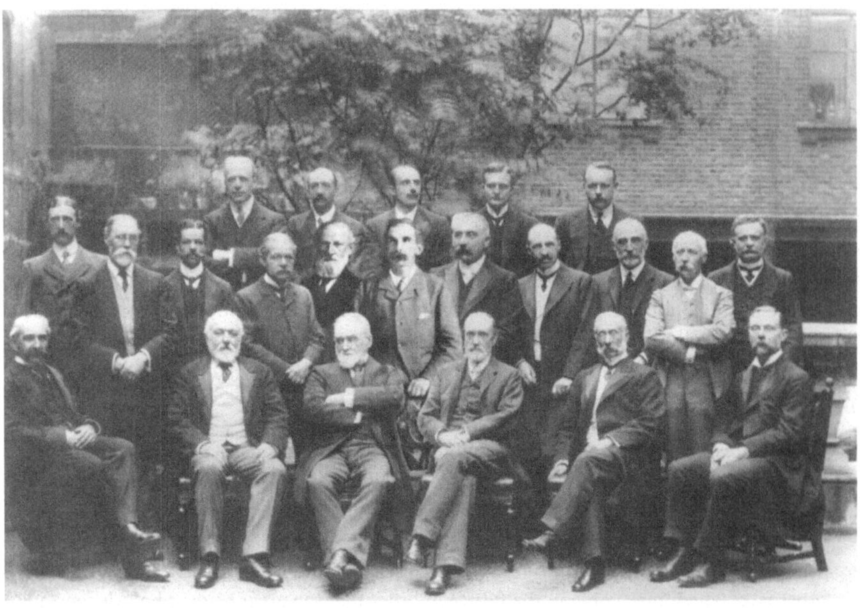

**Fig. 10.1** Staff of the National Hospital, 1906. Back, left to right: Armour, Batten, Collier, Sargent, E. F. Buzzard. Middle, left to right: Tate, Beevor, Risien Russell, Cumberbatch, Gowers, Horsley, Ballance, Aldren Turner, Taylor, Gunn, Tooth. Front, left to right: Semon, Thomas Buzzard, Hughlings Jackson, Bastian, Ferrier, Ormerod. Image courtesy of the Queen Square Library, Archive and Museum.

Gowers was extremely fortunate that Dr James Taylor became a colleague in 1893, at a time when his health was deteriorating and he desperately needed help in his practice. Taylor became a close personal friend and colleague of both Hughlings Jackson and Gowers, and worked closely with Ferrier, Horsley, and Gunn. He not only assisted Gowers in his consulting rooms, he prepared the index and helped revise and correct the proofs of the 1893 second edition of Volume 2 of the *Manual*. He played a major role in preparing the 1899 third edition of the first volume, and was listed on the title page. He probably helped Gowers to prepare the third (unpublished) edition of Volume 2.

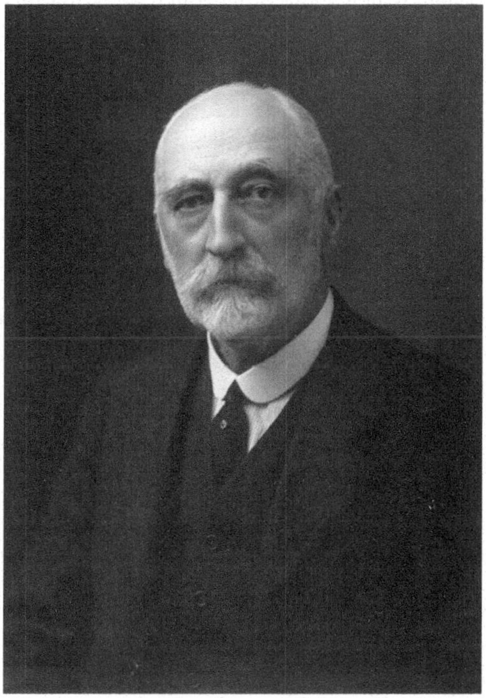

**Fig. 10.2** Dr James Taylor. Image courtesy of the Queen Square Library, Archive and Museum.

In 1905 J. & A. Churchill published Taylor's *Paralysis and other Diseases of the Nervous System in Childhood and Early Life*, in which he wrote in his Foreword:

> To Sir William Gowers' kindness and friendly advice I am indebted almost as much as to his teaching, and I have to thank him for the suggestion that I should write this book. I wish I could have brought it up to the high standard which I know he exacts from himself.[1]

Most of Hughlings Jackson's unpublished or personal papers were destroyed, on his instruction, when he died. In 1925 James Taylor edited the series 'Neurological fragments' that Hughlings Jackson had published in *The Lancet* between 1893 and 1909, for publication as a book, and played a major role in producing the two-volume publication, *The Selected Writings of John Hughlings Jackson*, in 1932.[2]

Another addition to the Queen Square staff was James Collier, who became clinical clerk to Thomas Buzzard in 1894. He was interested in the miscellaneous disorders which Gowers had described as 'ataxic paraplegia', and was probably responsible for introducing the term 'motor neuron disease'. James Risien Russell, born in Demerara (now part of Guyana), became resident medical officer in 1898. Early in his career he collaborated with Horsley on neurophysiological problems such as the cortical representation of the larynx, but later concentrated on his large clinical practice and on teaching. He was one of the few Queen Square physicians who took an interest in the care of patients with neurasthenia and other functional somatic syndromes. Risien Russell would have learned much from Gowers, both in the style of outpatient teaching and in the outstanding clarity of his writing. Risien Russell was appointed to the staff against close competition from Henry Head. Gowers wrote to Horsley about the appointment:

> A time at the museum, where the promise of original research is bright, & the important work of developing it, will be, I think, better for him [Risien Russell] than going straight on the staff. I have said nothing to anyone & have heard nothing from anyone except one about Head since I saw you. But the voting was a curious confirmation of my impression. Of this, indeed, I felt somewhat ashamed when I came to consider its cause. As far as I could discern it was simply that, whenever I spoke to Head about any subject (or rather he spoke to me) I always felt that I knew *nothing* about it & was only too glad to escape. I came little into contact with him. I think I remember hearing, formerly, that those who did had an analogous feeling about practical matters. Every one recognises his great ability. If you ask Russell I think he will say that he regards no one as a stauncher friend than I am.[3]

Head went on to have a distinguished career at the London Hospital, Whitechapel, and for 15 years was editor of *Brain*. Purdon Martin considered Risien Russell to be the brightest of all the staff, a phenomenal lecturer and an excellent diagnostician with a good bedside manner.[4]

Samuel Kinnier Wilson became Queen Square's resident medical officer in 1904, and remained on the staff there and at King's College Hospital for thirty years. He was an inspiring teacher with a particular interest in the basal ganglia (he coined the description 'the dark basement of the brain') and neuropsychiatry.

Gordon Holmes, who recorded much of the early history of Queen Square, was appointed in 1909, so barely overlapped with Gowers. Kinnier Wilson and Holmes were considered the greatest of the second generation of neurologists at Queen Square. Macdonald Critchley did not join the staff until 1929, fourteeen years after Gowers' death.

In 1893, Gowers, together with Hughlings Jackson, Ferrier, four other doctors, and a group of philanthropists, had been one of the founding members of the National Society for the Employment of Epileptics (now the National Society for Epilepsy), which planned to create a colony for people with epilepsy on the model of a similar institution in Bielefeld, Germany. By 1894 they had raised sufficient funds to buy a farm in Chalfont St Peter, north of London, as 'a home for such epileptic persons as are capable of work but unable to obtain regular employment on account of their

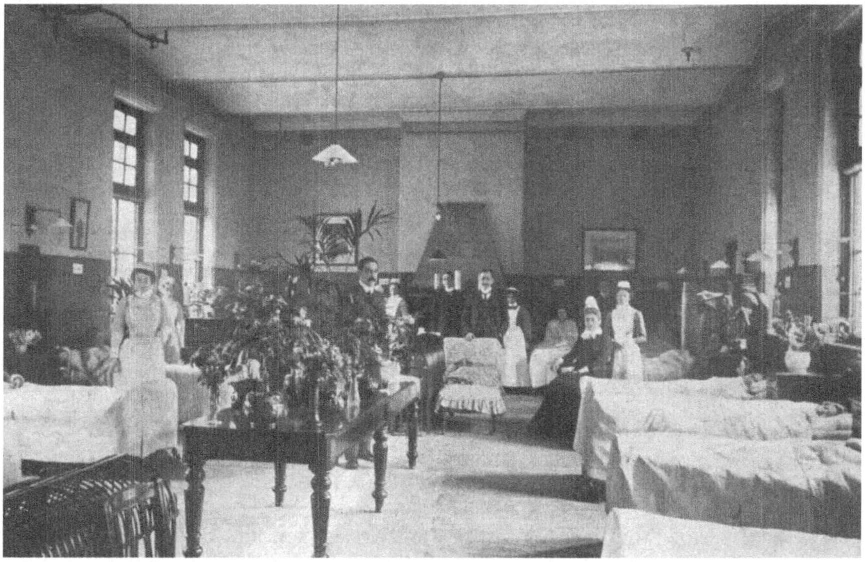

**Fig. 10.3** A Queen Square ward (1888). Image courtesy of the Queen Square Library, Archive and Museum.

liability to fit'. The Chalfont Centre for Epilepsy flourished, and now has the 'Sir William Gowers Assessment Centre', which offers inpatient assessment for patients with uncontrolled refractory epilepsy.

## Accommodating to new scientific discoveries

Gowers' intellectual curiosity never dimmed, and in later life he frequently applied new scientific discoveries outside his field to enhance the understanding of clinical neurology, in later life giving lectures on the 'new neurology', the 'dynamics of life', 'abiotrophy', and 'heredity'.

### *The Dynamics of Life* (1894)

In October 1894 Gowers addressed the Medical Society of Manchester on 'The dynamics of life'. His colleague Charlton Bastian's doomed and undying support for the notion of spontaneous generation (abiogenesis) may have influenced his choice of topic, but Gowers was much more interested in explaining the energy generated during an epileptic fit than solving the mysteries of evolution, and was intrigued by the recent research by physicists on atomic and molecular structure, and searched for the origins of the 'tremendous energy manifested in a typical epileptic seizure'.[5] He opened his lecture in his customary engaging fashion:

> At Manchester—second in England only to the metropolis as a medical centre and source of knowledge—it is, I conceive, superfluous for me to apologise for taking a theoretical

> subject for such an address as that which I have the honour to give tonight. I need hardly remind you that between what we term 'theory' and 'fact' the transition is gradual; that much of that which we regard as fact is only fact to our thought. Observation alone is certain—observation pure and simple. The interpretation of observation introduces uncertainty in proportion to the extent to which inference is involved; to this we are often blind—blind sometimes to its existence, generally to its amount. But there is a region in which we must recognise hypothesis as absolute. It is the region below the surface whence no reflected light can pass, but whence all observed phenomena proceed.

He declared himself a 'trespasser':

> I shall have to pass into regions where I have no strict right to be, but into which I go because from them come the streams that water our own province. ...
>
> The features of an epileptic fit make us ask, more than even the swift motion of the race-horse, whence and how is the intense manifestation of energy which by its violence makes the result so impressive and so alarming? But the wonder makes us ask a like question regarding analogous manifestations of energy in health equally marvellous in the humming-bird and the elephant.[6]

He briefly described the physical and chemical processes by which energy is generated in inanimate processes such as the burning of coal, then proceeded to consider the molecular mechanisms involved in muscle contraction. He pointed out how little was known about how nervous energy was transmitted, and suggested that Cajal's theory about neurons being composed of fibres indicated that the answer lay in a chemical action, rather than electricity (comparing the storage of electricity in batteries by chemical means). He explained the speed at which nerves could conduct by comparing it with the speed with which a train of gunpowder, when lit, causes an explosion.

Conscious that he was sailing on unfamiliar seas, for both the audience and himself, he proceeded slowly, avoiding jargon and technical terms, explaining the modern concepts of physics and atomic chemistry, before returning to more familiar anatomical ground. He concluded, based on the recent histological discoveries, that the dendrites of the spongy grey matter were the likely source of nervous vitality. He speculated that a distinct chemical process was also likely to be important in conducting nerve impulses from one nerve cell to the next.

He briefly considered disease states, and discussed the biophysics of excitation and inhibition in relation to epilepsy, anticipating the concept of kindling, suggesting that seizures were likely to result from a magnified discharge due to a subtle change in the molecular composition of the nerves:

> And so, gentlemen, in mystery we begin—and end. Was it not Coleridge who said, 'In wonder all knowledge begins, in wonder it ends, and admiration fills up the interspace'? Not altogether true, nor everywhere; and yet who is there that does not feel that an earnest effort to perceive that which is unseen leaves him on a higher level, and if he is still at his old standpoint, he has a better view. ... Search as we may, with eyes however earnest and however aided, that which we call 'Life' eludes our search and resists our efforts.
>
> We may, indeed, trace the relations to vitality of matter and of the energy it bears—their entrance into the domain of Life, their exit, their effects. We see them dimly shadowed

> now and then within the luminous mist, but the mist obscures our sight, and the light it radiates hides by its own brightness. We must be content with what knowledge we can gain, secure or insecure, and, while using it as best we may, should realise, in all humility, how much there is we cannot know, and yet we cannot doubt.[7]

## 'The new neurology' (1899)

Five years later, in 1899, Gowers delivered a lecture at Queen Square on 'The new neurology' in which he explained how his understanding of nervous disease had been radically changed by the new insights into neuronal histology revealed with the help of Golgi's silver stains and expounded by Ramon y Cajal in his 1895 Croonian lectures.[8]

In the introduction to his *Manual*, Gowers had written that nervous diseases had been divided, in an approach prevalent at the time, into either 'organic' or 'functional'. 'Organic' nervous diseases were identified by the presence of a visible macroscopic lesion, whereas 'functional' disorders were those in which where there was a physiological disturbance which could be transient or temporary. Gowers knew that a large number of diseases did not fit easily into either of these groups. He became convinced that this 'new neurology', which involved histopathological examination of the nervous system, would not only broaden the range of organic nervous disease but, significantly, shed light on hitherto cryptic pathogenic processes.

Ramon y Cajal had shown that the central nervous system was made up of a complex web of cells in which the cell processes of one nerve cell were linked functionally, but separated structurally, from those of another by small gaps. Each nerve cell (neuron) was made up of three units, the cell body, the long medullated fibrillary cylinder, the axon, with its fine collateral branches arising near its termination, and thirdly the branching dendrites in the grey matter arising from nerve cell bodies and with some of their ramifications covered in knob-like arrangements. Based on the observation that a relatively minor nerve impulse (for instance the afferent path of the knee-jerk) could elicit a much greater response, Gowers thught that the process of transmission from one nerve cell to the next must be chemical (and at times 'explosive') in nature.

Based on the idea that the nucleus of each cell is its 'life centre' and that the cell body is essential for the survival, maintenance, and repair of the nerve cell processes, Gowers thought that much of the normal working of the brain and some of its disorders could be explained by physical retraction and re-extension of nerve-cell processes. This was the idea he had used to explain the mechanism of inhibition in the production of epileptic seizures (as mentioned earlier). The demonstration of intracellular fibrils that could be seen to continue through the length of neurons also led him to the conclusion that small packets of atomic nerve impulses generated in the dendrites could travel along these fibrils to result in the whole neuron's output energy, while the gap between one neuron and the next allowed a flexibility in responding to external influences and thus could modify the behaviour of the nervous system.

## Abiotrophy

In February 1902 Gowers introduced the notion of loss of neuronal vitality to explain the causes of many cryptic neurological disorders.[9] He apologized for coining a new term, 'abiotrophy' (a lack of vital nutrition) to describe this process and drew an analogy with the development of grey hair or baldness. The cause of some nervous disorders had previously been ascribed to sclerosis, a fibrotic thickening of nervous tissue due to neuroglial proliferation, rather than the accompanying dying back of the nerve cells from their axonal terminals. 'Abiosis' was a convenient name for a process in which certain systems of structure had an essential defect of vital endurance leading to a slow but inexorable failure of function. Gowers singled out paralysis agitans (Parkinson's disease) as a particularly vivid example of a senile abiotrophy. The absence of a demonstrable lesion in the brain or spinal cord, and the apparent preservation of motor neurons, led him to speculate that disturbed chemical processes in the dendrites of the grey matter could lie at the root of the disease. He suggested that Friedreich's ataxia and muscular dystrophies were examples of abiotrophies presenting in early life, and a final group consisted of disorders like locomotor ataxia where a specific toxic agent was suspected.

Gowers was trying to explain the constitutional influence on disorders where biological inferiority of certain organs led them to wear out prematurely. The processes underlying selective vulnerability of regions of the brain remain an important line of scientific enquiry in neurological disease, and the dying back of the neuronal projections in the brainstem is believed to be involved in explaining neuronal death in both Alzheimer's and Parkinson's disease. The term is now restricted to veterinary medicine. A condition 'cerebellar abiotrophy', for example, is found in some breeds of horses and dogs.

## Heredity

The study of the role of genetics in human disease was in its infancy when Gowers was practising but he was aware of the potential importance of heredity in many nervous diseases, particularly for the group of conditions that he had described as early abiotrophies. He concluded that Huntington's disease and the heredo-ataxia described by Pierre Marie were indisputably genetic disorders. He wrote of the need to probe deeper into the family history and when appropriate examine supposedly unaffected siblings before rejecting genetic influences. Gowers anticipated monogenetic forms of paralysis agitans and Graves' disease, based on the strong family history present in some cases. He concluded that genetics, like histopathology, would inevitably lead to a new classification of nervous disease. He cautioned against thinking that genetics alone would elucidate the cause of a disease, suggesting that the underlying cell biology would also need to be understood:

> The difficulties of precision and fullness of knowledge are great and the chance fertilisation, from which the flowers of Mendel were guarded by his paper bags, is the rule in the human race, unalterable by us, however we may wish. Hence it seems useless even to apply the hereditarian terminology to facts that are in general inconsistent with its grounds. I can only hope to present a few of the general facts of heredity in some diseases of the nervous system, well known as they are, and I trust that they will be supplemented by others. We are only in the stage of random observation.[10]

## 'Gowers' eponyms

Like Hughlings Jackson, Gowers shunned the limelight (except when he was lecturing). He also disapproved of the practice of attaching eponyms to any medical discovery, particularly because of the difficulty it presented to students:

> This system of nomenclature is full of inconvenience, increasing the difficulties of the student, and leading to frequent mistakes in scientific writings. There are very few observations in medicine regarding which it is not obvious that they would speedily have been made by some one other than the actual observer: that it was very much of an accident that they were made by certain individuals. Scientific nomenclature should be itself scientific, not founded upon accidents. However, anxious [as] we may be to honour individuals, we have no right to do so at the expense of the convenience of all future generations of learners.[11]

Despite Gowers' disapproval, it is not possible to ignore the fact that his name is firmly fixed in the language of neurology.

### Gowers' sign

Using Gowers' sign to confirm proximal weakness of the extensor muscles of the thighs is still a standard component of neurological examination in the muscular dystrophies. The patient is asked first to lie on the floor, and then to rise. In attempting to get up the patient uses his hands and extended arms and literally climbs up his thighs and trunk from a squatting position. Gowers first described this in patients with pseudo-hypertrophic muscular dystrophy, regarding it as a defining characteristic of their condition.

### Gowers' tract

In 1880, in his *Diagnosis of Diseases of the Spinal Cord*, Gowers described a bundle of nerve fibres to the front of the pyramidal and direct cerebellar tracts in the lateral column of the spinal cord.[12] He had noticed that the tract degenerated upwards after a cord injury. Later, he traced the degeneration of this 'antero-lateral ascending tract' further.[13] It seemed to appear first in the lower part of the thoracic spinal cord, but Gowers did not know where it ended and thought it was a path for conveying pain sensation. It was realized later that he was the first person to identify the ventral spinocerebellar tract, as it is now known, at its spinal level. The Russian neurologist Bechterew named it 'Gowers' fasciculus' but this term is now little used.

### Local panatrophy of Gowers

Gowers seems to have maintained a considerable interest in skin disorders throughout his career. In 1885 he had first seen a patient in Wolverhampton with patches of morphoea (plaques on the skin) and the absence of subcutaneous tissue on the face, shoulder, and back, which he described in his *Manual*. Following the presentation of a second case by Dr Harry Campbell at the Clinical Society in 1902, Gowers (with the help of his house officer Stanley Barnes) wrote to and traced his original patient, whose details he then wrote up in the *Review of Neurology and Psychiatry* in 1903.[14] This condition is still known as 'local panatrophy of Gowers'.

### Gowers' mixture

Gowers' name was also given to a mixture he devised for treating migraine headaches. Gowers' mixture was composed of liquor trinitrini, sodium bromide, tincture of gelsemium, tincture of nux vomica (containing strychnine), dilute nitric or hypobromic acid, and chloroform water. It was widely prescribed in England for fifty years although it is uncertain if it had any real effect. Lord Brain included the formula in his *Diseases of the Nervous System* from 1933, and it remained in Walton's 1969 revision of the seventh edition of Brain's work.[15]

### Gowers, Paton, and Foster Kennedy syndrome

In 1909 *The Lancet* published a lecture Gowers had given reporting an instance of an apparently novel syndrome which could be diagnosed by applying knowledge of brain anatomy and pathophysiology.[16] The patient was a 37-year-old woman troubled by worsening headache for two or three years before she developed weakness on her left side, the beginnings of optic atrophy in her left eye and right-sided 'optic neuritis' (i.e. papilloedema). The reaction of her left pupil to light was impaired, and she also lost her sense of smell on the left. The patient did not recover from an operation to remove her tumour. Autopsy showed an 'indurated epithelioma' beneath the left frontal lobe. Gowers mentioned an earlier instance that had been recorded in 1905 by Schultz-Zebde. Dr Leslie Paton was credited by Gowers for his microscopic examination of the nerves. In 1911 the syndrome was reported in the USA by Foster Kennedy, one of Gowers' former house physicians.[17]

## Achievements recognized

In 1887, at the age of 42, Gowers had been elected a Fellow of the Royal Society. Not long before, the Royal Society had decided that its fellows would be elected solely on the merit of their scientific work. Gowers was recognized by his peers as a 'distinguished physiologist and physician' who was 'attached to science and anxious to promote its progress'. He must have been particularly pleased to be recognized by his peers in the scientific world for his career-long dedication to the scientific method. Amongst the men who proposed him were Jenner, Paget, Russell Reynolds, Erichsen, Lister, and Wilks.

The Royal Society held regular dinners at its headquarters in Burlington House (which also housed a number of learned societies, such as the Linnean Society, the Society of Antiquities, the Geographical Society, the Astrological Society, and the Chemical Society). Henson notes that Henry Head (for whose membership Gowers had been one of the proposers) found Gowers a congenial companion at the dinners.[18] In his later years Gowers also regularly attended the society's 'conversazione' meetings which featured presentations of 'objects of interest'.

The Canadian physician William Osler was one of Gowers' greatest friends and admirers. The feeling was mutual, and the men forged a strong and lasting bond.

Gowers' admiration for Osler was expressed in a reference he wrote to Weir Mitchell on Osler's behalf:

> There is, perhaps, no English physician of the same standing who has achieved a wider or higher reputation than Professor Osler of Montreal. His work at scientific and practical medicine is of highest character, exhibiting a rare combination of the power of exact observation, of estimating the value of evidence, and of critical judgment. As he is a clear thinker, so he is also a lucid and forcible teacher. The fact that he has worked assiduously not only at clinical medicine, but also at pathology, fits him in a peculiar way for the teaching of the former, since a basis of exact pathology is absolutely essential for the highest and best clinical teaching. A striking proof of the esteem in which he is held is afforded by the fact that he was elected a Fellow of the College of Physicians of London, almost as soon as he became eligible, an honour which, in the case of a physician residing out of England, is probably unique. As regards Dr Osler's personal character, I know him well, and know no one whom I should regard as more agreeable as a colleague, or in every respect, a more desirable acquisition to an important medical school.[19]

Osler paid tribute to Gowers' achievements in 1894, when he dedicated his *On Chorea and Choreiform Affections* to him:

> To the profession of the United States and Canada you stand as the most brilliant exponent of the complex science of neurology; please accept the dedication of this little volume as an earnest of the gratitude felt towards you by thousands of your kinsmen across the water, and as an expression of the personal attachment of your sincere friend.[20]

Gowers responded with a delightful letter describing the 'editorial sanctum' of the *Clinical Journal: a Weekly Record of Clinical Medicine and Surgery, with their Special Branches*. This journal had been launched in 1893 by a young doctor who died shortly afterwards at the age of 33, leaving an even younger widow who then took over as its editor. The journal published two volumes of medical lectures a year, and survived for over a decade. In his letter to Osler thanking him for his dedication, Gowers described a visit he paid to its offices.

> The dedication of your little book to me will be one of the pleasant things of life.
>
> I am sorry, very, you have not seen Mrs Cardew of the *Clinical Journal*. You would have loved her and your wife would have approved your love, thoroughly, if she too had seen the little Editress of 23, widow, two children, and the *Clin. Journal*. I shd. so much have like you to see her editorial sanctum—she has the top floor of a rather high house in Harley St and her room is at the back, looking over the western roofs towards America, with a window door opening on to a tiny round 'leads' where she sits a bit—a very little bit now and then when her head aches too badly to go on correcting proofs. Now you have got to send her a lecture soon too, and a good one. One to take with GPs. They read the *CJ* and read it carefully too. Since her husband's death the circulation has gone up from 3,000 to 4,000—so has she bowled us all over.
>
> How many things I have to say to you. Ah. Here is a grand idea. If I write to you in what they call in the USA 'Isaac Pitman' shorthand, can't your amanuensetical angel read it to you? I wd. write very plain. The difference or proportion of time of labour is from 1/6 to 1/10. You told me of a Baltimore med. phonographer. Please ask him to send me a shorthand postcard to say if I have written to him.[21]

Another admirer was the eminent American neurologist Silas Weir Mitchell. He wrote a letter of spontaneous praise from Philadelphia in March 1897:

> I may see you in England this summer, but cannot now say whether I shall reach London or not. I sail today for Le Havre and shall spend some time on the Continent. One of the last duties I have to fulfill is to write you a note which I have for some time been intending to dictate. I shall have to leave it for my son to sign as I am off in half an hour. I wish to express to you my obligation and thanks for the service which your work on *Diseases of the Nervous System* unfailingly gives me. When I am in doubt or perplexed with a difficult case I always find therein light for guidance, and I regard it both as a duty and a pleasure to say this to you. Moreover, I am of the belief that little new has been offered by later writers since your book was published, and all this shows how admirably your contribution to knowledge was thought out before it was given to the profession for counsel.[22]

## Queen Victoria's diamond jubilee honours

One of the events marking Queen Victoria's diamond jubilee in 1897 was the conferring of special jubilee year honours and awards. The Queen recognized Gowers' contribution to medical science that June by awarding him a knighthood. The announcement prompted many letters congratulating Gowers on his achievements, including those from neurologists he had never met, colleagues, ex-pupils, and friends. The letters have survived and provide an insight into how Gowers was viewed by some of his contemporaries.

Two of his National Hospital house physicians, Collier and Purves-Stewart, were unqualified admirers:

> How well that honour has been merited can only be fully appreciated by those who have enjoyed the immense advantages of your unique teaching and who have watched the work of a true master of his science. We feel ourselves deeply honoured to be at the present time associated with you in your work, and we beg to express the hope that you may long enjoy the distinctions which no one has more thoroughly earned than yourself.[23]

Dr Thomas Barlow had known Gowers since the 1870s, when both worked with Jenner at UCH:

> Your promotion will gain the unanimous approval of the whole profession because it represents the recognition of absolute work in the advancement of medical knowledge and is independent of any adventitious considerations whatever. When I think of the enrichment of English medicine by your volumes and their value in helping to make the crooked ways straight! I confess I think the title only a very moderate recognition of what has been done.[24]

Charles Beevor had also worked closely with Gowers over many years at Queen Square:

> I am writing to ask you to accept my warmest congratulations on the honour which will be conferred on you. It gives me an especial pleasure to do this as during the last twenty years, as student, house physician, assistant-physician and lastly co-lecturer at Queen Square, I have had the great pleasure of working under you and with you. I feel very indebted to you for all that you have taught me during this period and I have always taken you as my model in the way of teaching at Queen Square.[25]

Dr G. V. Poore, a physician at UCH who shared Gowers' interest in hand cramps, wrote:

> I am sure the profession will be unanimous in this opinion, for although few have known you personally so well as I, all of them equally, with myself, have been indebted to your monumental book which has shed abundant light and lucidity (and this is not tautology) where previously there was darkness and obscurity.[26]

Hughlings Jackson wrote 'I was pleased to see your name in the Honours List this morning—A well earned honour for splendid work honestly done'.[27] Lord Lister, by then in his seventies, was similarly succinct: 'Although your new title adds nothing to your eminence, may I beg to congratulate you cordially on this recognition by the Sovereign'.[28]

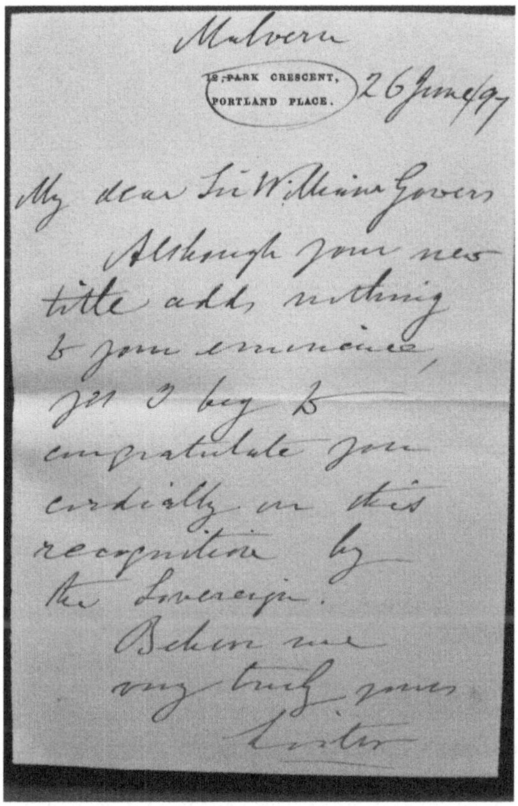

Malvern

12, PARK CRESCENT,
PORTLAND PLACE.

26 June/97

My dear Sir William Gowers

Although your new title adds nothing to your eminence, may I beg to congratulate you cordially on this recognition by the Sovereign.

Believe me
very truly yours
Lister

**Fig. 10.4** Congratulations from Lord Lister.

Physician Stephen Mackenzie described it as 'a fitting recognition of your most valuable work done under difficulties in the most quiet and unobtrusive manner'.[29] Thomas Wakley junior wrote from *The Lancet* congratulating Gowers, on behalf of his father and himself, on his 'well-deserved' honour.[30]

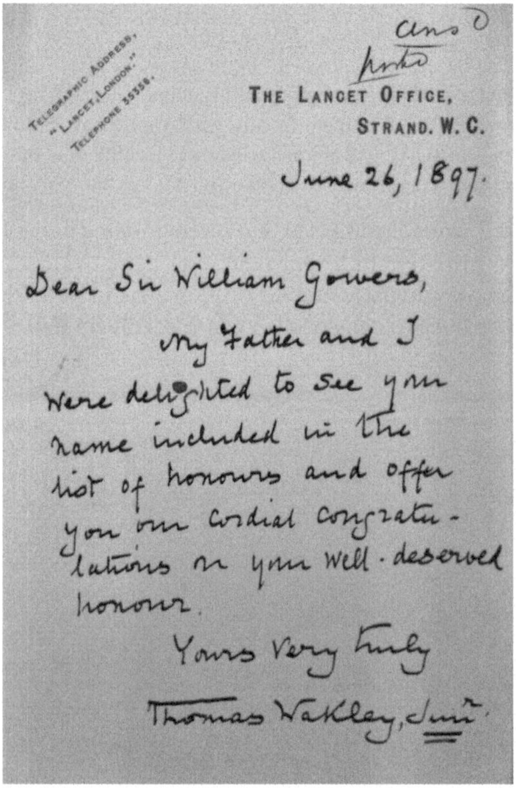

Telegraphic Address, "Lancet, London." Telephone 35358.

The Lancet Office,
Strand. W. C.

June 26, 1897.

Dear Sir William Gowers,

My Father and I were delighted to see your name included in the list of honours and offer you our cordial congratulations on your well-deserved honour.

Yours very truly
Thomas Wakley, Jun$^{r}$.

**Fig. 10.5** Congratulations from Thomas Wakley Jr.

Morrison wrote from Shanghai, saying that he had always regarded Gowers as his benefactor, sending his best wishes to all at 50 Queen Anne Street, and declaring himself 'very faithfully yours'.

Rudyard Kipling, who had been to the diamond jubilee celebrations himself, wrote a letter in his own distinctive style:

> We, and about five hundred various scalawags, have been down to Portsmouth in an excursion steamer looking at the Fleet—the most marvellous sight on earth. I had just time to drop you a line of congratulation—but that by no means did justice to my feelings. One can't say much at ½d a word. The honour in a case like yours is the outward and visible sign of a State's recognition of good work; and tho' Salisbury didn't know (there was never a Cecil that knew anything he was not coached into) it, it shows that he at least knows enough to do a sane thing when it is brought before him. What I chiefly value it for is that though it won't matter so much to those who know you, it gives you so to speak a better standing among the hidebound continental medicos.
>
> My sympathies are with Lady Gowers. From this minute every single solitary item in every one of her bills creeps up a little; and till the end of her days she will have to pay just a trifle more for everything she eats, wears or reads. She won't be able to lay her finger on

any precise item I fancy but from her cook to her dressmaker the conspiracy will be universal. That is the practical side of the matter but if the news gave you as much solid satisfaction as it did to me and the wife you should be completely enjoying yourself.

Yesterday being on a vile paddleboat steamer without proper refreshments, I did between the hours of 11am and 7pm eat three or four greasy ham sandwiches. Today I am very sad and tenderly mournful. Strange, isn't it? [31]

He added a postscript: 'What about the coat of arms?'

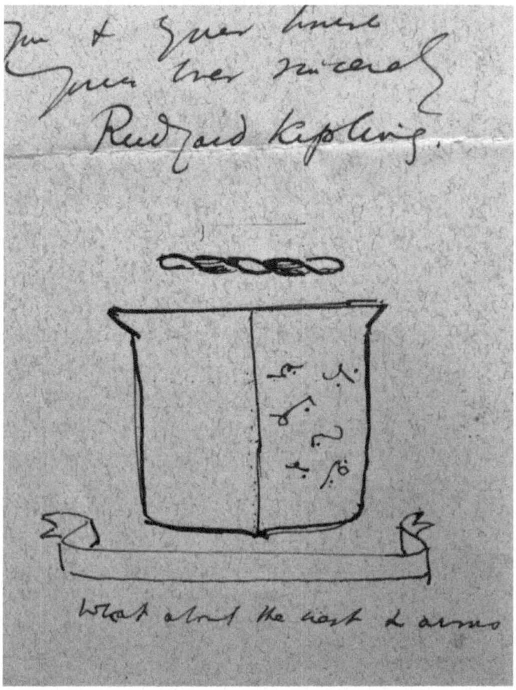


**Fig. 10.6** Kipling's mock coat of arms for Gowers.

The author of *A History of Coggeshall in Essex*, George Beaumont, was 'delighted to find the name of a Coggeshall worthy in the list of those receiving honours'.[32]

Dr Charles Mercier, 'psychologist, physician and logician', was an old friend who had worked closely with Hughlings Jackson, and was a friend of Osler's. He wrote in shorthand:

I hasten to send you my very sincere congratulations on your new honour, one which was a surprise to me, and I fancy to most people, for such honours are not often given to merit alone, nor indeed does merit easily account for much in the bestowal of them. Influence and official position are in the great majority of cases the only evidence of them, and it is therefore with no small surprise as well as pleasure that we see one occasion on which deserved recognition is given to scientific eminence pure and simple unaccompanied by these adventitious aids. It is something of a new departure, and a very welcome one. Of all things in this world I do most heartily detest reclamé and in this age of pushing and

> shoving and self-advertisement it is a compliment to the whole body of unobtrusive scientific workers that the most meritorious and least pushful of them should have had public recognition. One had begun to think that honours were given by the state only as a reward for precedent and successful advertisement, but when you and Dr Wilks are selected one feels that the titular honour has again become a real honour. So again I congratulate you.[33]

Gowers' friend Gregory wanted to contact Kipling:

> As the telegraph office refused to carry my congratulations I have to trust to the slower post. My wife and I were immensely delighted when your name welcomed us from the list of new knights. I had given no thought to anticipating to whom the honours would go, so it came as a surprise. You will have so many congratulations that I will make this very brief. If at any time you could send me R Kipling's address I should be grateful. I have a suggestion for him about 2-toed horses, and a message to him from A Russell Wallace.

On 3 August Gowers travelled to Osborne, the Queen's retreat on the Isle of Wight, for the investiture ceremony, and later described the day to Morrison:

> The reception by the profession has been most gratifying to me. My writings seem to have given such universal help as to cause a sense of personal satisfaction in all of this distinction, to have made men feel that it is what they would have picked on to be done, though they never anticipated it, because there are many undistinguished seniors. To me it is good because given purely for work, & timely—needed because my work has been so purely for the profession that it has hindered knowledge of me by the public & the money reward that is supposed to have come to me as it has not, and I could never save enough for a baronetcy.[34] Its chief personal satisfaction is naturally for the title it gives the wife—who was alarmed at first but has got reconciled to an appreciative degree I think. Of course the children were all delighted.

Gowers continued:

> I was unable to assume it until the Knighting at Osborne on August 3. A most interesting day. A batch of 10 of us went by a special train and boat for some Privy Councillors. Knowing Sir James Reid well, made the visit especially full of interest. He has a baronetcy—well deserved, indeed, considering how the Queen went thro' the Jubilee affair & his tremendous responsibility. She takes advice from no one else. He is splendidly straight honest good Scotchman & has a very close personal position outside professional relations. But he never initiates or suggests. No matter how much he deserves a thing, he always wants to be asked, wisely. This profession owes more to him than will ever be known. My Knighthood however is due to Acland & Broadbent—chiefly the latter whose earnestness and energy, tho' I have no claim on him, when Acland wrote about it were marvellous. Lord Salisbury had never heard my name!
>
> The Queen looked careworn but less wrinkled & less old than I expected. Her glance is keen but her voice soft & gentle, as she said, twice, 'Sir William' when she touched first one shoulder & then the other with the flat of an old carved light sword.

In November 1898, the Society of Medical Phonographers held a dinner to celebrate Gowers' knighthood, to which they invited Kipling, Sir Henry Howorth (president of the Royal Archaeological Institute), the Reverend Dr Augustus Jessopp, Professor Bonney, and Dr Bruce Dingwall. During the dinner the society presented Gowers with an illuminated manuscript, carrying their congratulations.

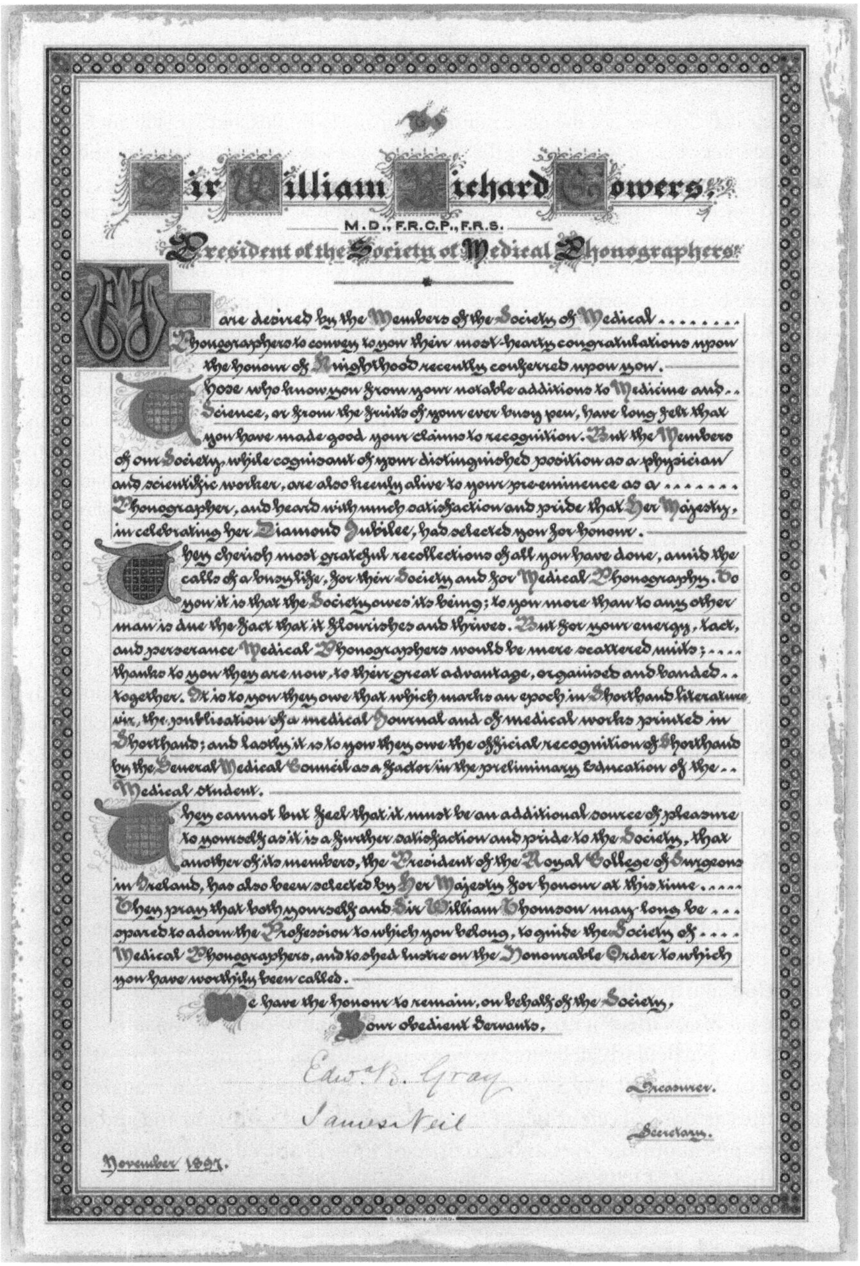

Sir William Richard Gowers,
M.D., F.R.C.P., F.R.S.
President of the Society of Medical Phonographers

We are desired by the Members of the Society of Medical Phonographers to convey to you their most-hearty congratulations upon the honour of Knighthood recently conferred upon you.

Those who know you from your notable additions to Medicine and Science, or from the fruits of your ever busy pen, have long felt that you have made good your claims to recognition. But the Members of our Society, while cognisant of your distinguished position as a physician and scientific worker, are also keenly alive to your pre-eminence as a Phonographer, and heard with much satisfaction and pride that Her Majesty, in celebrating her Diamond Jubilee, had selected you for honour.

They cherish most grateful recollections of all you have done, amid the calls of a busy life, for their Society and for Medical Phonography. To you it is that the Society owes its being; to you more than to any other man is due the fact that it flourishes and thrives. But for your energy, tact, and perseverance Medical Phonographers would be mere scattered units; thanks to you they are now, to their great advantage, organised and banded together. It is to you they owe that which marks an epoch in Shorthand literature viz, the publication of a medical Journal and of medical works printed in Shorthand; and lastly it is to you they owe the official recognition of Shorthand by the General Medical Council as a factor in the preliminary Education of the Medical student.

They cannot but feel that it must be an additional source of pleasure to yourself as it is a further satisfaction and pride to the Society, that another of its members, the President of the Royal College of Surgeons in Ireland, has also been selected by Her Majesty for honour at this time. They pray that both yourself and Sir William Thomson may long be spared to adorn the Profession to which you belong, to guide the Society of Medical Phonographers, and to shed lustre on the Honourable Order to which you have worthily been called.

We have the honour to remain, on behalf of the Society,
Your obedient Servants,

Edwd. B. Gray — Treasurer.
James Neil — Secretary.

November 1897.

**Fig. 10.7** The Society of Medical Phonographers' award of congratulation to Gowers on his knighthood.

Kipling replied to the toast of 'The visitors'. He began by praising the remarkable work of medical men he had seen practising in India, but said that he had to draw the line at the praise of phonography. The *BMJ* reported his speech:

> He knew that that was not the place nor the company to do this, but Sir William Gowers had said somewhere it was good for the nerves. Now it was not. He had tried it, and it led to incipient inflammation of the brain, the earliest symptoms of locomotor ataxy, paralysis, and one or two other things; and the trouble about it was that it was more or less like medicine, because, it might be remembered, someone in their profession—Aesculapius or Sir William Gowers or somebody—said a diagnosis was not worth a rap till it had been confirmed by a post mortem examination. It was the same with his phonography; he was perfectly splendid in the diagnosis, he could write a considerable amount of phonography, but when he came to the post mortem—that is to say, when he had to translate six or eight hours later what he had taken down in shorthand, it was—well, not a success. Moreover he had just taken the opportunity of asking Sir William Gowers how he wrote his name in shorthand, and he had given him an idiograph that looked remarkably like a dissolute Japanese dog. He had unbounded respect for the gentlemen present, and he had great appreciation of the kindness they had done him that evening, but he would be shot if he would write 'Sir William Gowers' like a dissolute dog.[35]

Kipling described the 'festive spread with electric lights and waiters and plush and flumdiddle', to his American friend Dr James Conlan:

> The other day I went up to town and was roped in to two public dinners—one of them a doctor's entertainment to congratulate Sir William Gowers (who is a crank on shorthand) upon his getting a knighthood. Gowers is the deuce and all of a neurologist but I believe he is simply a maniac on shorthand as a means to help Doctors put down their diagnoses.[36]

In December 1897 Gowers was elected honorary Fellow of the Royal College of Physicians of Ireland. In 1903 he was elected an honorary member of the Vienna Internal Medical Society. In 1906 he was awarded Hon.MD (Dublin), and in 1911 Hon.LLD (Edinburgh), and in 1909 the Moxon Medal, awarded by the Royal College of Physicians of London, for observation and research in clinical medicine. He was made an honorary member of the Russian Society of Medicine; the Royal Society of Science, Uppsala; the Netherlands Society of Psychiatry and Neurology; the Society for International Medicine, Vienna; and the American Neurological Association.

Gowers was particularly delighted to be awarded the 'Sloper award of merit', a regular feature in the journal *Ally Sloper's Half Holiday*, a comic Victorian magazine which carried little cartoons of celebrities of the day, embellished with amusing and imaginative paragraphs about the lives and activities of those featured. The favoured 'gentry' received the award of FOS (friend of Sloper). Sadly, Gowers' award has not survived.

## The turn of the century

By 1900 Gowers was prematurely ageing, and becoming increasingly difficult and eccentric. Many years later Ernest recalled his father in a letter to his own son, written on the centenary of Gowers' birth:

> He must have been rather terrifying to people he did not know well, because he always said what he thought, and what he thought, though generally right, was not always

> complimentary. I wish you had known him; he had many of the qualities of a really great man, including some of the faults that often go with greatness.

An era closed with the death of Queen Victoria in 1901, not only for England but also for the Gowers family. Willie and Ernest were embarking on their own careers. In 1902, the 'Zambezi boy', Willie, eventually joined the Colonial Civil Service. He came back to London regularly on annual leave. In 1904 he entered into what proved a disastrous first marriage, to Maud Lorraine, a woman he met in Nigeria. He remarried many years later, but had no children by either wife.

In May 1905 Ernest married Constance Greer from Ballycastle, a distant relative through the Baines family. Their first son, born in 1906, died in infancy. They had two daughters, born in 1907 and 1913. A second son, born in 1910, was christened William Richard (after his grandfather). Ernest had remained in London. He joined the Home Civil Service in 1903, and was allocated a position in the Inland Revenue office. But his father had not lost interest in the colonies. In 1904 Sir William wrote to the secretary of state for India asking whether Ernest could be 'offered removal' to a position that had become vacant in the India Office. The position was filled by open competition, and against a 'formidable competitor' from another office, Ernest was selected.[37]

The girls stayed at home with their parents, and became involved in various charitable works. They joined a group who were dressing dolls for 'the poor children belonging to the Children's Happy Evenings' (an after-school programme run by volunteers). The summer of 1911 was particularly hot, and they devoted their energies to a factory girls' country holiday fund appeal, to which their father added his name.[38] In May 1910 they invited Kipling to address a public meeting, but he could not, replying: 'We see the factory girls sometimes when they take a holiday at Hastings and a cheerful crowd of maidens they are'. Edith shared Gowers' enthusiasm for botany, and was elected to the Royal Botanical Society.

Gowers was ill for many years before he finally resigned from the National Hospital in 1910. The strife between the physicians and the board of management, and the hospital's severe financial hardship in 1904, made it a less congenial place of work than when he had been appointed to the staff nearly thirty-five years earlier.[39] He complained that the door to the museum had been locked during the absence of the director of the research fund. His suggestion that a history of the hospital might be commissioned was rejected on cost grounds.

He continued to work and to publish until 1910. He also became involved in a number of public campaigns and fund-raising activities. He retained his interest in church matters. Concerned about the High Church movement within the Anglican Church, the bishop of Hereford (John Percival, who at one time had been headmaster of Rugby) convened a conference of churchmen in April 1899 'with the object being to form a basis of common action between Moderate High Churchmen, Broad Churchmen, and Evangelicals'.[40] The meeting passed a number of resolutions rejecting Anglo-Catholic practices, such as the imposition of 'habitual' confession and subscribing to the belief in transubstantiation. There were 2700 signatories to the resolutions of whom the most eminent were listed in *The Times*. The list included Sir William Gowers, Dr Jessopp, Reverend Canon Bonney, Sir Francis Seymour Haden,

Lord Lister, and Sir Edward Sieveking.[41] Gowers continued to take an interest in contemporary ecclesiastical debates.

In 1902 he gave a talk on 'Lunacy and the law' to the Medico-Psychological Association, in which he argued that borderline insanity cases were suffering under the 1890 *Lunacy Act.* This received widespread coverage in both the medical journals and *The Times*, sparking a lively debate.[42]

In the same year Gowers wrote to *The Lancet* advocating the use of the metric system in pharmacy.[43] In 1949 this had still not been adopted: 'His advocacy of the metric system in pharmacy will engender melancholy thoughts, for the persistence, 60 years after the pleas of Gowers, in the middle of tremendous scientific developments of a backward, barbaric and dangerous mode of prescribing'.[44]

Gowers' father had been displaced from Hackney by the advent of the railway in the 1850s. By the beginning of the twentieth century motor traffic was beginning to be both a problem and a blessing to Londoners. Gowers was a member of the Metropolitan Street Ambulance Association, a lobby group of doctors pressing for the establishment of a more efficient ambulance service. In the 1890s the police and firefighters had taken the injured on wheeled stretchers, or 'litters', to the nearest hospital or doctor's surgery. A full-time ambulance service had been established in London in the late 1890s. The first petrol-driven ambulance (which could carry a single stretcher at up to fifteen miles per hour) appeared in 1904.[45] During the 1904 county council elections the association sent a postcard to every candidate asking whether, if elected, they would interest themselves in establishing an efficient street ambulance service, and kept a chart of the responses. They published the results in a letter to *The Times.*[46] In the same year Marylebone residents, including Gowers, petitioned the borough council about traffic noise in residential streets, suggesting that these streets should be paved with wood rather than macadam in order to decrease the noise, adding that: 'They had not only the noise of motor-cars to bear with but the terrible torture of traction engines'.[47]

It was 1904 when Gowers gave his lecture on lumbago. Towards the end he made revealing comments about the intractability of its pain, probably reflecting his own experience with back pain:

> The traumatic form of tendinous fibrositis, when it settles down to a stationary condition, with pain on any tension, and often some tenderness of pressure, resists almost all treatment.
>
> Rest is important, but it is not easy to maintain for an adequate time. Counter-irritation sometimes lessens the pain, and the actual cautery is certainly the most effective form. A local measure that often does good is the deep hypodermic injection of cocaine, repeated daily for two or three weeks. It unquestionably promotes the subsidence of the sensitiveness provided the ease obtained is not abused by increased exertion.[48]

Rumours still persist at Queen Square about Gowers and possible substance abuse. He was certainly not a teetotaller, and it is possible that he resorted to cocaine and opium to relieve his excruciating backache.

Hughlings Jackson, ten years older than Gowers, retired from the staff of Queen Square in 1906. Gowers was not too ill in November 1907 to unveil the bust that had been made to mark the event. At the end of his address, Gowers said: 'Let us look upon this bust and then turn to the living counterpart—our master!'[49] The bust was stolen from the front hall of Queen Square years later 'evidently by an unknown neurophilic kleptomaniac'[50] and rumours still circulate about the identity of the culprit and the whereabouts of the bust. Gowers acknowledged Jackson's brilliance again when he gave his Hughlings Jackson lecture in 1909, and said that 'facts are rare, and those already gathered have been made to yield their lessons by the master himself, beyond whom we cannot hope to go'.[51] Hughlings Jackson died in 1911.

In 1910, at the age of 65, Gowers retired. Enfeebled by 'generalized cerebrovascular degeneration', he was forced to leave Queen Anne Street the following year, moving to a more suitable house in Ladbroke Square.[52] The young Foster Kennedy, resident medical officer at Queen Square from 1906–10, wrote in October of 1908 that 'I saw Dr Ferrier today. He's as fit and as alive as ever ... He is wonderfully young compared with Gowers who I think has aged very much in the last few months, and shows it especially by the way he is beginning to lose grip of his cases'. A little later he wrote: 'I see a great change in the old man. He's breaking up badly and hardly thinks about his cases at all. It's a monstrous position for a man of his ability'.[53]

In 1908 Mary Gowers joined the planning committee for Queen Square's jubilee celebrations. The couple attended the jubilee dinner at the Mansion House the following June. Despite his frailty, Gowers continued to attend the Royal Society conversaziones until 1909, as well as functions at Queen Square. In October 1909, he joined the reception committee to greet the King when he opened the enlarged outpatients' hall, built in response to the recommendations of the 1901 Fry Inquiry.[54]

Gowers had been consulting physician to the Guardian Assurance Company for a number of years and was still occasionally called upon to provide medical opinions as an insurance assessor. In 1909, a man took out a negligence action for an electric shock from the electric conductor connected to a tramcar on which he was a passenger. He had been admitted to Queen Square after being diagnosed with traumatic neurasthenia, and treated by the use of a spinal douche combined with the 'Weir Mitchell treatment' of rest, preferably in isolation. He had insisted on leaving the hospital because he wanted fresh air and thought the spinal douche was killing him. Gowers and Horsley gave evidence that the treatment was appropriate and should have cured him in three to six months.[55]

Gowers gave the Hughlings Jackson lecture in 1909, and published a number of papers, but by this time he was extremely ill. Published in 1910, his last three papers dealt with poliomyelitis, gonococcal neuroretinitis, and the neurology of the eyelid, but these 'were penned with considerable difficulty'.[56] In December 1912 he resigned from the Athenaeum on the grounds of ill-health, and the secretary responded with regret 'the sad duty of erasing [his] name from the list on which it [had] occupied an honoured place for many years'.[57]

Gowers exchanged letters in shorthand with his friend (and possibly patient) Dr Charles Mercier. They discussed a wide range of topics from phonography to the problems of ageing. Mercier suffered a debilitating disorder and diagnosed himself as suffering from Paget's disease. In 1912 Gowers wrote to Osler about his case:

> Have you seen any more cases of Paget's disease since you wrote the last edition? I looked to you to learn about it for Dr Mercier says he is its victim. He is an alienist but the most

brilliant writer in the medical profession. He says half his bones soften, yield and bend and the other half harden and get knobby and bumpy. 'The consequence is that I am bent permanently double, a deformity that increases week by week and my legs assume more and more the shape of a pair of parentheses. I can't walk and I can't stand for more than a very few minutes and I have no activity left except that of my pen and tongue.'[58]

A few years earlier Mercier had described suffering from the disturbing loss of memory that comes with age:

> In experiencing defects of memory from which I suffer is as to where I put things. In fact I am constrained to believe that I am haunted by a devil who hoards all my things. If I lay down my pen and seal a letter it's a matter of an hour's search to find the pen again, and when I do find it, it is as likely to be upstairs or at least at the other end of the room as to be nowhere seen. I have very little memory for faces, and never remember or under what circumstances I have met them before. But I can always remember whereabouts in a book and on what particular page is the passage that I want, and I can learn a passage by heart with no great difficulty.[59]

Gowers, renowned for his excellent memory, had held that, provided accurate and instantaneous imprinting could be achieved, memories would harden and become as infallible as a photograph, and that writing things down could indelibly impress important facts on the mind. He believed that the brain could be trained to improve its ability to retain memories. Recollection simply involved a revival of the original stored brain trace rather than an imaginative inexact dynamic active process in which everything is being continually re-categorized and updated. Sacks, after comparing some of Gowers' own published recollections of a patient's symptoms, observed that some salient facts of the case had changed over time, and concluded that Gowers' own memory in the end refuted his early ideas of memory retention as a mechanical recording of brain traces.[60] It is a pity that Gowers' response to Mercier has not survived, as it may have shed further light on his latest ideas on how memory worked.

William Osler was appointed regius professor of medicine at Oxford in 1905, where he remained for the rest of his life. He visited Gowers in 1913, and wrote to Weir Mitchell: 'You will be sorry to hear that Gowers is very ill—his own disease, ataxic paraplegia, it looks like, and ascending, so that there are now bulbar symptoms'.[61]

The Gowers' had been in their new home for less than two years before, early in 1913, both Gowers and his wife were struck down by pneumonia. Mary Gowers died in February. Gowers outlived his wife by only two years. He died at home on 4 May 1915. His son Ernest was present, and Dr James Taylor certified the cause of death: coma resulting from arteriosclerosis. One of the first letters of condolence came from Sir William Osler, to which Ernest immediately replied describing the distressing last few hours, and ending:

> Now all pain is gone out of his face and he is more like his old self. I am so glad that you saw him and he knew you, as I am quite sure he did. You have indeed been a good friend to him all through.[62]

His funeral was held on 6 May at St Peter's Church, Vere Street. A memorial service was conducted at St Peter's shortly afterwards.

## In memoriam

William Frederick (Willie) Gowers had been posted to northern Nigeria to work under Frederick Lugard. Lugard was a figure who dominated colonial administration for a generation. A number of promising administrators served under him (nicknamed 'Lugard's young men'), of whom Willie was one. Lugard also married Flora Shaw, of *The Times*. When his father died Willie was serving as political advisor to the general commanding the Cameroons expeditionary force, for which he was mentioned in dispatches. He received a letter of condolence on his father's death, from Dr M. Cameron Blair, Zungeru, northern Nigeria:

> I should like, as a middle-aged member of your Father's profession, to tell you, out of my own knowledge, how he was regarded by the rank and file. He was to the average English-speaking medical man—both in the British dominions and in North America—what Lord Roberts was to the soldier. I know that he was highly esteemed in many foreign countries. ... For myself, personally, he has always been one of my heroes; I am not ashamed to acknowledge myself a hero-worshipper; and this letter is quite as much a wreath sent to his grave as a mark of friendship to his son.[63]

Willie was knighted when he became governor of Uganda in 1926. But he earned notoriety (as had Jameson) for his womanizing and gambling, and was referred to as 'naughty Willie' in official files.[64]

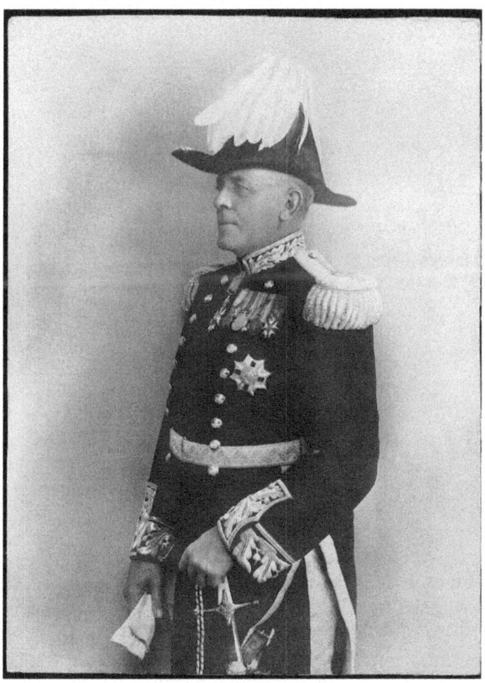

**Fig. 10.8** Sir William Frederick Gowers, governor of Uganda, 1925.

In 1915 Ernest was on his way to a highly successful civil service career. He had worked as Lloyd George's principal private secretary when the National Insurance Bill was being prepared against a chorus of protest from the medical profession, and then joined the National Insurance Commission when it was established to help in the difficult task of implementing the new Act. At the time of his father's death he had been moved into the secret World War I propaganda unit, Wellington House, through which his association with Kipling continued. Ernest's brother-in-law Kenneth served in the Irish Guards, as did Kipling's son John. John was killed in the battle and Kenneth died two months after from the wounds he received. Kipling, devastated that he had pressed his son to enlist, afterwards wrote the official history of the Irish Guards, in which he graphically described the horror of the battle.

Edith was 37 and Evelyn 31 when their father died. Neither daughter married. They were of the generation of young women whose marriage prospects were severely diminished by the carnage of World War I. They had another problem to contend with: they both began to develop the genetic eye disease retinitis pigmentosa. The disease first appeared when they were young adults and gradually progressed until they became almost totally blind.

The Gowers family maintained its links both with UCH and the National Hospital Queen Square. During World War II, Ernest was senior regional commissioner for London's civil defence, working from a concrete bunker under the Natural History Museum, South Kensington (the museum his father had often taken him to as a boy).

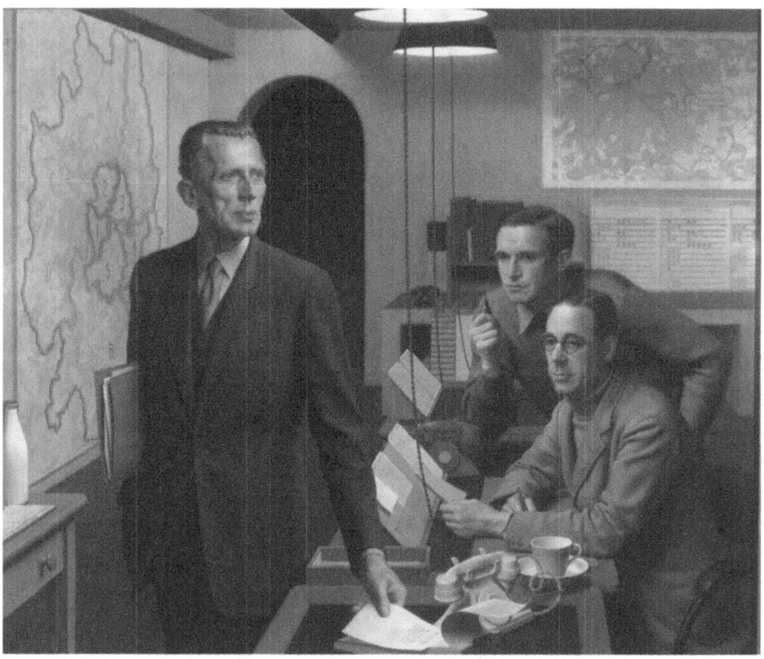

**Fig. 10.9** Sir Ernest Gowers, senior regional commissioner for civil defence, London region, at regional headquarters at the Natural History Museum, South Kensington (1944). Portrait by Meredith Frampton. By permission of the Imperial War Museums: IWM ART LD 2905.

Ernest contacted the National Hospital during a lull in the bombing to offer the hospital his support. His brother had by this time left Uganda, was living in London, and had become a governor of UCH. 'Not to be outdone in filial piety', Ernest said in a retirement speech, 'I made diffident approaches to Queen Square and was gratified to find myself welcomed with the utmost kindness'. He became a governor, and was elected chairman of the board in 1948, retiring in 1957. He also became chairman of the pension fund, established by Louisa Chandler in 1860, to help provide for the special needs of paralyzed patients, and remained its chairman after he had retired from the board. On 19 March 1945 Ernest dined with some younger members of the Queen Square staff to discuss future plans for the hospital, for which they had a programme that would cost 'a trifle of a million or so'. He wrote to his own son that, 'Father would have been thrilled beyond words to know that that was how I was celebrating the eve of his hundredth birthday'.

The anniversary of Gowers' birth was recognized in a ceremony at the hospital on 16 October 1946 when Princess Alice formally named the second floor ward in the Queen Mary wing, the Gowers ward. Family members were presented to her, and Sir William's 7-year-old great-granddaughter, his mother's namesake Ann Gowers, presented a bouquet.

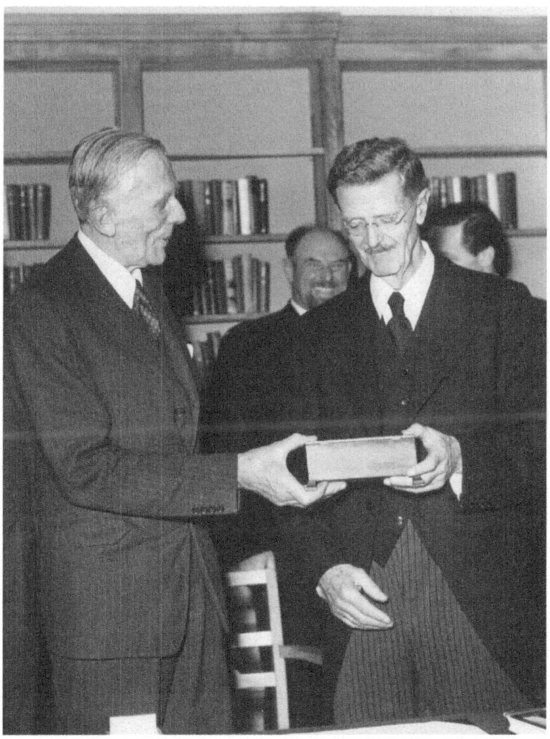

**Fig. 10.10** Sir Gordon Holmes being presented with a book by Sir Ernest Gowers after opening the Gowers Memorial Library on 29 November 1951. Image courtesy of the Queen Square Library, Archive and Museum.

Edith Gowers died January 1939 and Evelyn in 1946. The sisters left legacies of £500 each to Queen Square. The Gowers Memorial Library was built in 1951 as a general library and reading room containing 'library of books of all kinds, light and serious, ... meant for the use of both patients and staff', and equipped and run in association with the Holborn public library. It was opened by Sir Gordon Holmes on 29 November 1951.

The Gowers Memorial Library was later subsumed into the Rockefeller Medical Library, which then became the Queen Square Library.

The legacies were also used to fund a triennial 'Gowers lecture'. A special medal was struck, bearing a portrait of Gowers, for presentation to each lecturer.

The lecture was given in November 1956 by Sir Francis Walshe, FRS, on the 'Nature and dimensions of nosology in modern medicine'. Ernest Gowers was in the chair and Sir Russell Brain presented the medal. These lectures ceased temporarily when the funds were exhausted. However, the series was reinstated in 2007 when Andrew Lees gave a lecture entitled 'In search of the lost mystery of neurology' (and was presented with the Gowers medal). William Richard Gowers is still remembered at the hospital, now the National Hospital for Neurology and Neurosurgery, Queen Square, in the 'Gowers teaching grand round' which takes place in the Wolfson lecture theatre every Thursday afternoon.

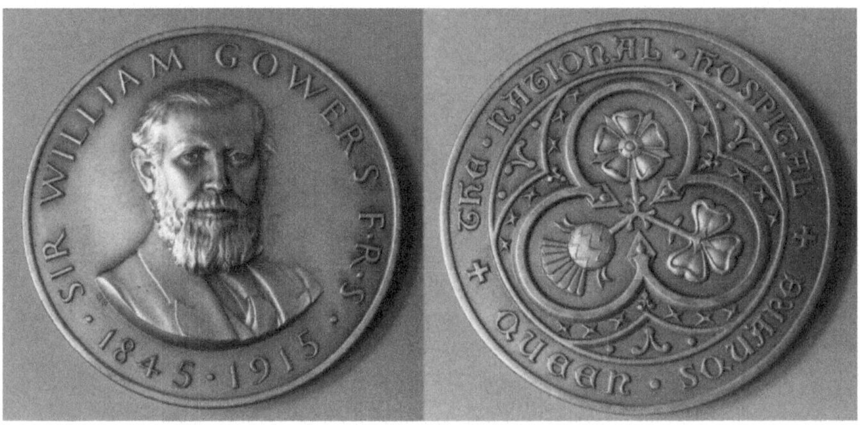


**Fig. 10.11** The Gowers medal. Image courtesy of the Queen Square Library, Archive and Museum.

Chapter 11

# Gowers: the man, his work, and his legacy

## Influences on Gowers' intellectual development

For the first ten years of his life, Gowers was a member of a small, close-knit, working-class family. From the age of 6, when his sister Letitia died, he must have been particularly treasured as the only one of his parents' four children to have survived. However, at the age of 11 Gowers' secure world was shattered by the death of his father, and his mother's decision to return from London to Yorkshire. After his father died, Gowers became an intensely lonely young man. He had to adjust to living with a large family of cousins in Oxford, and attending a new school. Fortunately, Christ Church College School provided the sound educational grounding that enabled him to study by correspondence when he eventually set his sights on gaining a place at the University of London. After deciding that he was unsuited to farming, he almost accidentally chose medicine as a career. However, he applied himself to his correspondence studies for the London matriculation examination with a single-minded sense of purpose from the moment he signed his apprenticeship indentures with Dr Simpson of Coggeshall. The chance advice he received from strangers—of the benefits of shorthand, the importance of statistics, and the need for clarity in his written English—he absorbed with enthusiasm, approaching each with characteristic perfectionism. These early lessons provided a sound foundation on which to build his work as a clinician, a researcher, a writer, and a lecturer. When he decided to teach himself to draw and to etch, he again approached the task as a perfectionist, achieving a standard of draughtsmanship that enabled to him to draw his own illustrations, including those in the *Manual of Diseases of the Nervous System*, and also provided a hobby from which he derived lifelong satisfaction.

Gowers received little intellectual guidance from Dr Simpson, but the Congregationalist ministers in Coggeshall, Bryan Dale and Alfred Philps, assumed this academic role, and it was Philps who introduced him to William Jenner, the man who Gowers always acknowledged as his most revered mentor. Jenner, in turn, provided support and guidance to his dedicated protégé throughout his brilliant career as a medical student. Another lecturer at UCL, John Russell Reynolds, not only recognized Gowers' academic potential but also nurtured him socially and introduced him to his future wife. But ultimately it was Gowers who was relentlessly self-driven both as a student and then throughout his career, undermining his own health as he did so.

Gowers' character was grounded in his Christian beliefs and the attitudes deeply embedded in the Victorian era. He started life in a strongly Nonconformist environment, and those values never left him. Nonconformists were amongst Britain's most active Christians at the time, and they were committed to the notion of service to the community at home or abroad: to the idea and missionary potential of the expanding British Empire as well as to social and political reform at home. He felt a strong obligation to justify having been 'spared' to survive his childhood. It is clear from his diary that he saw his medical career as a means of carrying out God's work.

## Gowers' personality

It has generally been agreed that Gowers was the consummate neurologist, but there have been sharply differing opinions about him as a man. In his later life, when he was chronically ill and had aged prematurely, he became a figure of fun to the students who had not known him in his prime, and who found his shuffling gait and high-pitched voice easy to mimic. It is their memories that have tended to dominate the stories that have been handed down to later generations.

Gowers was undoubtedly difficult, and became increasingly cantankerous as he aged. Ernest referred to his father's disconcerting outspokenness. Gowers did not conceal his pride in his own achievements. Humility was not one of his characteristics, at least not in later life, and in conversation he could leave other people feeling inferior. Ernest Jones left one of the most unflattering portraits of his former teacher:

> He had a peculiar personality and was reported to suffer from attacks of megalomania; a priceless saying attributed—*ben trovato* [even if it is not true, it is well invented]—to him in one of these was that every day he conceived an infinite number of original ideas, any one of which would make the reputation of an infinite number of neurologists.[1]

Opinion has differed about whether or not Gowers had a sense of humour. A comparison between the biographies of Gowers and Cushing concluded that Cushing had a sense of humour and Gowers did not.[2] There is plenty of evidence to the contrary. Despite Gowers' dry humour not always being well understood or received, it was frequently appreciated and enjoyed. H. H. Brown described it as 'pungent'.[3] Critchley tells the story of Gowers' response to physiologists who questioned whether there was any sensitivity in the Achilles tendon because they had discovered no nerve endings. When, in due course, they discovered the nerve endings, they conceded that the tendon might be sensitive. Gowers commented that it did not require a microscope to demonstrate this, as anyone might have discovered had they taken the trouble to give their own Achilles tendon a sharp pinch.[4]

Foster Kennedy was the butt of Gowers' humour on one occasion. He had joined the staff at Queen Square as Gowers' house physician shortly after graduating from Queen's University, Belfast. When Gowers was demonstrating a case in which his young house physician had recorded that the patient's knee-jerks were normal, Gowers found no knee-jerk. He announced to the class, 'Gentlemen, Dr Kennedy has the supreme distinction of having elicited this man's last knee-jerk'.[5] The story has variously been attributed to Ernest Jones and Foster Kennedy, both of whom worked with Gowers as young men, but Foster Kennedy is the more likely candidate. It was Foster Kennedy who wrote that no picture of Gowers could be appreciated without at the same time:

> having in the mind's eye his look of being a combination of one of the Wise Men of the East and the Ancient Mariner, and hearing too his harsh loud staccato voice speaking in sardonic humorous invective against the errors of the world.[6]

Another example of Gowers' caustic tongue was a story his son Ernest related of an American postgraduate student who had worked with Gowers for three months. When he left for a month of further study in Vienna, he told Gowers he would be examining disseminated sclerosis. Gowers responded that this was of personal interest to him as he had been studying it for thirty-five years, and he would be grateful if the student would send him a postcard with news of all he discovered.

A first-hand description of the way in which he was perceived by the nursing staff comes from a letter written in the 1950s by 87-year-old Lucy Holt, who had been at Queen Square in 1893, and remembered Gowers as a 'gruff old grizzly bear'.

Our discovery of new primary sources has allowed us to reassess earlier judgements about Gowers' personality. The suggestion that his aloof exterior was constructed to conceal his acute sensitivity seems to be confirmed by the content of his diaries and letters. Although Gowers may have claimed that he was not ashamed of having an artisan father, he was sensitive about his social status as a boy in Coggeshall, and he probably never lost an underlying sense of inferiority. His letters to Morrison reveal not only his kindness but also his vulnerability, hurt by being dropped by Morrison once the younger man he had befriended became famous and was being lionized by the aristocracy. His description of how he initiated his friendship with Kipling is almost childlike in its delight, and Kipling was another man upon whom he also bestowed many small kindnesses. His devotion to his family shines through the charm and wit of the diaries he wrote and illustrated for his children.

Howard and Willison have suggested that Gowers may have been the model for Dr Percy Trevelyan, 'the author of a book on obscure nervous lesions' who features in *The Resident Patient* by Conan Doyle.[7] The patient suffers from a cataleptic state. The doctor, Trevelyan, came from an impoverished background. He had a manner that 'was nervous and shy, like that of a sensitive gentleman, and the thin white hand which he laid on the mantelpiece as he rose was that of an artist rather than of a surgeon'. In the late nineteenth century forensic medicine and neurology were just emerging as scientific specialities. The painstaking assembly of seemingly disconnected clues (neurological signs) that often appeared insignificant to the layperson were decoded and used to form a diagnosis or solve a mystery. Indeed, neurologist David Ferrier started his medical career in forensic medicine.

Conan Doyle had been trained as an ophthalmologist and wrote his doctoral thesis on tabes dorsalis, and may have attended Gowers' lectures, which were open to any postgraduates. Conan Doyle modelled Sherlock Holmes himself on his Edinburgh mentor, surgeon Joseph Bell. A connection between Gowers and Trevelyan seems possible.

## Gowers and Charcot

It is interesting to compare Gowers with the great French neurologist Jean-Martin Charcot, born in 1825, and 20 years Gowers' senior. One of Charcot's great legacies as a clinician was his contribution to the development of systematic neurological examination. Charcot attempted to link clinical signs to specific anatomical lesions in the nervous system, and Gowers followed his lead. Through scrupulous attention to detail and eventual pathological correlation at autopsy both men were able to provide a new classification of neurological disease and put the clinico-anatomical approach firmly at the forefront of clinical method.

In 1869 Charcot had accompanied Brown-Séquard to a meeting of the British Medical Association at which he heard Russell Reynolds give a talk entitled 'Paralysis and other disorders of motion and sensation dependent on idea'. Reynolds conceded that although he disliked the label because of the stigma attached to it, many of the disorders he was describing could be labelled hysterical.[8] Charcot acknowledged Reynolds' paper as the impetus for his school's later extensive research on hysteria.

Both Charcot and Gowers were visionaries who were aware of the importance of illustration as an aid to neurological teaching . Both were also outstanding lecturers and laid down many of the teaching methods that continue to this day. However, Charcot had an audience, whereas Gowers took a class; Charcot used Gallic intuitiveness and showmanship to great effect, while Gowers emphasized attention to detail. Although it is clear that Gowers recognized Charcot's achievements, he expressed reservations about using on English women Charcot's method of terminating hysterical phenomena by ovarian compression.[9] Gowers also insisted that symptoms should not be dismissed as hysterical because they were strange. For example, when in 1907 he described in his *Borderland of Epilepsy* the subjective sensation of vasovagal attacks, he wrote: 'To dismiss it as a hysterical fancy is simply to push it out of sight with the foot. So definite a feeling must have a definite origin'. Symonds, in his 1960 Gowers lecture, 'Disease of the mind and disorder of brain' summed up Gowers' approach:

> Gowers was also an ardent collector of cases in which the phenomena of nervous disorder were mainly or wholly subjective but presented features sufficiently distinct to be clearly recognizable in a group of such cases. This for him was convincing evidence of a physical, as opposed to a psychogenic basis.[10]

## Gowers and Hughlings Jackson

It is also interesting to compare Gowers with John Hughlings Jackson, who was born ten years after Charcot, in 1835. Francis Walshe compared these two pioneer English neurologists:

> What greater contrast could be found between any two of the masters of our discipline than between Gowers and Hughlings Jackson: the first a born naturalist, an accurate and retentive observer and recorder of the phenomena of disease that came before him, a supreme artist in the field of nosography. The second with a dominating passion for wresting from phenomena the principles they exemplify, and thus concentrating upon a smaller field of inquiry and to a different end.
>
> Here we see two orders of genius, that of the naturalist and that of the philosopher, both essential to a living discipline of knowledge; the one primarily absorbed in irreducible and stubborn facts, the other using facts primarily for the derivation of scientific generalizations. Of course, to make an absolute antithesis here would be to simplify unduly, since

> for every good naturalist facts must yield some meaning, and every true philosopher must be concerned with experience, but that the two types exist no-one will dispute.[11]

Gowers helped to disseminate Hughlings Jackson's great insights. In his own lucid prose Gowers interpreted for the medical world the dense and confusing writings of his 'master'. In 1925 James Taylor wrote how difficult it was to realize the chaotic state of knowledge of nervous diseases which had existed before Hughlings Jackson's time, and how great a part Hughlings Jackson's work and stimulus played in evolving order out of this chaos:

> The extraordinary work of Gowers in this classification is universally recognized, and by no one was it more generously acknowledged and appreciated than by Jackson.[12]

When Gowers' personality was compared against that of Hughlings Jackson, Gowers always came out worst. Hughlings Jackson was seen as easy-going where Gowers was intolerant, and warm-hearted where Gowers was difficult.[13] However, these two men, Gowers a devout Congregationalist who saw nature as part of God's work, and Hughlings Jackson an agnostic philosopher, held one another in the greatest esteem. It was fortunate for the development of the science of neurology that for nearly forty years they worked so closely and harmoniously together at Queen Square.

## Twentieth-century assessments of Gowers' contributions to neurology

When Gowers died in 1915, his obituary in *The Times* singled out his 1879 lecture on 'Diseases of the spinal cord' as ground-breaking:

> The lecture was really epoch-making because of the manner in which pathological anatomy and clinical symptomatology were brought into relation, and it laid the foundation of the wonderful complete knowledge which we now possess of the organic diseases of the spinal cord.

The obituary then commented on 'Diagnosis of diseases of the brain':

> By this time [1885] the clinical and pathological observations of Hughlings Jackson and the experimental work of Fritsch, Hitzig and Ferrier had completely altered the conceptions of cerebral physiology and functions, and Gowers' acute mind readily grasped the significance of their observations. In the volume referred to … principles were laid down and rules enunciated which at the present day are perhaps a little extended but scarcely in any way altered.
>
> If he lacked the originality and inspiration of Hughlings Jackson, Gowers was nevertheless a great clinical neurologist and through his writings enriched the wider understanding of scientific neurology in the medical world of his time.[14]

*The Lancet* noted that Hughlings Jackson 'often remarked that he would always be grateful to Gowers because of the manner in which Gowers had expounded the Jacksonian theories' and concluded its obituary with the words: 'It may be mentioned without impertinence that Sir William Gowers was peculiarly happy in his married life and a devoted husband and father'.[15]

The American *Journal of Nervous and Mental Disease* rated Gowers as one of the most notable figures of the English medical field, 'distinguished by a certain dynamic forcefulness which manifested itself in his thought and in his vigorous methods of activity, combined with breadth of observation, clear perception and constructive imagination'.[16]

In 1945, to mark the centenary of Gowers' birth, the *BMJ* carried a reassessment of his contribution:

> In medical literature we have our English classics, but we regard them too little. Among them the published works of Gowers hold a distinguished place. Of particular value to those not specially interested in neurology are his published clinical lectures, which reveal a perfect balance of observation and of judgment, and a broad outlook that every clinical teacher might take as an example.[17]

The same article described him as one of the greatest clinicians and teachers of clinical medicine in the nineteenth century.

Macdonald Critchley's biography was published four years later. When he considered the (unattributed) statement that Gowers 'was probably the greatest clinical neurologist of all time', Critchley concluded that while he was only one among many great pioneering neurologists, what singled him out was his clinical method, but that to Gowers' great achievement as a scientific observer of natural morbid phenomena and as a field worker must be added his skill as an exponent.[18] He described Jackson and Gowers as the 'benevolent Gog and Magog' of Queen Square:

> Very different in their personalities and achievement, they were complementary. Each held the other in high esteem. ... Whereas Jackson was inclined to be untidy, and at times vague, Gowers was obsessional, perfectionist, and exacting. Equally astute as a clinician, Gowers recorded punctiliously.[19]

Critchley's concluding assessment was based on frequency of citation, terminology of nervous disorders, therapies, and the disorders themselves:

> In turning over the Index of such a fully documented work as Kinnier Wilson's *Neurology*[20] we find that Gowers' contributions to the subject are referred to in 132 separate items. What this means is shown by a comparison with other names: Oppenheim 93; Pierre Marie 77; Spiller 72; Van Bogaert 60; Guillain 56; Cushing 55; Déjérine 50; Marinesco 48; Lhermitte 45; Foerster 42; and Hughlings Jackson 21.
>
> If we turn to the terminology of nervous disorder we cannot escape his influence. The words 'amyotatic', 'abiotrophy', 'knee-jerk', 'fibrositis', were all his coinage. Gowers' tract, Gowers' mixture are expressions in daily use today. In neurological therapy, priority is due to him for advocating borax in epilepsy, aluminium chloride in tabes, and nitroglycerine in headache—though these remedies are largely forgotten today. We should never forget, however, that the early descriptions - if not the earliest - of many of the nervous diseases which we today recognize with confidence, are due to the acumen of Gowers: progressive lenticular degeneration; myasthenia gravis; ataxic paraplegia; paramyoclonus multiplex; Schilder's disease; the syndrome of the frontal tumour; musicogenic epilepsy; geniculate herpes[21]; sleep paralysis; dystrophia myotonica; local panatrophy[22]; vasovagal attacks.
>
> Among the classical physical signs which Gowers was the first to recognize are the nasal smile of myasthenics, fixation spasm and pharyngolaryngeal nystagmus[23]. Gowers also recognized early postero-median sclerosis in the tabetic spinal cord.[24]

Two years after Critchley's biography was published, Gordon Holmes wrote an assessment of Gowers career at Queen Square, concluding:

> Though in subsequent years many important papers appeared from his pen, the *Manual* remains his chief monument, but to those who knew him and worked with him he was obviously greater than his monument. To him the National Hospital is largely indebted for the high level of its clinical practice; few have added so much to its reputation as a centre of scientific medicine or contributed more to its policy as a teaching school.[25]

In 1969, in *Garrison's History of Neurology*, McHenry wrote:

> To Gowers we owe the earliest and in many cases the original descriptions of many disorders, including dystrophia myotonia, encephalitis periaxalis diffusa, ataxia paraplegia, vasovagal attacks, musicogenic epilepsy, paramyoclonus multiplex, the syndrome of subfrontal tumors, sleep paralysis, local panatrophy and palatal myoclonus. His studies on posthemiplegic movement disorders (1869), pseudohypertrophic muscular dystrophy (1879), and distal myopathy (1902) are classic.[26]

Some writers have suggested that he was the first to describe dystrophia myotonica (now known as Steinert's disease), which Gowers described as a distal myopathy.

## Reassessment of Gowers' legacy to British neurology

To the very end of his career Gowers reconstructed, updated, and recategorized his case material, and it is this which creates the freshness and pleasure neurologists have in reading the *Manual*, particularly where he reflects on his earlier clinical observations.

Medicine for Gowers was a personal science that must be applied to human need. He searched for commonalities and exceptions that would allow him to deduce where and why a particular area of the nervous system had become dysfunctional. After the patient's death his enquiry would continue through post-mortem examination of the brain and spinal cord.

Gowers was quick to learn both from chance advice and from his mentors and to apply these lessons to his exploration of the nervous system. His impeccable shorthand became a powerful research tool, enabling him to make immediate and comprehensive records of clinical events and to maintain detailed records of his clinical practice. His case notes were sometimes clarified by his own quick sketches. His methodical approach to collecting and analysing his statistics gave scientific validity to his research findings. The emphasis he placed on accurate recording is reflected in neurological practice today, distinguishing it from some other 'technique driven' medical specialities. Gowers never lost his enthusiasm for materia medica, to which he was first introduced when mixing potions in Coggeshall for Mr Simpson, and then reinforced by 'botanizing' during his studies for the new Preliminary Scientific Examination. This lifelong interest led to his strong commitment to improving the therapeutic options for his patients through effective medication. He also recognized the potential of brain and spinal cord surgery, and was not afraid to suggest likely tumour sites to his colleague Victor Horsley when localization was still in its earliest stages.

He was as committed to passing on knowledge as he was to acquiring it, and put as much care and thought into his lectures as he did into everything else he turned his hand to. He was renowned in his day as an outstanding lecturer. The importance he attributed to teaching was demonstrated by the priority he gave to clinical demonstrations for both undergraduate and postgraduate medical students and physicians, as well as by the quality of his undergraduate lectures at UCL.

Gowers' constant quest for improvements in diagnostic tools led him to invent devices such as the haemoglobinometer and to embrace new technology such as the ophthalmoscope. He was quick to grasp that the new developments in histological staining of the brain would lead to a revolution in the definition of nervous disease.

His exquisite medical writing is a lasting legacy, and set an exacting standard for those who followed him. Given the level of knowledge at the time, Gowers' *Manual of Diseases of the Nervous System* remains the greatest single-author comprehensive textbook of clinical neurology ever published, and many of his original publications continue to influence current thinking in the fields of epilepsy, migraine, Parkinson's disease, and writer's cramp.

Gowers' wonderful ability to create order was recognized by Sir William Broadbent, who said that Gowers had 'taken up the raw material of knowledge wherever it was to be found, and had worked it up into a piece of most beautiful texture, presenting the difficult problems of nervous physiology and nervous disease in the clearest way'.[27]

The impeccable clinical method that he applied to his work led to the description of many previously unrecognized phenomena and a greater understanding of the mechanisms responsible for neurological illnesses. Gowers was undoubtedly a superb diagnostician, and his clear, logical, and analytical approach to diagnosis established the model that is still used today in British neurology.

In November 1956, Sir Francis Walshe gave the first Gowers lecture at Queen Square on 'The nature and dimensions of nosography in modern medicine'. It seems fitting to repeat his conclusion which was a tribute not only to the man himself, but also to the hospital which appointed him its first medical registrar in 1870, and to which he devoted 40 extraordinarily productive years:

> And if, as we rightly do, we look upon Gowers' superb clinical writings as his monument, they are also the monument of the special hospital in which he laboured, and without which he could never have attained the rich achievement by which his name will live wherever neurological medicine is studied.[28]

# Bibliography

Many of the sources listed below are rare, and in some cases it has not been possible to verify either the number of editions of each, or the page sequences for sections in books. Many are now becoming available in digital reproductions. No attempt has been made to try to list these recent re-issues which are easily discovered through online searches. Nor does the list include books translated from English originals into other languages.

## Contributions by Gowers to edited works


'Carditis', 'Atrophy', 'Hypertrophy', 'Dilatation', 'Fatty disease', and 'Fibroid disease of the heart', in Reynolds, J R (ed.) *A System of Medicine*, 4 (London: Macmillan, 1868).

'Cases of convulsion from organic brain disease', in Hughlings Jackson, *J* (ed.) *On the Anatomical and Physiological Localisation of Movements in the Brain* (London: J & A Churchill, 1874).

'The central nervous system', in Sharpey-Schafer, E A, Sharpey, W, and Thomson, A (ed.) *Quain's Elements of Anatomy*, 8th edn (London: Longmans Green & Co., 1876).

Hughlings Jackson, J, Gowers, W R, and Tweedy, J, *Case of large cerebral tumour without optic neuritis, and with left hemiplegia and imperception* (London: Harrison and Sons, 1876).

'Splenic leucocythaemia', in Reynolds, J R (ed.) *A System of Medicine, 5* (London: Macmillan, 1879).

'Carditis', 'Atrophy', 'Hypertrophy',' Dilatation', 'Fatty disease', and 'Fibroid disease of the heart', in Reynolds, J R (ed.) *A System of Medicine*, 4 (London: Macmillan, 1877).

'Paralysis agitans', in Allbutt, T C (ed.) *A System of Medicine*, 8, pp.73–82 (London: Macmillan, 1899).


## Books by Gowers


(translated by Gowers) *Atlas of Pathological Anatomy of the Eyeball* [translation of Pagenstecher and Genth's *Atlas der pathologischen Anatomie des Gaugapfels*] (Wiesbaden: Kreidel, 1875).

*Diagrams for the record of physical signs* [*of thoracic and abdominal disease*] (in books of 12 sets of figures) (London: H. K. Lewis, 1878).

(with Foster, M) *Pathologischer Beweis einer unvollständigen Kreuzung der Sehnerven beim Menschen* (Berlin: Schumacher, 1878).

*A Manual and Atlas of Medical Ophthalmoscopy*, 1st edn (London: J & A Churchill, 1879).

*Pseudo-Hypertrophic Muscular Paralysis* (London: J & A Churchill, 1879).

*The Diagnosis of Diseases of the Spinal Cord* (London: J & A Churchill, 1880).

*Epilepsy and Other Chronic Convulsive Disorders, their Causes, Symptoms and Treatment* (London: J & A Churchill, 1881).

*The Diagnosis of Diseases of the Spinal Cord* [revised and partly rewritten, with additions and illustrations], 2nd edn (London: J & A Churchill, 1881).

*A Manual and Atlas of Medical Ophthalmoscopy*, 2nd edn (London: J & A Churchill, 1882).

*The Diagnosis of Diseases of the Spinal Cord*, 2nd edn (Philadelphia: Presley, Blakiston, 1882).

*The Diagnosis of Diseases of the Spinal Cord*, 3rd edn (London: J & A Churchill, 1884).

*Introductory Lecture Delivered on the Opening of the Medical Session at University College, London, October 1st, 1884* (London: HK Lewis, 1884).

*Lectures on the Diagnosis of Diseases of the Brain*, 1st edn (London: J & A Churchill, 1885).

*Diagnosis of the Diseases of the Brain and of the Spinal Cord*, 1st edn (New York: William Wood & Co, 1885).

*A Manual of Diseases of the Nervous System*, Vol 1, 1st edn (London: J & A Churchill, 1886).

*Lectures on the Diagnosis of Diseases of the Brain*, 2nd edn (London: J & A Churchill, 1887).

*A Manual of Diseases of the Nervous System*, Vol 2, 1st edn (London: J & A Churchill, 1888).

(with Horsley, V and Brandis, K J B) *Ein Fall von Rückenmarkgeschwulst mit Heilung durch Exstirpation* (Berlin: August Hirschwald, 1889).

(with Gunn, R M) *A Manual and Atlas of Medical Ophthalmoscopy*, 3rd edn (London: J & A Churchill, 1890).

*Syphilis of the Nervous System* [being a revised reprint of the Lettsomian Lectures for 1890] (London: J & A Churchill, 1892).

*A Manual of Diseases of the Nervous System*, Vol 1, 2nd edn (London: J & A Churchill, 1892).

*Syphilis and the Nervous System* [being a revised reprint of Lettsomian Lectures for 1890] (Philadelphia: Blakiston, 1892).

*A Manual of Diseases of the Nervous System*, Vol 2, 2nd edn (London: J & A Churchill, 1893).

*The Dynamics of Life: an Address Delivered Before the Medical Society of Manchester October 3rd, 1894* (London: J & A Churchill, 1894).

*The Dynamics of Life: an Address* (Philadelphia: Blakiston, 1894).

*The Element of Art in Phonography: an Address Delivered to the Phonetic Shorthand Writers' Association, London, 22 November 1894* (London: Phonetic Institute, 1894).

*Clinical Lectures on Diseases of the Nervous System* (London: J & A Churchill, 1895).

*The Use of Shorthand by the Practitioner: with Examples* (London: Society of Medical Phonographers, 1895).

*The Use of Shorthand by the Student: with Examples* (London: Society of Medical Phonographers, 1895).

*Clinical Lectures on Diseases of the Nervous System* (Philadelphia: Blakiston, Son & Co, 1895).

*The Use of Shorthand by the Practitioner*, 2nd edn (London: Society of Medical Phonographers, 1896).

*The Use of Shorthand by the Student*, 2nd edn (London: Isaac Pitman, 1896).

*Diagnosis of the Nature of Organic Brain Disease* (London: Isaac Pitman, 1897).

*A Manual of Diseases of the Nervous System*, 2, 2nd edn (Philadelphia: Blakiston, 1898).

(edited with Taylor, J) *A Manual of Diseases of the Nervous System*, Vol 1, 3rd edn (London: J & A Churchill, 1899).

*The Work of the Life Assurance Examiner* (London: Pitman, 1899).

*Epilepsy and Other Chronic Convulsive Diseases*, 2nd edn (London: J & A Churchill, 1901).

*Lunacy and the Law: an Address on the Prevention of Insanity* [delivered before the Medico-Psychological Association of Great Britain and Ireland, with an appendix note] (London: J & A Churchill, 1903).

*Subjective Sensations of Sight and Sound, Abiotrophy and Other Lectures* [including a note on the designation of musical notes in science and medicine] (Philadelphia: Blakiston, 1904).

*Subjective Sensations of Sight and Sound, Abiotrophy and Other Lectures* (London: J & A Churchill, 1904).

(with Gunn, R M) *A Manual and Atlas of Medical Ophthalmoscopy*, 4th edn, (London: J & A Churchill, 1904).

*The Borderland of Epilepsy: Faints, Vagal Attacks, Vertigo, Migraine, Sleep Symptoms, and Their Treatment* (London: J & A Churchill, 1907).

*Problems in Practical Diagnosis* [printed in shorthand] (London: Pitman, 1909).

(with Church, W S, Latham, A, and Bashford, E F) *The Influence of Heredity on Disease: with Special Reference to Tuberculosis, Cancer and Diseases of the Nervous System* (London: Longman, 1909).

## Journal articles by Gowers

### 1870–9

'A safety hypodermic syringe', *Lancet*, **99**:2526, 27 January 1872, 113.

'Cancer of the liver', *Transactions of the Pathological Society of London*, **23**, 1872, 145–51.

'On the influence of posture in "pre-systolic" cardiac murmurs', *Practitioner*, **2**, 1873, 401–7.

(with Hughlings Jackson, J) 'Cases of convulsion from organic brain disease', *Medical Times and Gazette*, 3 January 1874.

'Cases of convulsion from organic brain disease (lecture, BMA)', *BMJ*, **2**:717, 26 September 1874, 398–400.

'Notes on facial paralysis', *Lancet*, **103**:2641, 11 April 1874, 507–9.

(with Lockhart-Clarke, J) 'On a case of pseudo-hypertrophic muscular paralysis', *Medico-Chirurgical Transactions*, **57**, 1874, 247–59.

'A case of convulsion from brain injury', *Lancet*, **106**:2723, 6 November 1875, 655–7.

'On a case of simultaneous embolism of the central retinal and middle cerebral arteries', *Lancet*, **106**:2727, 4 December 1875, 794–6.

(with Hughlings Jackson, J) 'Right-sided fits, most of them limited to the right arm; subsequently hemiplegia; double optic neuritis; tumours of the left cerebral hemisphere', *Medical Times and Gazette*, 21 July 1875.

'Pathological: double memory (consciousness)', *Mind*, **1**:4, October 1876, 552–4.

'Philosophical and pathological: functions of the optic thalami', *Mind*, 3, July 1876, 412–14.

'Athetosis and post-hemiplegic disorders of movement', *Journal of Nervous and Mental Disease*, **3**:3, July 1876, 510.

'The state of the arteries in Bright's disease' [a lecture to the BMA], *BMJ*, **2**:832, 9 December 1876, 743–5.

'On "athetosis" and post-hemiplegic disorders of movement', *Medico-Chirurgical Transactions*, **59**, 1876, 271–327.

'On the development of spindle-cells in "nested sarcomas"', *Medico-Chirurgical Transactions*, **59**, 1876, 217–26.

'Reports: mental automatism in epileptics', *Mind*, **1**:2, April 1876, 272–3.

'Shoulder-joint friction' [clinical memoranda], *BMJ*, **2**:829, 18 November 1876, 652.

'Glioma of the left cerebral hemisphere', *Transactions of the Pathological Society of London*, **27**, 1876, 13–17.

'Myo-lipoma of spinal cord', *Transactions of the Pathological Society of London*, **27**, 1876, 19–22.

'Posterior sclerosis and posterior median sclerosis of the spinal cord', *Transactions of the Pathological Society of London*, **27**, 1876, 30–3.

'Cerebral aneurysms associated with endocarditis', *Transactions of the Pathological Society of London*, **27**, 1876, 33–9.

'The diagnosis and treatment of auditory nerve vertigo' [summary, presented to BMA], *BMJ*, **2**:271, 26 August 1876, 274–5.

'The diagnosis and treatment of auditory nerve vertigo' (1), *BMJ*, **1**:845, 10 March 1877, 287–9; (2) *BMJ*, **1**:849, 7 April 1877, 418–20; (3) *BMJ*, **1**:851, 21 April 1877, 477–8.

'Report of paper on the arteries in Bright's disease' [lecture, BMA], *BMJ*, **2**:816, 19 August 1876, 238.

'A case of lymphatic leucocythaemia and allied diseases treated by phosphorus' [report, Clinical Society of London], Lancet, **108**:2779, 1876, 786.

'Lymphatic leucocythaemia treated by phosphorus', *Transactions of the Clinical Society of London*, **10**, 1877, 33–43.

'The automatic action of the sphincter ani', *Proceedings of the Royal Society of London*, **26**:1 January 1877, 77–84.

'On saltatoric spasm' (1), *Lancet*, **110**:2811, 14 July 1877, 42–5; (2), *Lancet*, 110:2814, 4 August 1877, 152–5.

'The morbid changes in chronic Bright's disease' [letter], *Lancet*, **109**:2797, 7 April 1877, 515.

'On the numeration of blood-corpuscles', *Lancet*, **110**:2831, 1 December 1877, 797–8.

'On the use of iron in epilepsy', *Practitioner*, **19**, 1877, 241–6.

'The pathological anatomy of hydrophobia (with four cases)', *Transactions of the Pathological Society of London*, **28**, 1877, 10–23.

'Local cerebral anaemia—bilateral symmetry in neurovascular disease', *Medical Times and Gazette*, **2**, 1877, 491.

'Remarks on two cases of writer's cramp', *Medical Times and Gazette*, **2**, 1877, 536–8.

'Cases of paralysis of the musculo-spinal nerve', *Medical Times and Gazette*, **1**, 1877, 474–5.

'Hypertrophy of the heart with primary renal disease', *Transactions of the Pathological Society of London*, **28**, 1877, 44–7.

'Mitral disease, compensatory enlargement of the anterior flap, high arterial tension', *Transactions of the Pathological Society of London*, **28**, 1877, 51–7.

'Cerebral syphiloma: mode of growth', *Transactions of the Pathological Society of London*, **28**, 1877, 280.

'Syphilomata of brain and spinal cord, syphilitic thickening of membranes around nerves, etc', *Transactions of the Pathological Society of London*, **28**, 1877, 281–5.

'Syphilitic disease of cerebral artery', *Transactions of the Pathological Society of London*, **28**, 1877, 286–7.

'Syphilitic disease of the lungs', *Transactions of the Pathological Society of London*, **28**, 1877, 330–1.

'Heart with mitral disease and dilatation and hypertrophy of both ventricles', *Lancet*, **109**:2784, 6 January 1877, 12.

'Visceral syphilis' [Pathological Society], *BMJ*, **1**:838, 20 January 1877, 86–7.

(with Sankey, H R O) 'The pathological anatomy of canine "chorea"', *Medico-Chirurgical Transactions*, **60**, 1877, 229–48.

(with Sankey, H R O) 'On the pathological anatomy of canine chorea' [report of paper read to the Medical Chirurgical Society], *Lancet*, **109**:2794, 1877, 388.

'Observations in specimens illustrating lymphatic diseases', *Transactions of the Pathological Society of London*, **29**, 1878, 304–13.

'A case of unilateral gunshot injury to the spinal cord', *Transactions of the Clinical Society of London*, **11**, 1878, 24–32.

'On some symptoms of organic brain disease', *Brain*, **1**:1, 1 April 1878, 48–59.

'The brain in congenital absence of one hand', *Brain*, **1**:3, 3 October 1878, 388–90.

'Empyema complicated with pneumonia; repeated aspirations; recovery', *Lancet*, **111**:2844, 2 March 1878, 310–11.

'Cases illustrating the treatment of bromide rash with arsenic', *Lancet*, **111**:2859, 15 June 1878, 866–7.

'On a peculiar form of albumen in urine', *Lancet*, **112**:2862, 6 July 1878, 3–4.

'On a case of anaemia, observed with the haemacytometer', *Lancet*, **111**:2854, 11 May 1878, 675–7.

'The numeration of blood-corpuscles', *Lancet*, **112**:2886, 21 December 1878, 901.

'The history of leucocythaemia' [letter], *Lancet*, **111**:2850, 13 April 1878, 550.

'The numeration of blood corpuscles and the effect of iron and phosphorus on the blood', *Practitioner*, **21**, 1878, 1–17.

'On some points in the clinical history of chorea: I The irritability of nerve and muscle in chorea; II On the relation of the muscular disturbance in chorea to voluntary movements', *BMJ*, **1**:900, 30 March 1878, 447–9; 'III The distribution of hemichorea', *BMJ*, **1**:901, 6 April 1878, 479–81.

'The estimation of haemoglobin in the blood' [Clinical Society of London], *Lancet*, **112**:2886, 21 December 1878, 882.

'A study of the so-called tendon-reflex phenomena', *Medico-Chirurgical Transactions*, **62**, 1879, 269–305.

'The movements of the eyelids' [Royal Medical Chirurgical Society], *Medico-Chirurgical Transactions*, **62**, 1879, 429–40.

'Syphilitic neuroses' [lecture, BMA], *BMJ*, **1**:948, 1 March 1879, 303–5.

'Cases of cerebral tumour illustrating diagnosis and localisation (cases 2 and 3)', *Lancet*, **113**:2898, 15 March 1879, 363–5.

'A study of the so-called tendon reflex phenomena' [Royal Medical and Chirurgical Society], *BMJ*, **2**:944, 1 February 1879, 169.

'A study of the so-called tendon reflex phenomena' [Royal Medical Chirurgical Society], *Lancet*, **113**:2892, 1 February 1879, 156–7.

'The movements of the eyelids' [Royal Medical and Chirurgical Society], *BMJ*, **1**:963, 14 June 1879, 894.

'The movements of the eyelids' [Royal Medical and Chirurgical Society], *Lancet*, **113**:2911, 14 June 1879, 844–5.

'An apparatus for the clinical estimation of haemoglobin', *Transactions of the Clinical Society of London*, **12**, 1879, 64–7.

'A note on the examination of the brain in Hutchinson, J "An ophthalmoplegia externa, or symmetrical immobility (partial) of the eyes, with ptosis", *Medico-Chirurgical Transactions*, **62**:44 (2nd series), 1879, 316–18.

'Note on a reflex mechanism in the fixation of the eyeballs', *Brain*, **2**:1, 1 April 1879, 39–41.

'The diagnosis of diseases of the spinal cord' [an address to the Medical Society of Wolverhampton], *Medical Times and Gazette*, 2:Nov-Dec 1879, 524–6, 575–7, 657–9, 683–5.

'Pseudo-hypertrophic muscular paralysis' [clinical lectures], (1) *Lancet*, **114**:2914, 5 July 1879, 1–2; (2) *Lancet*, **114**:2915, 12 July 1879, 37–9; (3) *Lancet*, **114**:2916, 19 July 1879, 73–5; (4) *Lancet*, **114**:2917, 26 July 1879, 113–16.

'Cases of cerebral tumour illustrating diagnosis and localisation (case 1)', *Lancet*, **113**:2897, 8 March 1879, 327–9.

### 1880–9

'Illustrations of diseases of the pons varolii', *Brain*, **2**:4, 4 January 1880, 466–77.

'The Ophthalmological Society' [letter], *BMJ*, **2**:1023, 7 August 1880, 233.

'A note on an outbreak of rubeola' [Rotheln], *Lancet*, **116**:2970, 31 July 1880, 169.

'The Gulstonian Lectures on epilepsy' [abstracts], *Brain*, **3**, 1880, 268–82.

'Contribution to discussion on hysterical anaesthesia' [opened by Dr Bristowe], *BMJ*, **2**:1026, 28 August 1880, 331.

'On paralytic chorea', *BMJ*, **2**:1026, 28 August 1880, 332–3.

'Optic neuritis in chlorosis' [lecture, BMA], *BMJ*, **2**:1037, 13 November 1880, 780.

'Five cases of locomotor ataxy in members of the same family' [Clinical Society of London], *BMJ*, **2**:1033, 16 October 1880, 623.

'The Gulstonian Lectures on epilepsy' [abstracts], *Medical Times and Gazette*, **1**, 1880, 227–448.

'The Gulstonian Lectures on epilepsy' [abstracts], *Medical Press and Circular*, **80**, 1880, 63–4, 85–6, 143–4.

'The Gulstonian Lectures on epilepsy', *Lancet*, **115**:2948, 28 February 1880, 315–18; *Lancet*, **115**:2949, 6 March 1880, 353–5; *Lancet*, **115**:2950, 13 March 1880, 391–3; *Lancet*, **115**:2951, 20 March 1880, 433–6; *Lancet*, **115**, 2952; *Lancet*, **115**:2953, 3 April 1880, 515–17; *Lancet*, **115**:2954, 10 April 1880, 552–4.

'The Gulstonian Lectures on epilepsy' (1) *BMJ*, **1**:1001, 6 March 1880, 353–7; (2), *BMJ*, **1**:1002, 13 March 1880, 393–5; (3), *BMJ*, **1**:1003, 20 March 1880, 427–30; (4), *BMJ*, **1**:1004, 27 March 1880, 465–7; (5), *BMJ*, **1**:1005, 3 April 1880, 503–4; (6), *BMJ*, **1**:1006, 10 April 1880, 547–9.

'On psoriasis from borax', *Lancet*, **118**:3030, 24 September 1881, 546.

'Syphilis and locomotor ataxy', *Lancet*, **117**:2994, 15 January 1881, 94–5.

'Subsequent history of a young woman suffering from cerebral tumour and double optic neuritis, shown last session' [Ophthalmic Society of the United Kingdom], *Lancet*, **118**:3042, 17 December 1881, 1046.

'A family affected with locomotor ataxy', *Transactions of the Clinical Society of London*, **14**, 1881, 1–5.

'Gowers' remarks at the discussion on the relation between optic neuritis and intracranial disease' [opened by J Hughlings Jackson], *Transactions of the Ophthalmological Society*, **1**, 1881, 102–8.

'Case of slight optic neuritis with paresis of sixth nerve, probably due to transient meningitis', *Transactions of the Ophthalmological Society*, **1**, 1881, 115–17.

'Case of intracranial disease with optic neuritis and paralysis of the upward movement of both eyes', *Transactions of the Ophthalmological Society*, **1**, 1881, 117–19.

'Gowers' remarks on paper by J. W. Hulke in ophthalmoplegia externa', *Transactions of the Ophthalmological Society*, **1**, 1881, 160–4.

'On paralytic chorea' [lecture, BMA], *BMJ*, **1**:1060, 23 April 1881, 636–7.

'Optic neuritis in chlorosis', *BMJ*, **1**:1064, 21 May 1881, 796–7.

'A case of loss of taste from disease of the fifth nerve', *Journal of Physiology*, **3**:3–4, 1 January 1882, 229–31.

'Remarks on acute spinal paralysis', *BMJ*, **1**:1116, 20 May 1882, 729–31.

'Report of the committee appointed to examine Dr Harbinson's specimens (diffuse changes in the brain, possibly sclerosis)', *Transactions of the Pathological Society of London*, **33**, 1882,

'Sequel to a case of cerebral tumour', *Transactions of the Ophthalmological Society*, **2**, 1882, 84–5.

'Gowers' remarks on a paper by W. Lang and W. A. FitzGerald on the movements of the eyelids in association with the movements of the eyes', *Transactions of the Ophthalmological Society*, **2**, 1882, 226–9.

'Epilepsy: auditory aura', *BMJ*, **1**:1115, 13 May 1882, 696.

'Eye symptoms in diseases of the spinal cord' [opening remarks, Ophthalmological Society], *Transactions of the Ophthalmological Society*, **3**, 1883, 190–204.

'Eye symptoms in diseases of the spinal cord' [address, Ophthalmological Society], *Medical Times and Gazette*, **1**, 1883, 661–4.

'Eye symptoms in spinal disease' [memoranda, Ophthalmological Society], *Medical Times and Gazette*, 1, 10 May 1883.

'Eye symptoms in diseases of the spinal cord' [address, Ophthalmological Society], *Lancet*, **121**:3120, 16 June 1883, 1031–4.

'Eye symptoms in spinal disease' [memoranda, Ophthalmological Society], *Lancet*, **121**:3116, 19 May 1883, 869–70.

'Tetany' [clinical lecture, UCH], *Lancet*, **122**:3125, 21 July 1883, 91–3.

(with Savage, G H and Payne, J F) 'Report of the committee appointed to investigate the changes exhibited by specimens of the nervous centres in cases of diabetes submitted for examination by Drs Dickinson, F. Taylor and Goodhart, Seymour Taylor, S. Mackenzie and Hale White', *Transactions of the Pathological Society of London*, **34**, 1883, 397.

'Introductory lecture' [lecture, UCH], *Lancet*, **124**:3188, 4 October 1884, 582–86.

'On certain forms of spasm of the ocular muscles', *Transactions of the Ophthalmological Society*, **4**, 1884, 306–9.

'Introductory address delivered at University College' [abstract], *Medical Times and Gazette*, **2**, 1884, 466–9.

'The diagnostic value of the so-called "tendon-reflexes"' [presented to Medical Society of London], *Lancet*, **126**:3245, 7 November 1885, 839–42.

'Lectures on the diagnosis of diseases of the brain', *Mind*, **11**, 1886, 438.

'Notes on diseases of the nervous system: (2) On the antero-lateral ascending tract of the spinal cord', *Lancet*, **127**:3277, 19 June 1886, 1153–4.

'Ataxic paraplegia' [clinical lectures, UCH]: (1) *Lancet*, **128**:3279, 3 July 1886, 1–3; (2) *Lancet*, **128**:3280, 10 July 1886, 61–3.

'Notes on diseases of the nervous system: (1) On a case of miliary sclerosis of the brain', *Lancet*, **127**:3256, 23 January 1886, 145–6.

'Bemerkungen uber die antero-laterale aufsteignende Degeneration im Ruckenmark', *Neurologisches Centralblatt*, **5**, 1886, 97–9.

'Weitere Bemerkunger uber den aufsteigenden antero-lateralen Strang', *Neurologisches Centralblatt*, **5**, 1886, 150.

(with Barker, A E) 'On a case of abscess of the temporo-sphenoidal lobe of the brain, due to otitis media, successfully treated by trephining and drainage', *BMJ*, **2**:1345, 11 December 1886, 1154–6.

'Shorthand teaching in medical schools' [letter], *Lancet*, **130**:3349, 5 November 1887, 935.

'The value of shorthand to the student and to the practitioner of medicine', *Lancet*, **130**:3345, 8 October 1887, 703–4.

'Conjugate palsy of ocular muscles with nystagmus' [brief report of Gowers' presentation to the Ophthalmological Society], *BMJ*, **1**:1368, 19 March 1887, 624.

'Birth palsies' [clinical lectures, UCH]: (1) *Lancet*, **131**:3372, 14 April 1888, 709–11; (2) *Lancet*, **131**:3373, 21 April 1888, 759–60.

(with Horsley, V) 'A case of tumour of the spinal cord, with removal and recovery' [Royal Medical and Chirurgical Society], *Lancet*, **131**:3381, 16 June 1888, 1194.

(with Horsley, V) 'A case of tumour of the spinal cord. Removal, recovery', *Medico-Chirurgical Transactions*, **71**, 1888, 377–430.

'Blindness by disability', *Lancet*, **134**:3456, 23 November 1889, 1083.

'The Lettsomian lectures on syphilis and the nervous system': (1) *BMJ*, **1**:1463, 12 January 1889, 57–64; (2) *BMJ*, **1**:1465, 26 January 1889, 169–71; (3) *BMJ*, **1**:1466, 2 February 1889, 235–8; (4) *BMJ*, **1**:1467, 9 February 1889, 283–5; (5) *BMJ*, **1**:1468, 16 February 1889, 345–8.

'The Lettsomian lectures on syphilis and the nervous system', (1) *Lancet*, **123**:3411, 12 January 1889, 59–66; (2), *Lancet*, **133**:3413, 26 January 1889, 159–61; (2), *Lancet*, **133**:3414, 1889, 207–10; (3), *Lancet*, **133**:3415, 9 February 1889, 259–61; (3), *Lancet*, **133**:3416, 16 February 1889, 313–16.

'Notes on the functions of the nervous system: (i) How does the cerebellum co-ordinate?', *Lancet*, **135**:3479, 3 May 1890, 955–6; '(ii) The dual activity of the nerve cells', *Lancet*, **135**:3480, 10 May 1890, 1006–7; '(iii) Automatic reflex co-ordination', *Lancet*, **135**:3482, 24 May 1890, 1113–14; '(iv) Muscular adaptation and hypnotic catalepsy', *Lancet*, **135**:3483, 3 May 1890, 1167–8.

'Die funktionen des kleinhirm', *Neurologisches Centralblatt*, **9**, 1890, 194–5.

'Consultants and general practitioners' [letter], *Lancet*, **138**:3561, 28 November 1891, 1249.

'The convulsive cough of puberty' [letter], *BMJ*, **1**:1567, 10 January 1891, 88.

'Atrophic spinal paralysis and multiple neuritis' [Clinical Society of London], *Lancet*, **137**:3525, 21 March 1891, 662–3.

'A case of anterior poliomyelitis and multiple neuritis', *Transactions of the Clinical Society of London*, **24**, 1891, 127–33.

'General principles of the diagnosis of diseases of the nervous system' [lecture, Queen Square], *Lancet*, **139**:3573, 20 February 1892, 403–5.

'Neurology and therapeutics' [address, Medical Society of London], *BMJ*, **1**:1685, 15 April 1893, 781–2.

'Locomotor ataxy' [two clinical lectures, Queen Square], *Clinical Journal*, **2**, 1893, 353–8, 369–76.

'A case of syringomyelia' [clinical lecture, Queen Square], *Clinical Journal*, **2**, 1893, 65–70.

'Acute ascending myelitis' [clinical lecture, Queen Square], *Clinical Journal*, **3**, 1893, 113–16.

'Facial paralysis' [clinical lecture, Queen Square], *Clinical Journal*, **3**, 1893, 241–8.

'The nervous sequelae of influenza' [post-graduate lectures, Queen Square], (pt 1) *Lancet*, **142**:3645, 1 July 1893, 1–3; (pt 2), *Lancet*, **142**:3644, 8 July 1893, 73–6.

(with Coupland, S) 'Dr Wilson Fox's plates of diseases of the lung' [letter], *Lancet*, **144**:3700, 28 July 1894, 226–7.

'The dynamics of life in relation to the nature of epilepsy' [paper, Manchester Medical Society], (pt 1) *Lancet*, **144**:3714, 3 November 1894, 1015–19; (pt 2) *Lancet*, **144**:3715, 10 November 1894, 1080–5.

'Out-patient hospital abuse' [letter], *BMJ*, **1**:1735, 3 March 1894, 716–17.

'Pernicious anaemia at 21', *BMJ*, **1**:1739, 28 April 1894, 904.

'Mistaken diagnosis' [post-graduate lecture, Queen Square], *BMJ*, **2**:1749, 7 July 1894, 1–3.

'Silver and syphilis' [clinical lecture, Queen Square], *BMJ*, **2**:1770, 1 December 1894, 1221–3.

'Chapel of S. Margaret, Mells', *Proceedings of the Suffolk Institute of Archaeology and Natural History*, **8**, 1894, 334–79.

'Optic neuritis' [clinical lecture, Queen Square], *Clinical Journal*, **5**, 1894, 85–90.

'A postgraduate lecture on the treatment of muscular contractions', *Clinical Journal*, **5**, 1894, 293–6.

'Bulbar paralysis' [post-graduate lecture, Queen Square], *Clinical Journal*, **4**, 1894, 1–8.

'The infantile causes of epilepsy', *Clinical Journal*, **4**, 1894, 309–12, 13–16.

'Facial contraction after paralysis', *Clinical Journal*, **4**, 1894, 329–33.

(with Gray, E B and Neil, J) 'Shorthand in medicine' [letter], *Lancet*, **144**:3700, 28 July 1894,

'The Society of Medical Phonographers', *BMJ*, **2**:1803, 1895, 175.

'Colour vision and accidents' [letter], *Lancet*, **145**:3731, 2 March 1895, 576–7.

'Is meteorology a science?' [letter], *Lancet*, **146**:3750, 13 July 1895, 122.

'An address on the use of drugs' [Harlesden Medical Society], *Lancet*, **146**:3769, 23 November 1895, 1271–4.

'Subjective visual sensations' [the Bowman Lecture], *Transactions of the Ophthalmological Society*, **15**, 1895, 1–38.

'Severe optic neuritis' [lecture, Queen Square], *Clinical Journal*, **6**, 1895, 81–6.

'Lead palsy' [lecture, Queen Square], *Clinical Journal*, **6**, 1895, 12–16.

'Anterior poliomyelitis' [lecture, Queen Square], *Clinical Journal*, **7**, 1895, 241–5.

'Caries in the spine' [two lectures, Queen Square], *Clinical Journal*, **7**, 1895, 17–21, 33–5.

'The old and the new in therapeutics', *Practitioner*, **54**, 1895, 209–10.

'What is shorthand?', *Medical Magazine*, January 1895, 383.

'The art of writing in relation to medical and scientific work', *BMJ*, **2**:1814, 5 October 1895, 817–19.

'A post-graduate lecture on acute myelitis' [Queen Square], 27 November 1895, manuscript, Queen Square Library, Archive and Museum.

(with Hutchinson, J) 'Discussion on the affections of the nervous system occurring in the early (secondary) stages of syphilis', *Medico-Chirurgical Transactions*, **7**, 1895, 68–111.

'Medical spelling', *BMJ*, **1**:1833, 1896, 439.

'An address on some aspects of diseases of the nervous system and their study', *BMJ*, **2**:1870, 1896, 1310.

'The Bradshaw Lecture on subjective sensations of sound', *BMJ*, **2**:1872, 14 November 1896, 1429–36.

'Medical spelling: an epicriticism', *BMJ*, **1**:1830, 1896, 244(b).

'Medical and other spelling', *BMJ*, **1**:1832, 1896, 375–6.

'Shorthand in medicine', *Lancet*, **147**:3796, 30 May 1896, 1523–4.

'Some aspects of diseases of the nervous system and their practical study' [inaugural address, first session of instruction at the National Hospital Queen Square as a recognized clinical school], *Lancet*, **148**:3818, 31 October 1896, 1205–10.

'Slight multiple neuritis' [lecture, Queen Square], *Clinical Journal*, **8**, 1896, 21–4.

'Anaemia or anemia?' [letter], *Lancet*, **147**:3375, 4 January 1896, 68.

(with Gray, E B, Neil, J, and Thomson, W) 'Shorthand and the General Medical Council', *BMJ*, **2**:1877, 1896, 1804, 228.

'Should epileptics marry?' [letter], *Lancet*, **149**:3834, 20 February 1897, 554.

'A note from the clinic: habit spasm', *Clinical Journal*, **10**, 1897, 401–2.

'A case of paralysis of the fifth nerve', *Edinburgh Medical Journal*, January 1897, 229–31.

'The neuron and its relation to disease' [lecture, Queen Square], *Lancet*, **150**:3871, 6 November 1897, 1172–5.

'Annotation: the marriage of female epileptics', *Lancet*, **149**:3830, 23 January 1897, 260.

'An appreciation of Sir William Jenner as a clinical teacher and physician', *BMJ*, **2**:1981, 17 December 1898, 1852.

'Remarks on the pathology of tabes in relation to general paralysis of the insane' [Pathological Society of London], *BMJ*, **2**:2032, 9 December 1899, 1597–8.

'Polymyositis' [lecture, Queen Square], *BMJ*, **1**:1985, 14 January 1899, 65–7.

'The new neurology' [lecture, Queen Square], *Lancet*, **153**:3933, 14 January 1899, 71–3.

**1900–9**

'Minor epilepsy' [clinical lecture, Queen Square], *BMJ*, **1**:2036, 6 January 1900, 1–5.

'The late Sir James Paget', *Lancet*, **155**:3985, 13 January 1900, 131.

'Contribution to a discussion on the pathological identity of tabes and general paralysis', *Transactions of the Pathological Society of London*, **51**, 1900, 352–6.

(with Hughlings Jackson, J, Buzzard, T, Carter, R B, Bastian, H C, and Ferrier, D) 'The medical staff and the management of the National Hospital for the Paralysed and Epileptic, Queen Square' [letter], *Lancet*, **156**:4014, 4 August 1900, 351–2.

(with Hughlings Jackson, J, Buzzard, T, Carter, R B, Bastian, H C, and Ferrier, D) 'The National Hospital for the Paralysed and Epileptic' [letter], *BMJ*, **2**:2066, 1900, 333.

'The outbreak of arsenical poisoning among beer drinkers' [letter to Medical Chirurgical Society], *BMJ*, **1**:2089, 12 January 1901, 87.

'A case of syphilitic arterial disease' [lecture, Queen Square], *BMJ*, **2**:2135, 30 November 1901, 1581–4.

'Metallic poisoning' [lecture, Queen Square], *Lancet*, **158**:4079, 2 November 1901, 1173–6.

'Tuberculosis and heredity' [letter], *Lancet*, **158**:4076, 1901, 1007.

'A question of spelling' [letter], *Lancet*, **158**:4080, 9 November 1901, 1298.

'Letter contributing to discussion (opened by E S Reynolds) on arsenical poisoning in beer drinks', *Medico-Chirurgical Transactions*, **8**, 1901, 431.

'Myopathy and a distal form' [lecture, Queen Square], *BMJ*, **2**:2167, 12 July 1902, 89–92.

'Myasthenia and ophthalmoplegia' [English version of a contribution to the special issue of the Deutsche Medizinische Wochenschrift, 28, 278–80, in honour of the 70th birthday of Professor von Leyden], *BMJ*, **1**:1253, 24 May 1902, 1253–6.

'The metric system in pharmacy' [letter], *Lancet*, **160**:4127, 4 October 1902, 956.

'Right-handedness and left-brainedness' [letter], *Lancet*, **160**:4138, 20 December 1902, 1719–20.

'Abiotrophy' [lecture, Queen Square], *Lancet*, **159**:4102, 12 April 1902, 1003–7.

'Taste and the fifth nerve', *Journal of Physiology*, **28**:4, 21 July 1902, 300–3.

'Further remarks on myasthenia', *BMJ*, **1**:1323, 31 May 1902, 1323–4.

'Inflammation of the caecum and appendix' [extract from notes of Sir William Jenner's lecture in 1862], *BMJ*, **2**:2169, 1902, 293.

'Lunacy and the law' [address, Medico-Psychological Association], *BMJ*, **2**:2186, 22 November 1902, 1633–8.

'Discussion on Gowers' paper on lunacy and the law' [Medico-Psychological Association], *Lancet*, **160**:4135, 29 November 1902, 1463–4.

'Gowers' remarks on C. O. Hawthorne's paper on intracranial thrombosis as the cause of double optic neuritis in cases of chlorosis', *Transactions of the Ophthalmological Society*, **22**, 1902, 281–3.

'Lunacy and the law' [address, Medico-Psychological Association], *Lancet*, **160**:4134, 22 November 1902, 1369–73.

'Myasthenie und Ophthlamoplegie', *Deutsche Medizinische Wochenschrift*, **28**, 1902, 278–80, 305–6.

(with Morris, H and Gairdner, W T) 'Perityphlitis' [letter], *Lancet*, **160**:4115, 12 July 1902, 107–9.

(with Ferrier, D, Gray, E V, Thomson, W, Woodhead, G S, and Porritt, N) 'The Society of Medical Phonographers' [letter], *Lancet*, **162**:4185, 14 November 1903, 1394.

'Syringal haemorrhage into the spinal cord' [lecture, Queen Square], *Lancet*, **162**:4180, 10 October 1903, 993–7.

'Local panatrophy', *Transactions of the Clinical Society of London*, **36**, 1903, 240–1.

'Local panatrophy', *Review of Neurology and Psychiatry (Edinburgh)*, **1**, 1903, 3–4.

'Note on syringal haemorrhage into the spinal cord', *Review of Neurology and Psychiatry (Edinburgh)*, i, 1903, 155–7.

'The designation of musical notes in science and medicine', *Review of Neurology and Psychiatry (Edinburgh)*, i, 1903, 228–31.

'Appendix to lecture on lunacy and the law', *BMJ*, **1**:2197, 7 February 1903, 323–3.

'The prognosis and treatment of syphilitic diseases of the nervous system' [lecture, Medical Graduates' College and Polyclinic], *BMJ*, **1**:2205, 4 April 1903, 773–8.

'The Flintwork Inscription in Blythburgh Church', *Proceedings of the Suffolk Institute of Archaeology and Natural History*, II, 1903, 51–8.

'The rate of nerve impulses', *Nature*, **69**:1038, 3 December 1903, 105.

'Insanity and epilepsy in relation to life assurance' [lecture, Association of Life Assurance Medical Officers], *Lancet*, **164**:4233, 15 October 1904, 1061–4.

'A triple-wick candle', *Lancet*, **163**:4200, 27 February 1904, 586.

'A standard dynamometer', *Lancet*, **164**:4223, 6 August 1904, 381.

'Lumbago: its lessons and analogues' [lecture, Queen Square], *BMJ*, **1**:2246, 16 January 1904, 117–21.

'Lumbago' [letter], *BMJ*, **1**:2251, 20 February 1904, 459.

(with Evans, W G) 'The treatment of blood poisoning by perchloride of iron' [letter], *Lancet*, **164**:4235, 29 October 1904, 1248–9.

'Heat a mode of motion in the seventeenth century', *Nature*, **73**:1038, 21 December 1905, 175.

'A metastatic mystery' [lecture, UCH], *Lancet*, **166**:4792, 2 December 1905, 1593–6.

'Influence of facial hemiatrophy on the facial and other nerves', *Review of Neurology and Psychiatry (Edinburgh)*, **4**, 1905, 1–5.

'The pains of tabes' [lecture, Queen Square], *BMJ*, **1**:2297, 7 January 1905, 1–5.

'The nature of tabes' [lecture, Queen Square], *BMJ*, **2**:2323, 8 July 1905, 57–61.

'Dendrites and disease' [lecture, Queen Square], *Lancet*, **168**:4324, 14 July 1906, 67–9.

'On tetanoid chorea and its association with cirrhosis of the liver', *Review of Neurology and Psychiatry (Edinburgh)*, **4**, 1906, 249–71.

'The borderland of epilepsy' [clinical lectures, Queen Square]: I 'Vertigo', *BMJ*, **2**:2375, 7 July 1906, 7–11; II 'Vertigo', *BMJ*, **2**:2377, 21 July 1906, 128–31; III 'Migraine', *BMJ*, **2**:2397, 8 December 1906, 1617–22.

'A new haemocytometer', *Lancet*, **167**:4307, 17 March 1906, 767.

'The dystrophy of tabes and the problem of trophic nerves' [lecture, Queen Square], *BMJ*, **1**:2370, 2 June 1906, 1267–9.

(with Allbutt, C T) 'Prodromata' [letter], *Lancet*, **168**:4341, 10 November 1906, 1304.

'Vagal attacks' [letter], *Lancet*, **169**:4374, 29 June 1907, 1804–5.

'A case of cervical myelopathic trichosis', *Medico-Chirurgical Transactions*, **90**, 1907, 455–67.

'The estimation of sugar' [letter], *Lancet*, **169**:4372, 15 June 1907, 1673.

'Tabetic atrophy of the auditory nerve', *Review of Neurology and Psychiatry (Edinburgh)*, **5**, 1907, 169–71.

'Psycho-epilepsy', *Review of Neurology and Psychiatry (Edinburgh)*, **5**, 1907, 529–31.

'A case of narcolepsy', *Review of Neurology and Psychiatry (Edinburgh)*, **5**, 1907, 615–16.

'Report of paper on cervical myelopathic trichosis' [Royal Medical and Chirurgical Society], *BMJ*, **1**:2422, 1 June 1907, 1304.

'Cervical myelopathic trichosis' [Royal Medical and Chirurgical Society], *Lancet*, **169**:4370, 1 June 1907, 1492–3.

'Sudden cerebral lesions: their diagnosis and immediate treatment' [lecture, Queen Square], *BMJ*, **2**:2427, 6 July 1907, 1–6.

'Faints and fainting' [lecture, Queen Square], *Lancet*, **169**:4357, 2 March 1907, 565–8.

'Vagal and vasovagal attacks' [lecture, Queen Square], *Lancet*, **169**:4371, 8 June 1907, 1551–4.

'The needs of London medical students' [letter], *Lancet*, **170**:4395, 23 November 1907, 1493–4.

(with McCall Anderson, T, Barrs, A G, Bennett, W H, Crichton-Browne, J, Dixon, W E, and Duckworth, D) 'The use of alcoholic beverages' [letter], *Lancet*, **169**:4361, 30 March 1907,

'The mechanism of nystagmus', *Proceedings of the Royal Society of Medicine (Neurological Section)*, **1**, 6 May 1908, 71–83.

'Heredity in diseases of the nervous system: introduction to a discussion on heredity at the Royal Society of Medicine', *BMJ*, **2**:2499, 21 November 1908, 1541.

'Shorthand in medical work' [letter], *BMJ*, **1**:2459, 15 February 1908, 417.

(with Cathcart, G. and Sims Woodhead, G) 'The Society of Medical Phonographers' [letter], *Lancet*, **171**:4404, 25 January 1908, 262.

'Pseudo-myasthenia of toxic origin (petrol fumes)', *Review of Neurology and Psychiatry (Edinburgh)*, **6**, 1908, 1–5.

'The mechanism of nystagmus: abstract by the author (paper, Neurological Section, Royal Society of Medicine)', *Review of Neurology and Psychiatry (Edinburgh)*, **6**, 1908, 359–61.

'Heredity in diseases of the nervous system' [Royal Society of Medicine], *Lancet*, **174**:4498, 14 November 1908, 1467–8.

'Gowers' remarks on L. Paton's paper on "Optic Neuritis in Cerebral Tumours"', *Transactions of the Ophthalmological Society*, **28**, 1908, 138–40.

(with Cathcart, C W, Woodhead, G S, and Gruner, O C) 'The Society of Medical Phonographers' [letter], *BMJ*, **1**:2456, 25 January 1908, 235.

'Science and shorthand', *The Shorthand Gazette*, **15**, 1909, 112–15.

'A case of unilateral optic neuritis from intracranial tumour' [lecture, UCH], *Lancet*, **174**:4480, 10 July 1909, 67–8.

'Myopathy and syringomyelia' [lecture, Queen Square], *BMJ*, **1**:2523, 8 May 1909, 1101–4.

'Discussion on the influence of heredity on disease, with special reference to tuberculosis, cancer, and diseases of the nervous system: introductory address', *Proceedings of the Royal Society of Medicine*, 2, Gen Rep, 11 November 1909, 15–22.

'The prodromas of migraine' [address, Westminster Division, BMA], *BMJ*, **1**:2528, 12 June 1909, 1400–3.

'A magnifying otoscope', *Lancet*, **173**:4460, 20 February 1909, 552.

'Special sense discharges from organic disease' [Hughlings Jackson Lecture, Neurological Section of the Royal Society of Medicine], *Lancet*, **174**:4503, 18 December 1909, 1803–8.

### 1910–15

'Special sense discharges from organic disease' [Hughlings Jackson Lecture], *Brain*, **32**:4, 4 March 1910, 303–26.

'Some aspects of poliomyelitis' [lecture, Queen Square], *BMJ*, **1**:2562, 5 February 1910, 305–8.

'Special sense discharges from organic disease' [Hughlings Jackson lecture], *Proceedings of the Royal Society of Medicine (Neurology Section)*, **3**, 25 November 1910, 1–16.

'Gonococcal neuroretinitis', *Medical Press and Circular*, **89**, 1910.

## *Phonographic Record of Clinical Teaching and Medical Science*

The list below is derived from the tables of contents of *Phonographic Record for Clinical Teaching and Medical Science.* The list was developed as part of the current research, in order to create as complete a record as possible of the various authors who wrote for the journal, and the subjects they wrote about. However, the entries in the tables of contents were often sparse, especially in the early years of the journal's development, so the list reflects these inconsistencies. In addition, the list was compiled from the holdings in the British Library, which are incomplete.

### Anon

'The progress of the Society', 5:March 1895, 1.

'The late Dr John Carslaw, of Glasgow', 1:9, October 1895.

'Remarks on West Africa and palustral fever', 3:5, May 1897, 72–6.

'Sir William Gowers, MD FRS', 3:7, July 1897, 97–8.

'Mirror writing in phonography', 3:7, July 1897, 106–8.

'Aphorisms', 3:7, July 1897, 109–10.

'Professional infelicities', 3:10, October 1897, 156–7.

'Review, "The diagnosis of the nature of organic brain disease (by W R Gowers)"', 3:10 October, 1897, 158–9.

'The "digraphic" series of school copy books', 3:11, November 1897, 174.

'The sexagenary of phonography', 3:11, November 1897, 175.

'Humours of patients', 3:12, December 1897, 182–3; 4:5, May 1898, 77; 4:8, August 1898, 124; 5:8, August 1899, 136; 5:4, April 1899, 72; 5:9, September 1899, 152; 5:10, October 1899, 167; 6:2, February 1900, 31; 6:5, May 1900, 79.

'The Pitman memorial', 3:12, December 1897, 190.

'Congratulatory dinner to Sir Wm R Gowers, MD, FRS', 3:12, December 1897, 191.

'Dr Byron Bramwell and shorthand writers', 4:1, January 1898, 14–15.

'Death of John Foster, FRCS', 4:2, February 1898, 28.

'The Phonographic Magazine, Cincinnati, Ohio', 4:3, March 1898, 45–6.

'Some medical word histories', Pt 1, 4:4, April 1898, 55–6; Pt 2, 5:6, June 1899, 97–9.

'Mr Thomas Allen Reed', 4:6, June 1898, 95.

'Anecdotes from "The Quarterly Medical Journal for Yorkshire and Adjoining Counties"', 4:7, July 1898, 109–10.

'Discussion on Dr Benson Cooke's paper "Chronic disease of the uterine appendages",' 4:11, November 1898, 161–6.

'Reporters' errors and mis-hearing', 5:1, January 1899, 14–18.

'The light side of medicine', 5:1, January 1899, 22.

'The late Mr Thomas Allen Reed', 5:5, May 1899, 82–5.

'Obituary—T L Webster, MRCS, LRCP', 5:9, September 1899, 151.

'Heredity', 5:12, 1899, 194–5.

'The continental method of jumping to conclusions', 6:5, May 1900, 79.

'Obituary', 6:6, June 1900, 92.

'Shorthand for medical students (preliminary notice)', 6:7, July 1900, 112.

'Shorthand for medical students (amended notice)', 6:8, August 1900, 131–2.

'Resignation of Dr Neil', 6:9, September 1900, 146–7.

'Shorthand for medical students', 6:9, September 1900, 149.

'Obituary—W D Donald', 6:9, September 1900, 148.

'Omnia sanitas', 6:9, September 1900, 151.

'Obituary—Philip Henry Fearnsides MB ChB (Vict)', 6:12, December 1900, 193.

'Some medicinal names', 12:2, April 1906, 60–1; 12:4, October 1906, 122.

'Frostbite in the Antarctic regions', 12:4, October 1906, 125–8.

'Medical thrift', 12:4, October 1906, 129–30.

'Idle rhymes of an idle beggar', 12:4, October 1906, 130–4.

### A

Adam, J, 'Pharyngeal abscess not connected with spinal disease', 4:3, March 1898, 35–7.

Atchley, G F, 'The "cancer cure" in the eighteenth century', 4:9, September 1898, 142–3.

——— 'Post-mortem examination of King George II. An extract from the Royal Magazine of 1760', 4:10, October 1898, 156.

——— 'What are the duties of the medical examiner towards the proposer?', 5:1, January 1899, 9–12.

——— 'Condensed notes of cases occurring in private practice: a neurotic family', 5:7, July 1899, 114–16.

## B

Bannister, M, 'Peripheral neuritis during pregnancy. Necrosis of the finger', 5:3, March 1899, 51–3.

Barlow, T, 'Clinical notes', 1:8, July 1895,

Beach, F, 'Remarks on the etiology and treatment of sporadic cretinism', 1:9, October 1895,

——— 'Observation of mentally deficient children (1)', 4:7, July 1898, 98–104.

——— 'Observation of mentally deficient children (2)', 4:8, August 1898, 113–19.

——— 'Observation of mentally deficient children (3)', 4:9, September 1898, 129–36.

——— 'The treatment of epileptics and imbeciles', 6:1, January 1900, 1–9.

Beale, P T B, 'The treatment of naevi in infants', 1:6, May 1895.

——— 'Hints to the student on passing urethral instruments', 2:4, May 1896.

——— 'Flat foot', 3:4, April 1897.

Beale, P T B, 'Remarks on cases of ulceration of the vermiform appendix, with very acute symptoms', 3:6, June 1897.

——— 'Notes on genu valgum, or knock-knee', 3:11, November 1897, 168–71.

——— 'Purifying the skin prior to surgical operations', 3:8, August 1897, 120–3.

——— 'Notes on the hernial truss; its use and abuse in inguinal and ventral herniae', 4:5, May 1898, 67–71.

——— 'On the use of alcohol applied locally in dressing wounds', 4:9, September 1898, 136–7.

——— 'Notes on varicose veins', 5:8, August 1899, 126–9.

——— 'When should a transverse fracture of the patella be treated by wiring?', 6:2, February 1900, 17–22.

Bernard, H W, 'Nature's methods of curing disease', 6:6, June 1900, 91.

——— 'Hysterical contraction of knee-joint and its treatment', 6:11, November 1900, 179.

Bird, M M, 'The treatment of facial erysipelas with ice bags', 2:1, January 1896.

Bristow, A T, 'The opportunities and responsibilities of modern medicine [an extract from the US Phonographic Magazine]', 6:3, March 1900, 42–5.

Broadbent, W, 'Notes on clinical teaching', 1:8, July 1895.

Brown, W G S, 'Some of nature's barriers to the dissemination of tubercle', 5:10, October 1899, 159–63.

Burn, D H, 'Notes on a case of puerperal mania, with mild symptoms, proving rapidly fatal', 5:2, February 1899, 25–7.

Burton, L L, 'Points of interest in a ship surgeon's life', 3:4, April 1897, 52.

——— 'The light and dark sides of an assistant's and locum tenens' life', 4:7, July 1898, 105–8.

——— 'A few cases of interest on a recent voyage to and from the Cape', 6:4, April 1900, 60–3.

Bury, J, 'Functional aphasia', 1:7, June 1895.

## C

Caiger, H, 'Notes on country practice in South Africa', 1:8, July 1895.

——— 'An obscure case', 3:11, November 1897, 166–7.

——— 'Tapeworm complicating typhoid fever', 5:4, April 1899.

——— 'The war in South Africa', 6:8, August 1900, 113–30.

——— 'Case of cyst (probably hydatid) in cerebral hemisphere' [paper from Burghersdorp, Cape Colony], 12:2, April 1906, 44–7.

——— 'Notes of a railway medical officer's work in South Africa', 12:4, October 1906, 105–17.

Cathcart, C W, 'Thirst and enemata', 1:4, February 1895.

——— 'On the ambulant treatment of fractures of the lower limb', 5:9, September 1899, 137–44.

——— 'Cranial surgery— some recent instruments and their application', 6:4, April 1900, 49–59.

——— 'On the conservative treatment of tubercular joints and cold abscesses, as practised by Mikulicz, of Breslau, 1890 to 1896 transcribed from the Scottish Medical and Surgical Journal', (Pt 1) 6:6, June 1900, 81–7; (Pt 2) 6:7, July 1900, 97–104.

——— 'On Bier's method of treating acute suppuration by passive congestion', 7:1, January 1906, 1–11.

Clifford, M, 'How to learn phonography by devoting one hour a day to it for a month', 5:6, June 1899, 100–2.

Colborne, W W, 'On memory', 12:3, July 1906, 98–9.

——— 'Notes on medical work in China', 3:6, June 1897, 89–93.

——— 'Notes on opium smoking', 3:7, July 1897, 98–101.

Collier, J, 'Spontaneous occurrence of vesical fistula in the groin in a case of paraplegia with retention of urine. Under the care of Sir W R Gowers, FRS', 4:8, August 1898, 120–3.

Colman, W S, 'Mercurial stomatitis', 1:2, October 1894.

——— 'Note on a case of traumatic neuralgia of the arm, treated by rest and continuous cold', 3:8, August 1897, 113–15.

Conway, A, 'Over-treatment', 6:3, March 1900, 36–8.

Cooke, B, 'A case of intestinal obstruction presenting some unusual features', 4:1, January 1898, 10–11.

——— 'Chronic disease of the uterine appendages—its palliative treatment', 4:10, October 1898, 145–9.

——— 'Neurasthenia: brief notes with some suggestions for treatment', (Pt 1) 5:5, May 1899, 73–81; (Pt 2) 5:6, June 1899, 89–96.

Crocker, R, 'Arsenic in skin diseases', 1:2, October 1894.

## D

Daly, 'Some remarks on life assurance', 6:2, February 1900, 23–30.

Davies-Colley, N, 'Notes on clinical teaching', 1:9, October 1895.

——— 'Part of a clinical lecture on umbilical hernia delivered at Guy's Hospital on 19 October 1898', 5:8, August 1899, 121–5.

Deanesly, E, 'Remarks on intestinal obstruction', 4:3, March 1898, 43.

——— 'Remarks on operations for stone in the kidney and ureter', 5:11, November 1899, 169–74.

——— 'A case of primary epithelioma of common bile duct—abdominal section—death', 5:12, December 1899, 189–91.

Donkin, H B, 'Clinical remarks on a case of partial hemiplegia and complete hemianaesthesia, occurring in the course of a case of heart disease', 4:2, February 1898, 25–7.

——— 'Clinical remarks upon a supposed case of pseudo-hypertrophic muscular paralysis occurring in an adult', 4:5, May 1898, 72–4.

Dreschfeld, J, 'Tubercular peritonitis', 1:5, March 1895.

## E

Eastes, T, 'A case of diabetes insipidus', 5:1, January 1899, 13.

——— 'The open-air treatment of consumption', 5:4, April 1899, 57–66.

——— 'Paracentesis of the membrana tympani for acute suppurative otitis media', 6: 5, May 1900, 73–5.

## F

Fausset, 'Remarks on the administration of gas and ether', 1:11, December 1895.

Fearnley, W, 'Lord Lister— a reminiscence', 12:4, October 1906, 121.

Friel, A R, 'The Irish hospital in South Africa', 6:10, October 1900, 153–8.

——— 'A case of infantile scurvy', 12:3, July 1906, 88–93.

## G

Gee, 'Cerebro-spinal meningitis', 2:2, February 1896.

Given, J C M, 'Paralysis of the II, V, VI cranial nerves', 3:6, June 1897, 84–9.

——— 'The relation of myxoedema and chronic kidney disease', 5:11, November 1899, 175–9.

Godlee, R J, 'Notes of clinical teaching', 1:5, March 1895.

Gowers, W R, 'The ophthalmoscope in general practice', 1: June 1894, 6–8.

——— 'The treatment of infantile paralysis' (Pt 1) 1: June 1894, 9; (Pt 2) 1: 2, October 1894, 31.

——— 'Problems in practical diagnosis': (1) 'A sudden cerebral lesion' 1:7, June 1895; (2) 'An abdominal mystery' 1:8, July 1895; (3) 'An unknown disease' 1:10, November 1895; (4) 'Brain, or spinal cord?' 2:1, January 1896; (5) 'Prognostic diagnosis in sudden hemiplegia' 2:1896, 70; (6) 'Heart and brain' 2:8, November 1896; (7) 'Haemoptysis; a mistake' 3:4, April 1897, 49–51; (8) 'The lead line' 3:8, August 1897, 116–19; (9) 'Paroxysmal unconsciousness' 3:9, September 1897, 129–31; (10) 'Embolic hemiplegia: unusual initial headache complicating the diagnosis' 4:1, January 1898, 1–3; (11) 'Juvenile cerebral failure' 4:3, March 1898, 33–4; (12) 'Significance of a single symptom' 4:6, June 1898, 81–2; (13) 'Cerebellar disease' 5:10, October 1899, 153–8; (14) 'Right hemiplegia and loss of speech' 7:1901; (15) 'Arsenical neuritis' 7:1901, 104; (16) 'Functional or organic disease?' 9:1903, 33; (17) 'Sensory aphasia' 9:1903, 49; (18) The impracticable' 9:1903, 65; (19) 'No solvent analysis' 9:1903, 105; (20) 'Mysterious palsy' 9:1903; (21) 'Transient hyperpyrexia and its sequel' 12:1, January 1906, 12–18; (22) 'Query-amputation?' 12:2, April 1906, 48–50.

——— 'The treatment of infantile paralysis (pt 3)', 1:3, January 1895.

——— 'President's annual address, Society of Medical Phonographers', 2:6, July 1896, 81.

——— 'The ophthalmoscope as otoscope', 2:3, March 1896.

——— 'Collective investigations', 2:3, March 1896.

——— 'Some fallacies in auscultation', 2:1896, 74.

——— 'The cure of epilepsy', 2:3, March 1896.

——— 'Petition to the General Medical Council', 2:3, March 1896.

——— 'St Bartholomew and his hospital', 1896.

——— 'Collective investigations: chorea, the cure of epilepsy', 2:43, 1896.

——— 'Notes: chlorotic anaemia', 3:1897, 16.

——— 'Diagnosis of hysterical hemiplegia', 3:12, December 1897, 177–9.

——— 'Results of treatment: no 1—complications of tabes', 3:7, July 1897.

——— 'Sir Isaac Pitman', 3:2, 1897, 17–21.

——— 'Results of treatment: (2) established indifference', 4:5, May 1898, 65–6.
——— 'An obscure disorder', 4:7, July 1898, 97.
——— 'Syphilitic disease of the cerebral arteries', 4:9, September 1898, 136–7.
——— 'A note on the lead line', 4:10, October 1898, 150–1.
——— 'Polyneuritis', 4:12, December 1898, 177–8.
——— 'The work of the life assurance examiner: part I—examination and report', 5:7, July 1899, 117–18.
——— 'Valedictory address by the late president', 5:1, January 1899, 1–6.
——— 'Parental consanguinity—a query', 5:4, April 1899, 69.
——— 'Cases and comments—sleep palsy', 6:3, March 1900, 33–5.
——— 'Questions and answers', 6:6, June 1900, 88–90.
——— 'Chronic myelitis' [lecture, Queen Square], 6:7, July 1900, 105–11.
——— 'Rheumatic fever and obscure heart disease' (Pt 1), 6:9, September 1900, 140–5.
——— 'Rheumatic fever and obscure heart disease' (Pt 2), 6:10, October 1900, 153–8.
——— 'Tuberculosis and heredity', 7:1901, 188.
——— 'Insurance notes. Examiner, report and assessment', 8:1902, 28.
——— 'Insurance notes. The expectation of life', 8:1902, 43.
——— 'Persistence of the lead line: an appeal', 8:1902, 46.
——— 'Ocular indications of old syphilis', 8:1902, 77.
——— 'Insurance notes. A phthisical family', 8:1902, 81.
——— 'The lead line' [letter], 8:1902, 134.
——— 'Note appended to H. Caiger's article "A case for diagnosis"', 8:1902, 176.
——— 'Notes and queries: (1) the disappearance of albuminuria in Bright's disease', 8:1902, 178.
——— 'Notes and queries: (2) symptoms of renal calculus', 8:1902, 190.
——— 'On tests for albumen', 9:1903, 9.
——— 'Notes on clinical teaching: (1) paralysis agitans and senile cerebellar degeneration', 9:1903, 24.
——— 'Notes on clinical teaching: (2) syphilitic vascular hemiplegia', 9:1903, 121.
——— 'Rectal feeding: a query and a remark', 9:1903, 89.
——— 'Incontinence of urine', 9:1903, 145.
——— 'Albuminuria and life assurance', 9:1903, 183–5.
——— 'Visual spectra', 10:1904, 12.
——— 'Treatment of gall stones', 10:1904, 17.
——— 'A lecture on chorea and its neuronic aspect', 10:1904, 113, 129.
——— 'Syphilitic disease of the brain' [postgraduate lecture, Queen Square], ii:1904, 18.
——— 'Fatigue', ii:1905, 33.
——— 'Adult poliomyelitis' [postgraduate lecture, Queen Square], ii:65, 1905.
——— 'Epilepsy', ii:1905, 116.
——— 'A lecture on a case of intracranial tumour', 13:1907, 83.
——— 'Abstract of a lecture on sudden cranial lesions', 13:1907, 111.
——— 'The president and members (Society of Medical Phonographers)', 14:1908, 1–3.
——— 'The murmurs of mitral constriction', 14:1908, 33–40.
——— 'The nervous system in old age' [abridged lecture], 14:1908, 33–40.
——— 'Pseudo-hypertrophic paralysis' [lecture, Queen Square], 14:1908, 89–92.

——— 'Clinical teaching', 14:1908, 113–18.

——— 'Note by Gowers on a case for diagnosis (by Henry Whitley)', 14:1908, 121–2.

——— 'Out-patient teaching', 14:1908, 137–9.

——— 'Clinical teaching: alcoholic pseudo-tabes', 15:1909, 1.

——— 'Clinical teaching: facial contracture after paralysis; general paralysis; and disseminated sclerosis', 15:1909, 25.

——— 'Clinical teaching: general paralysis of the insane', 15:1909, 73.

——— 'Science and shorthand (from the *Shorthand Gazette* August 1909)', 15:1909, 112.

——— 'The neurology of the eyelids', 16:6, 1910.

Gray, E B, 'Our Society's vocabulary', 2:7, October 1896.

——— 'The new edition of the List of Outlines', 4:11, November 1898, 171–3.

——— 'Misadventures in medicine', 5:9, September 1899, 149–50.

Greer, W J, 'Succinate of iron', 4:1, January 1898, 8–9.

——— 'The treatment of appendicitis', 5:12, December 1899, 185–8.

Grey, S G, 'A case of spontaneous evolution with a living child', 5:10, October 1899, 164–5.

Griffith, P G, 'Acute rheumatism, followed by pericarditis and double pneumonia—recovery', 3:10, October 1897, 152–5.

Gruner, O C, 'Medical students in the Middle Ages. i—At Salerno', 7:1, January 1900, 12–18.

Gunn, R M, 'How to examine the eyes of children', 1:6, May 1895.

## H

Heath, C, 'Lateral curvature of the spine', 1:3, January 1895.

Hodgson, M, 'Shorthand in the army', 3:12, December 1897, 184.

Huggard, 'Points determining the selection of climate in phthisis' (Pt 1), 2:1, January 1895.

——— 'Points determining the selection of climate in phthisis' (Pt 2), 2:2, February 1896.

## I

Irving, J, 'A bladder problem' (Pt 1), 6:10, October 1900, 166–8.

——— 'A bladder problem' (Pt 2), 6:11, November 1900, 178.

## J

Jenner, W, 'On some diseases of the mouth, acute glossitis', 1:1, June 1894, 3–5.

——— 'Stomatitis', 1:2, October 1894.

Johnson, R, 'Belladonna poisoning', 1:5, March 1895.

Johnston, J, 'The St John Ambulance Brigade. A tribute to the ambulance volunteers in the South African war', 6:9, September 1900, 149–50.

Joseph, A H, 'Notes on cases illustrating the influence of one disease upon another', 3:11, November 1897, 172–4.

——— 'Note on the duration of a "lead line on the gums"', 4:1, January 1898, 12–13.

——— 'A case of spina bifida presenting some unusual features', 4:6, June 1898, 83–7.

——— 'Enamelled tinware as a cause of plumbism', 5:12, December 1899, 192–3.

——— 'Stray notes from practice', 12:2, April 1906, 51–5.

## L

Little, 'The use of digitalis', 1:4, February 1895.

Lundie, R A, 'The therapeutic use of phosphorus', 4:4, April 1898, 49–51.

## M

Mallam, E, 'Granuloma of the nose', 12:2, April 1906, 58–9.

Martin, J W, 'Delayed desquamation in scarlet fever', 1:10, November 1895.

——— 'Clinical notes', 2:2, February 1895.

——— 'A note on vaginal douching', 5:8, August 1899, 132–3.

——— 'Permanent amenorrhoea', 5:11, November 1899, 183.

——— 'A case of purulent cyst in Douglas' pouch, and double salpingitis', 6:9, September 1900, 137–9.

Mercier, C, 'Sane lunatics', 2:9, December 1896.

Mitchell, M, 'Methylal in delirium tremens', 5:9, September 1899, 145–8.

Moynihan, B G A, 'Drainage of the intestine in acute obstruction', 12:4, October 1906, 117–20.

## N

Neil, J, 'Three cases of recovery from melancholia after unusually long periods', 1:10, November 1895.

——— 'A case of insanity associated with gout', 12:3, July 1906, 88–93.

Nettleship, E, 'Blinding by electric light', 1:5, March 1895.

——— 'Neurasthenic asthenopia', 1:7, June 1895.

## O

Osler, W, 'The diagnosis of malignant endocarditis', 1:6, May 1895.

## P

Parker, A P, 'Four cases to illustrate the value of X-rays in diagnosis', 12:2, April 1906, 56–7.

Patrick, H C, 'Two cases of malignant abdominal tumour', 3:11, November 1897.

Paul, M E, 'The cause of periodicity in malarial fever', 5:3, March 1899, 41–50.

Poore, G V, 'Notes of a lecture on writer's cramp', 3:5, May 1897, 66.

Porritt, N, 'The toxic action of coal tar derivatives', 3:10, October 1897, 145–51.

——— 'Septic cellulitis of the neck, causing fatal spasm of the glottis', 3:12, December 1897, 180–1.

——— 'The light side of medicine', 4:1, January 1898, 4–7.

——— 'The light side of medicine II', 4:4, April 1898, 52–4.

——— 'The duration of a "lead line on the gums"', 4:5, May 1898, 75.

——— 'Gunshot wound of head—autopsy', 4:10, October 1898, 152–3.

——— 'Two instructive examples of abdominal surgery: (i) perforation of gastric ulcer', 4:11, November 1898, 167–70; '(ii) Ruptured tubal pregnancy—abdominal section', 4:12, December 1898, 179–82.

——— 'Notes on a case of artificially induced scurvy', 5:11, November 1899, 180–2.

——— 'On taking things for granted', 6:10, October 1900, 163–5.

Poulter, R, 'A case of ranula—spontaneous cure', 4:5, May 1898, 76.

## R

Reynolds, E S, 'Some curious aortic aneurisms', 4:2, February 1898, 17–24.

Riddell, S, 'Six cases of remarkable injuries', 2:5, June 1896.

Ritchie, J, 'The therapeutic pathology of diphtheria', 1:5, March 1895.

Rogers, L, 'A case illustrating a haemorrhagic diathesis secondary to malaria', 5:2, February 1899, 37–8.

——— 'Medical work in India', 5:7, July 1899, 105–13.

——— 'India as a field for medical research', 12:3, July 1906, 81–7.

Ross, J M, 'The relation of medical officers of health and general practitioners', 5:2, February 1899, 28–36.

——— 'Impressions of a visit to the cases of plague in Belvidere, Glasgow', 6:11, November 1900, 169–77.

### S

Spencer, H R, 'Chancres in women', 1:4, February 1895.

——— 'The diagnosis between ovarian tumours and uterine fibroids', 1:8, July 1895.

Spooner, F H, 'Phonographic notes', 3:12, December 1897, 189; 4:4, April 1898, 57–9.

——— 'Influenza, followed by epileptoid fits and persistent pyrexia', 4:10, October 1898, 154–5.

Stewart, T G, 'A case of renal disease', 1:7, June 1895.

Swanzy, 'Clinical notes', 1:8, July 1895.

### T

Taylor, J, 'Alcoholic neuritis', 1:2, October 1894.

——— 'On treatment by electricity', 3:9, September 1897, 132.

——— 'The treatment of acute peritonitis' [paper read to the Chester Medical Society] (Pt 1), 12:2, April 1906, 33–43; (Pt 2) 12:3, July 1906, 73–80.

Thompson, W, 'Address to members' [by incoming President], 5:1, January 1899, 7–8.

——— 'Some diseases of the rectum and anus', 5:8, August 1899, 130–1.

Treves, F, 'Abdominal section in private practice', 1:9, October 1895.

### W

Wallace, R, 'Medical practice in America', 6:12, December 1900, 185–92.

Ward, E, 'Actinomycosis', 1:5, March 1895.

Wethered, 'Haemoptysis', 2:3, March 1896.

Whitaker, S, 'Esperanto', 12:2, 1906, 67–70.

Whitby, H, 'Stokers' cramp', 12:3, July 1906, 100–4.

Wilks, S L B, 'The treatment of influenza', 6:5, May 1900, 65–72.

Williams, R, 'The pathogenesis of cancer', 1:11, December 1895.

Wilson, T, 'Backward displacement of the gravid uterus', 1:4, February 1895.

——— 'Transient spasmodic torticollis in a case of intraperitoneal haemorrhage due to tubal abortion', 4:12, December 1898.

——— 'On some varieties of metritis and their treatment', 6:1, January 1900, 10–14.

## Correspondence

Personal correspondence cited in the references comes from a limited range of sources. All the letters from Kipling come from Gowers family records, as do almost all the letters received by Gowers. The letters from Gowers to Morrison are held in the George Ernest Morrison Papers 185–1932, Series 01, MLMSS 312, Mitchell Library, Sydney, Australia. Exchanges with Burford Rawlings, and other Queen Square correspondence are held by the University of London, Queen Square Archives. Correspondence between Osler and Gowers is held in the Osler Library of the History of Medicine, McGill University, Montreal, Canada.

## Sources cited in text


A.P.C., 'Sir William Gowers', *Postgraduate Medical Journal*, **25**:288, October 1949, 507.

Adams, F, *The genuine works of Hippocrates* (London: Sydenham Society, 1849).

Airy, H, 'On a distinct form of transient heniopia', *Philosophical Transactions*, **159**, 1870, 247–64.

Allbutt, C T (ed.), *A System of Medicine* (London: Macmillan, 1899).

Altholz, J L, *Anatomy of a Controversy: the Debate over Essays and Reviews 1860–1864* (Aldershot: Scholar Press, 1994).

Angus, J, *Handbook of the English Tongue: for the Use of Student and Others* (London: Religious Tract Society, 1862).

Annotation, 'A fruitful century', *Lancet*, **275**:7138, 18 June 1960, 1305–8.

Anon, 'Recent works on nervous diseases', *American Journal of the Medical Sciences*, **93**:185, January 1887, 204–7.

Anon, 'Discussion on Dr Benson Cooke's paper "Chronic disease of the uterine appendages"', *Phonographic Record*, **4**:11, November 1898, 161–6.

Anon,'Sir William Gowers, 1845–1915' [leading article], *BMJ*, **1**: 4395, 31 March 1945, 452.

Anon, *Queen Square and the National Hospital 1860–1960* (London: Edward Arnold, 1960).

Arnold, T, *Principles of Church Reform*, 2nd edn (London: Fellowes, 1833).

Babington, C C, *Manual of British Botany, Containing the Flowering Plants and Ferns Arranged According to the Natural Orders* (London: J Van Voorst, 1851).

Babinski, J, 'Sur le réflexe cutané plantaire dans certains affections organiques du système nerveux centrale', *Comptes-Rendus Hebdomadaires des Séances et Mémoires de la Société de Biologie*, **3**:1896, 207–8.

Bailey, J B, 'The medical societies of London', *BMJ*, **2**:1802, 13 July 1895, 100–4.

Bartrip, P W J, 'Churchill, John Spriggs Morss (1801–1875) medical publisher', *Oxford Dictionary of National Biography* (Oxford: Oxford University Press, 2004).

Beaumont, F G, *A History of Coggeshall, in Essex*, (Coggeshall: Marshall Brothers and Edwin Potter, 1890).

Beckett, I F W, 'Wolseley, Garnet Joseph, first Viscount Wolseley (1833–1913)', *Oxford Dictionary of National Biography* (Oxford: Oxford University Press, 2004).

Bellot, H H, *University College London, 1816–1926* (London: University of London Press, 1929).

Birken, W, 'The Dissenting tradition in English medicine of the seventeenth and eighteenth centuries', *Medical History*, **39**, 1995, 197–218.

Birkenhead, *Rudyard Kipling* (London: Weidenfeld and Nicolson, 1978).

Boyd, A K H, *Leisure Hours in Town: a Selection from the Contributions of A.H.K.B. to Fraser's Magazine* (London: Longmans Green, 1862).

Brain, W R and Walton, J N, *Diseases of the Nervous System*, 7th edn (Oxford: Oxford University Press, 1969).

Briggs, A, *Victorian People* (London: Odhams Press, 1954).

Brown, H B, 'UCH and Sir William Gowers', *BMJ*, **1**:4400, 5 May 1945, 645.

Butterfield, E K, *The Making of a Neurologist: the Letters of Foster Kennedy 1884–1952 to his Wife* (Cambridge: private, 1981).

Buzzard, E F, 'Hughlings Jackson and his influence on neurology', *Lancet*, **224**:5800, 27 October 1934, 909–13.

Cain, P, *Examination Registers of the University of London 1838–1889* (London; University of London Archives, 1982).

Carey, H M, *God's Empire: Religion and Colonialism in the British World,* c.1801–1908 (Cambridge: Cambridge University Press, 2011).

Carpenter, M, *Health, Medicine, and Society in Victorian England* (Santa Barbara, CA: Praeger, 2010).

Carswell, R, *Pathological Anatomy: Illustrations of the Elementary Forms of Disease* (London: Longman, Rees, Orme, and others, 1835–8).

Cassell's, *Cassell's German Pronouncing Dictionary, Consisting of Extracts in Prose and Verse, with Appropriate Vocabularies* (London: Cassell's, 1853).

Charcot, J M, *Lectures on Diseases of the Nervous System*, Vol 1 (transl. Sigerson, G) (London: New Sydenham Society, 1877).

Clarke, J F, *Autobiographical Recollections of the Medical Profession* (London: J & A Churchill, 1874).

Clarke, K, *Ruskin Today* (London: John Murray, 1964).

Compston, A, 'Editorial', *Brain*, **130**:7, 2007, 1709–11.

Cook, E T, *The Life of Florence Nightingale: Vol 2 1862–1910* (London: Macmillan, 1913).

Critchley, M, *Sir William Gowers 1845–1915: a Biographical Appreciation* (London: William Heinemann Medical Books, 1949).

Critchley, M, 'The Beginnings of the National Hospital, Queen Square (1859–1860)', BMJ, **1**:5189, 18 June 1960, 1829–37.

Cruveilhier, J, *Anatomie Pathologique du Corps Humaine*, Vol 2 (Paris: Balliere, 1835–42).

Cullen, W, *First Lines of the Practice of Physic* (New York: Duyckinck, Swords, Falconer *et al.*, 1805 [originally 1789]).

Dale, B, *The Annals of Coggeshall, otherwise Sunnedon, in the County of Essex* (London: A G Coventry, 1863).

De Lehoczky, T, 'On recent biographies of two great physicians: Gowers and Cushing', *Journal of Nervous and Mental Disease*, **166**:6, December 1952, 506–10.

De Watteville, A, 'Review: *A Manual of the Diseases of the Nervous System*', *Brain*, **2**:1, 1888, 131–3.

Delasiauve, L J F, *Traité de l'Épilepsie* (Paris: Masson, 1854).

Desmond, A and Moore, J, *Darwin* (London: Michael Joseph, 1991).

Dobson, J and Wakely, C, *Sir George Buckston Browne* (Edinburgh: Livingstone, 1957).

Du Bois-Reymond, E H, 'De l'hémicrânie ou migraine', *Journal de la Physiologie de l'Homme et des Animaux*, **4**:1861, 130–7.

Duchenne, G B A, 'Recherches sur la paralysie musculaire pseudohypertrophique ou paralysie myosclérotique', *Archives Générales de Médicine*, **11**,1869, 5–25; 179–209; 305–21; 421–43; 552–88.

Duncan, D, *Life and Letters of Herbert Spencer*, Vol 2 (New York: Appleton, 1908).

Easton, P G, 'Sir William Gowers', *BMJ*, **2**:5191, 2 July 1960, 72.

Editorial, 'Continence *versus* syphilis', *Lancet*, **133**:3430, 25 May 1889, 1042–3.

Erichsen, J E, *Science and Art of Surgery: Being a Treatise on Surgical Injuries, Diseases, and Operations* (London: Walton and Maberly, 1853).

Fitzgerald, C P, 'An appreciation', in Hui-Min, L (ed.) *The Correspondence of G E Morrison* (Cambridge: Cambridge University Press, 1976).

Flourens, M J P, *Recherches Expérimentales sur les Propriétés et les Fonctions du Système Nerveux dans les Animaux Vertébrés* (Paris: Crevot, 1824).

Fournier, J-A, 'De l'ataxie locomotorice d'origine syphilitique', *Annales de Dermatologie et de Syphilologie*, **7**, 1875, 187–97.

Froggatt, P, '*The Lancet*: Wakley's instrument for medical education reform', *Journal of the Society of Occupation Medicine*, **29**, 1979, 45–53.

Gibson, G S, *The Flora of Essex* (London: William Pamplin, 1862).

Gilmour, D, *The Long Recessional: the Imperial Life of Rudyard Kipling* (London: Pimlico, 2002).

Godlee, R J, *Lord Lister* (Oxford: The Clarendon Press, 1924).

Gowers, E A, Notes for Macdonald Critchley, unpublished, 1948.

Gowers, E A, *Plain Words: a Guide to the Use of English* (London: HMSO, 1948).

Gowers, W R, Shorthand diary, 1862–3.

Gregory, G S, 'Morrison, George Ernest (Chinese) (1862–1920)', Australian Dictionary of Biography (Melbourne: Melbourne University Press, 1986).

Haden, F S, 'About etching', *Fine Arts Quarterly Review*, new series:1, 1866, 145–60.

Haley, B, *The Healthy Body and Victorian Culture* (Harvard, MA: Harvard University Press, 1978).

Hall, M, 'On the reflex function of the medulla oblongata and medulla spinalis', *Philosophical Transactions*, **123**, 1833, 635–65.

Hall, M, *Lectures on the Nervous System and its Diseases* (London: Sherwood, Gilbert & Piper, 1836).

Hall, M, 'On the theory of convulsive diseases, and especially of epilepsy', *Lancet*, **50**, 1847, 460–67.

Hall, M, *Synopsis of Apoplexy and Epilepsy with Observations on Trachelismus, Laryngismus, and Tracheostomy; and a Proposal for a Hospital for Epileptics* (London: Mallett, 1852).

Hamilton, G H, *Queen Square: its Neighbourhood and its Institutions* (London: Leonard Parsons, 1926).

Hammond, W A, *A Treatise on Disease of the Nervous System* (New York and London: Appleton & Co, and Turner & Co, 1871).

Handfield Jones, C, 'Clinical lectures on cases of paralysis agitans', *BMJ*, **1**:635, 1 March 1873, 221–3.

Helly, D O and Callaway, H, 'Lugard [nee Shaw], Dame Flora Louise, Lady Lugard (1852–1929)', *Oxford Dictionary of National Biography* (Oxford: Oxford University Press, 2004).

Henson, R A, 'Commentary on de Watteville review', *Brain*, **110**:4, August 1987, 1082–3.

Herpin, T, *Des Acces Incomplets d'Epilepsie* (Paris: Ballière, 1867).

Hind, A M and Chambers, E, 'Haden, Sir Francis Seymour (1818–1910)', *Oxford Dictionary of National Biography* (Oxford: Oxford University Press, 2004).

Holmes, G, 'Sir William Gowers at the National Hospital', *BMJ*, **2**:4744, 8 December 1951, 1397–8.

Holmes, G, *An Introduction to Clinical Neurology*, 2nd edn (Edinburgh: Livingstone, 1952).

Holmes, G, *The National Hospital Queen Square* (Edinburgh: E & S Livingstone, 1954).

Howard, R and Willison, H, 'The nature of catalepsy and the model for Percy Trevelyan', *The Sherlock Holmes Journal*, **20**:4, 1992, 128–30.

**Hughlings Jackson**, J, 'Case of large cerebral tumour without optic neuritis and with left hemiplegia and imperception', in Taylor, J (ed.) *Selected Writings of John Hughlings Jackson*, Vol 2, pp. 146–52 (London: Hodder & Stoughton, 1931).

Hughlings Jackson, J, Buzzard, T, Carter, R B, Bastian, H C, Gowers, W R, Ferrier, D, et al., 'The medical staff and the management of the National Hospital for the Paralysed and Epileptic, Queen Square' [letter], *Lancet*, **156**:4014, 4 August 1900, 351–2.

Hughlings Jackson, J and Purves Stewart, J, 'Epileptic attacks with a warning of a crude sensation of smell and with the intellectual aura (dreamy state) in a patient who had symptoms pointing to gross organic disease of the right temporo-sphenoidal lobe', *Brain*, **22**:4, 1899, 534–49.

Hui-Min, L (ed.), *The Correspondence of G E Morrison* (Cambridge: Cambridge University Press, 1976).

Hunting, P, *The History of the Royal Society of Medicine* (London: Royal Society of Medicine Press, 2001).

J.H.L, 'Recent works on diseases of the nervous system', *American Journal of the Medical Sciences*, **104**:4, October 1892, 450–3.

Jacyna, L S, A tale of three cities, *Medical History*, Supplement No 9 (London: Wellcome Institute for the History of Medicine, 1989).

Jensen, J V, 'Return to the Wilberforce–Huxley debate', *The British Journal for the History of Science*, **21**:2, June 1988, 161–79.

Jessopp, A, *Arcady, for Better for Worse* (London: T Fisher Unwin, 1887).

Jones, E, *Free Associations: Memories of a Psycho-Analyst* (London: The Hogarth Press, 1959).

Kennedy, F, 'Retrobulbar neuritis as an exact diagnostic sign of certain tumors and abscesses in the frontal lobes', *American Journal of Medical Science*, **142**, 1911, 355–68.

Kennedy, F, 'William Gowers (1845–1915)', in Haymaker, W and Schiller, F (eds) *The Founders of Neurology* (Springfield, IL: Charles C Thomas, 1953).

Kinnier Wilson, S A, *Neurology* (London: Edward Arnold, 1940).

Kussmaul, A and Tenner, A, *On the Nature and Origin of Convulsions Caused by Profuse Bleeding, and Also Those of Epilepsy* (transl. Bronner, E) (London: New Sydenham Society, 1859).

Lane, J, *A Social History of Medicine: Health, Healing and Disease in England, 1750–1950* (London: Routledge, 2001).

Latham, P W, 'Clinical lecture nervous or sick-headaches' (Pt 1), *BMJ*, **1**:586, 23 March 1872, 305–6.

Latham, P W, 'Clinical lecture on nervous or sick-headaches' (Pt 2), *BMJ*, **1**:587, 30 March 1872, 336–7.

Latham, P W, *On Nervous or Sick Headache, its Varieties and Treatment* (Cambridge: Deighton, Bell & Co, 1873).

Lawrence, C, 'Lister, Joseph, Baron Lister (1827–1912)', Oxford Dictionary of National Biography (Oxford: Oxford University Press, 2004).

Lees, A J, Woodward, R M P, Scott, A E M, and Eadie, M J, 'W R Gowers 1895: two unpublished postgraduate lectures', *Brain*, 2012, doi: 10.1093/brain/aws029.

Liddell, E G T, 'Gowers, Sir William Richard (1845–1915)', Oxford Dictionary of National Biography (Oxford: Oxford University Press, 2004).

Liveing, E, *On Megrim, Sick-Headache, and some Allied Disorders: a Contribution to the Pathology of Nerve-Storms* (London: Churchill, 1873).

Lockhart-Clarke, J and Gowers, W R, 'On a case of pseudo-hypertrophic muscular paralysis', *Medico-Chirurgical Transactions*, **57**, 1874, 247–59.

Lowry, D, 'Jameson, Sir Leander Starr, baronet (1853-1917)', Oxford Dictionary of National Biography (Oxford: Oxford University Press, 2004).

Lyons, J B, 'Correspondence between Sir William Gowers and Sir Victor Horsley', *Medical History*, **9**:3, 1965, 260–7.

M.A.S, '*A Manual of Diseases of the Nervous System*, by W R Gowers', *American Journal of the Medical Sciences*, **95**:6, June 1888, 603–5.

McHenry, L C, *Garrison's History of Neurology* (Springfield, IL: Charles C Thomas, 1969).

Masters, M T, 'Teaching of botany in medical schools', *BMJ*, **2**:1136, 24 September 1864, 374–5.

Maudsley, H, 'Insanity', in Reynolds, J R (ed.), *A System of Medicine*, 2nd edn (Philadelphia: Henry C Lea's Son & Co, 1879).

Mercier, C, 'The late Dr Hughlings Jackson: recollections by Dr Mercier', *BMJ*, **1**:2663, 13 January 1912, 85–6.

Merrington, W R, *University College Hospital and its Medical School: a History* (London: Heinemann, 1976).

Merskey, H, 'Some features of medical education in Great Britain during the first half of the nineteenth century', *British Journal of Medical Education*, **3**:2, 1969, 118–21.

Meryon, E, 'On granular and fatty degeneration of the voluntary muscles', *Medico-Chirurgical Transactions*, **35**, 1851, 73–84.

Möllendorf, 'Ueber Hemikranie', *Virchow's Archives*, **47**, 1867, 385–95.

Morrison, G E, *An Australian in China: Being the Narrative of a Quiet Journey across China to Burma* (London: Horace Cox, 1895).

Musgrove, F, 'Middle-class education and employment in the nineteenth century', *The Economic History Review*, **2**:1, 1959, 99–111.

Neuberger, M, *The Historical Development of Experimental Brain and Spinal Cord Physiology before Flourens* (transl. and ed. Clarke, E) (Baltimore and London: Johns Hopkins Press, 1981) [originally 1897].

Newbolt, S F, *The History of the Royal Society of Painter-Etchers & Engravers* (London: The Print Collectors' Club, 1930).

Newman, C, *The Evolution of Medical Education in the Nineteenth Century* (London: Oxford University Press, 1957).

Nightingale, F, *Notes on Nursing: What it is and What it is Not* (London: Harrison and Sons, 1860).

Northcote, S H and Trevelyan, C E, *Report on the Organisation of the Permanent Civil Service*, paper number 1713, xxvii, 1 (London: Parliamentary Sessional Papers, 1854).

Nothnagel, H, 'Die Entstehung allgemeiner Convulsionen vom Pons und der Medulla oblongata aus', *Virchow's Archives*, **44**, 1868, 1–12.

Obituary, 'Sir J Russell Reynolds, MD, FRCP, FRS', *BMJ*, **1**:1849, 6 June 1896, 1422–5.

Obituary, 'Death of Sir W Gowers: a famous nerve specialist', *The Times*, 5 May 1915.

Obituary, 'Sir William Gowers, MD, FRCP, FRS', *BMJ*, **1**:2836, 8 May 1915, 828–30.

Obituary, 'Sir William R Gowers, FRS', *Nature*, **95**:2376, 1915, 296–7.

Obituary, 'Sir William Richard Gowers, MD Lond and Dub, FRCP Lond, LL.D Edin. FRS', *Lancet*, **185**:4785, 15 May 1915, 1055–7.

Obituary, 'William Richard Gowers', *Journal of Nervous and Mental Diseases*, **43**:5, May 1916, 485–6.

Osler, W, *On Chorea and Choreiform Affections* (Philadelphia: Blakiston, 1894).

Paget, J and Paget, C, *Sketch of the Natural History of Yarmouth and its Neighbourhood: Containing Catalogues of the Species of Animals, Birds, Reptiles, Fish, Insects, and Plants, at Present Known* (London: Longman Rees, 1834).

Perlman Lorch, M, 'The unknown source of John Hughlings Jackson's early interest in aphasia and epilepsy', *Cognitive and Behavioral Neurology*, **17**:3, September 2004, 124–32.

Pernet, G, 'Sir William Gowers on the nature of tabes', *BMJ*, **1**:2837, 1915, 871.

Peterson, M J, *The Medical Profession in Mid-Victorian London* (Los Angeles: University of California Press, 1978).

Picard, L, *Victorian London: the Tale of a City 1840–1870* (New York: St Martin's Griffin, 2005).

Pinney, T, *The Letters of Rudyard Kipling*, Vol *2 1890–99* (London: Macmillan, 1990).

Poore, G V, 'Notes of a lecture on writer's cramp', *Phonographic Record*, **3**:5, May 1897, 66.

Purdon Martin, J, 'Reminiscences of Queen Square', *BMJ*, **284**:6307, 1981, 1640–2.

Purdon Martin, J, 'Medicine and books: personal account of a career in neurology', *BMJ*, **284**:6329, 1982, 1624.

Quain, J and Wilson, W J E, *Anatomical Plates of the Human Body* (London: Taylor and Walton, 1836–42).

Radcliffe, C B, *Epilepsy and other Convulsive Affections, their Pathology and Treatment* (London: Churchill, 1858).

Radcliffe, C B, 'Diseases of the spinal cord', in Reynolds, J R (ed.) *A System of Medicine*, 2nd edn, (Philadelphia: Lea's Son & Co, 1879).

Rawlings, B B, *A Hospital in the Making: a History of the National Hospital for the Paralysed and Epileptic* (London: Pitman, 1913).

Reader, W J, *Professional Men: the Rise of the Professional Classes in Nineteenth-Century England* (New York: Basic Books, 1966).

Reed, T A, *A Biography of Isaac Pitman (Inventor of Phonography)* (London: Griffith, Farran, Okeden & Welsh, 1890).

Reid, S J, *Memoirs of Sir Wemyss Reid 1842 to 1885* (Whitefish, MT: Kessinger Publishing) [originally self-published, London: 1905].

Report, 'Regulations concerning degrees, diplomas, etc in medicine', *BMJ*, **2**:91, 27 September 1862, 323–32.

Report, 'Apparatus for the clinical estimation of the haemoglobin in blood', *BMJ*, **2**:938, 1878, 939.

Report, 'Dr Gowers', *Lancet*, **133**:3413, 26 January 1889, 186.

Report, 'Sir William Gowers and the Society of Medical Phonographers', *BMJ*, **2**:1927, 1897, 1657–8.

Report, 'The Savile Club', *BMJ*, **2**:3272, 15 September 1923, 472–3.

Review, '*A Manual and Atlas of Medical Ophthalmoscopy*', *Lancet*, **114**:2932, 8 November 1879, 694–5.

Review, '*A Manual of Diseases of the Nervous System*', *BMJ*, **2**:1347, 30 October 1886, 824.

Review, '*A Manual of the Diseases of the Nervous System*', *Lancet*, **128**:3294, 16 October 1886, 729.

Review, 'Gowers, W R: *Epilepsy and other Chronic Convulsive Diseases* (2nd edn)', *BMJ*, **1**:2140, 4 January 1902, 27.

Reynolds, H R and Reynolds, J R, *Yes and No; or, Glimpses of the Great Conflict* (London: Macmillan, 1860).

Reynolds, J R, *The Diagnosis of Diseases of the Brain, Spinal Cord, Nerves and their Appendages* (London: Churchill, 1855).

Reynolds, J R, *Epilepsy: its Symptoms, Treatment, and Relation to Other Chronic Convulsive Disease* (London: J & A Churchill, 1861).

Reynolds, J R, *A System of Medicine*, Vol 2, 1st edn (London: Churchill, 1868).

Reynolds, J R, 'Paralysis and other disorders of motion and sensation dependent on idea', *BMJ*, **2**:462, 1869, 483–5.

Reynolds, J R, *Lectures on the Clinical Uses of Electricity* (London: J & A Churchill, 1871).

Richardson, R, *The Making of Mr Gray's Anatomy* (Oxford: Oxford University Press, 2008).

Ringer, S, 'A suggestion concerning the condition of the nervous centres in migraine, epilepsy, and other explosive neuroses', *Lancet*, **109**, 1877, 228–9.

Rolleston, H D, *The Right Honourable Sir Thomas Clifford Allbutt* (London: Macmillan, 1929).

Romberg, M H, *A Manual of the Nervous Diseases of Man* (transl. Sieveking, E H) (London: New Sydenham Society, 1853).

Rosenthal, M and Putzel, L, *A Clinical Treatise in the Diseases of the Nervous System* (New York: Wood & Co, 1879).

Ross, J, *A Treatise on the Diseases of the Nervous System*, 1st edn (London: J & A Churchill, 1881).

Ross, J, *A Treatise on the Diseases of the Nervous System*, 2nd edn (London: J & A Churchill, 1883).

Ruskin, J, *The Queen of the Air: being a Study of the Greek Myths of Cloud and Storm* (London: George Allen, 1908).

Ruskin, J, *Lectures on Art: delivered before the University of Oxford in Hilary Term, 1870* (London: George Allen & Sons, 1910).

Russell, J S R, Batten, F E, and Collier, J, 'Subacute combined degeneration of the spinal cord', *Brain*, **23**, 1900, 39–110.

Sacks, O, 'Gowers' memory', *Neurology*, **46**, 1996, 1467–9.

Smith, W (ed.), *Dictionary of Greek and Roman Biography and Mythology* (London: Taylor and Wootton, 1842).

Smith, W (ed.), *Dictionary of Greek and Roman Antiquities* (London: John Murray, 1844).

Snow, J, 'Cholera, and the water supply in the south districts of London', BMJ, **1**:42, 17 October 1857, 864–5.

Spillane, J D, *The Doctrine of the Nerves: Chapters in the History of Neurology* (Oxford: Oxford University Press, 1981).

Stein, J F and Stoodley, C J, *Neuroscience: an Introduction* (Chichester: Wiley, 2006).

Steinert, H, 'Uber das klinische und anatomische Bild des Muskelschwunds der Myotoniker', *Deutsche Zeitschrift Nervenheilkunde*, **37**, 1909, 38–104.

Strümpell, A, *Lehrbuch der speciellen Pathologie und Therapie der innern Krankheiten* (Leipzig: Vogel, 1883–4).

Swash, M, 'John Hughlings Jackson: a sesquicentennial tribute', *Journal of Neurology,* Neurosurgery, and Psychiatry, **49**, 1986, 981–5.

Symonds, C, 'Disease of the mind and disorder of brain' [Gowers Memorial Lecture given 23 June 1960], *BMJ*, **2**:5191, 1960, 1–5.

Taylor, J, *Paralysis and other Diseases of the Nervous System in Children and Early Life* (London: J & A Churchill, 1905).

Taylor, J (ed.), *Neurological Fragments (John Hughlings Jackson)* (London: Oxford University Press Medical, 1925).

Taylor, J (ed.), *Selected Writings of John Hughlings Jackson*, Vols 1 and 2 (London: Hodder & Stoughton, 1932).

Temple, F, Williams, R, Baden-Powell, R, Wilson, H B, Goodwin, C W, Pattison, M, *et al.*, *Essays and Reviews* (London: Parker, 1860).

Thornton, D, *Mr Mercury: the Life of Edward Baines 1774–1848* (Chesterfield: Merton Priory Press, 2009).

Tissot, S A, *Traité des Nerfs et de Leurs Maladies* (Paris: 1840) [originally Paris: Didot, 1780].

Todd, R B, 'On the pathology and treatment of convulsive diseases', *London Medical Gazette*, **8**, 1849, 661–71; 724–9; 66–72; 815–22; 37–46.

Todd, R B, *The Student's Guide to Systematic Botany: including the Classification of Plants and Descriptive Botany* (London: J & A Churchill, date unknown).

Tyler, K L, 'Pioneers in Neurology: William Richard Gowers (1845–1915)', *Journal of Neurology*, **250**, 2003, 1012–13.

Tyler, K L, Roberts, D, and Tyler, H R, 'The shorthand publications of Sir William Richard Gowers', *Neurology*, **55**, 2000, 289–93.

Vora, S K and Lyons, R W, 'The medical Kipling—syphilis, tabes dorsalis, and Romberg's test', *Emerging Infectious Diseases*, **10**:6, June 2004, 1160–2.

Waller, A D, 'The velocity of a nervous impulse', *Nature*, **69**, 1903, 151.

Walshe, F, 'The nature and dimension of nosography in modern medicine' [first Gowers Memorial Lecture given on 15 November 1956], *Lancet*, **268**:6952, 24 November 1956, 1059–63.

Watson, T, *Lectures on the Principles and Practice of Physic delivered at King's College*, 4th edn (London: John W Parker & Son, 1857).

Wilks, S, 'On syphilitic affections of the internal organs', *Guy's Hospital Reports*, **9**: 1863, 1–16.

Wilks, S, *Lectures on Diseases of the Nervous System* (London: Churchill, 1878).

Wilks, S, 'Syphilis and tabes dorsalis', *BMJ*, **1**:1310, 6 February 1886, 273–4.

Wilks, S, *Biographical Reminiscences of Sir Samuel Wilks* (London: Alard & Son, 1911).

Wilson, J V K and Reynolds, E H, 'Translation and analysis of a cuneiform text forming part of a Babylonian treatise on epilepsy', *Medical History*, **34**, 1990, 185–98.

Wilson, S A K, 'Progressive lenticular degeneration: a familial nervous disease associated with cirrhosis of the liver', *Brain*, **34**, 1912, 295–509.

Woodham-Smith, C, *Florence Nightingale 1820–1910* (New York: McGraw-Hill, 1951).

Worboys, M, 'Bastian, (Henry) Charlton (1837–1915), physician and neurologist', *Oxford Dictionary of National Biography*, (Oxford: Oxford University Press, 2004).

Young, G M, *Victorian England: Portrait of an Age* (London: Oxford University Press, 1953).

Zeigler, P, *Legacy: Cecil Rhodes, the Rhodes Trust and Rhodes Scholarships* (New Haven and London: Yale University Press, 2008).

von Ziemssen, G, *A Cyclopaedia of the Practice of Medicine* (New York: Wood & Co, 1878).

## References

### Preface

1 Critchley, M, *Sir William Gowers 1845–1915: a Biographical Appreciation* (London: William Heinemann Medical Books, 1949).

2 Leader, 'Sir William Gowers, 1845–1915', *BMJ*, **1**:4395, 31 March 1945, 452.

3 Critchley, p.96.

4 Critchley, p.12.

5 Henson, R A, 'Commentary on de Watteville review', *Brain*, **110**:4, August 1987, 1082–3.

6 Lees, M J, Woodward, R M P, Scott, A E M, and Eadie, M J, 'W R Gowers: 1895: two unpublished post-graduate lectures', *Brain*, doi 10.1093, March 2012; and Eadie, M J, Scott, A E M, Lees, A J, and Woodward, R M P, 'William Gowers' 'Bible of Neurology': the never completed third edition', *Brain*, 2012 (forthcoming).

### Chapter 1: Family and schooling

1 Briggs, A, *Victorian People* (London: Odhams Press, 1954), p.1.

2 Northcote, S H and Trevelyan, C E, *Report on the Organisation of the Permanent Civil Service*, paper number 1713, xxvii, 1 (London: Parliamentary Sessional Papers, 1854).

3 W.E.A., *The History of Coggeshall 1700–1914* (Coggeshall: Workers' Educational Association and Coggeshall Museum, 1999).

4 Beaumont, F G, *A History of Coggeshall, in Essex* (Coggeshall: Marshall Brothers and Edwin Potter, 1890).

5 Gowers, E A, 'Reminiscence of William Richard Gowers', 1948. [All references to Ernest Gowers' recollections refer to this document in the Gowers family archives.]

6 Critchley, M, *Sir William Gowers 1845–1915: a Biographical Appreciation* (1949), p.14.

7 Report, 'Funeral of Dr Thomas Simpson of Coggeshall' (unknown: Coggeshall, 1893). [Copy provided by the Coggeshall Museum.]

### Chapter 2: Apprentice years 1861–2

1 Peterson, M J, *The Medical Profession in Mid-Victorian London* (Los Angeles: University of California Press, 1978), p.5

2 Gowers, W R, 'Science and shorthand', *The Shorthand Gazette*, **15**, 1909, 112–15.

3 Reed, T A, *A Biography of Isaac Pitman (Inventor of Phonography)* (London: Griffith, Farran, Okeden & Welsh, 1890), p.32.

4 Gowers, W R, Letter to the Members, 1894. [Included with first issue of the *Phonographic Journal of Clinical Practice and Medical Science.*]

5 Dale, B, *The Annals of Coggeshall, otherwise Sunnedon, in the County of Essex* (London: A G Coventry, 1863)

6 Dale, B, p.3.

7 Gowers, W R, Shorthand diary, 1862. [All diary extracts are taken from this document, held by the Gowers family.]

8 Report, 'Regulations concerning degrees, diplomas, etc in medicine', *BMJ*, **2**:91, 27 September 1862, 323–32.

9 Angus, J, *Handbook of the English Tongue: for the Use of Student and Others* (London: Religious Tract Society, 1862).

10 Erichsen, J E, *Science and Art of Surgery: Being a Treatise on Surgical Injuries, Diseases, and Operations* (London: Walton and Maberly, 1853).

11 Smith, W (ed.), *Dictionary of Greek and Roman Biography and Mythology* (London: Taylor and Wootton, 1842); Smith, W (ed.), *Dictionary of Greek and Roman Antiquities*, (London: John Murray, 1844).

12 Report, 'University Matriculation Examination, January 1863', *The Times*, London, 1863.

13 Gowers, W R, 'Science and shorthand' p. 112.

## Chapter 3: Apprentice year 1863

1 Newman, C, *The Evolution of Medical Education in the Nineteenth Century* (London: Oxford University Press, 1957), p.79.

2 Watson, T, *Lectures on the Principles and Practice of Physic delivered at King's College*, 4th edn (London: John W Parker & Son, 1857).

3 Todd, R B, *The Student's Guide to Systematic Botany: including the Classification of Plants and Descriptive Botany* (London: J & A Churchill, date unknown).

4 Boyd, A K H, *Leisure Hours in Town: a Selection from the Contributions of A.H.K.B. to Fraser's Magazine* (London: Longmans Green, 1862).

5 Cassell's, *Cassell's German Pronouncing Dictionary, Consisting of Extracts in Prose and Verse, with Appropriate Vocabularies* (London: Cassell's, 1853).

6 Newman, C, *The Evolution of Medical Education in the Nineteenth Century* (1957), p.96.

7 Paget, J and Paget, C, *Sketch of the Natural History of Yarmouth and its Neighbourhood: Containing Catalogues of the Species of Animals, Birds, Reptiles, Fish, Insects, and Plants, at Present Known* (London: Longman Rees, 1834).

8 Quoted in Newman, p.97.

9 Masters, M T, 'Teaching of botany in medical schools', *BMJ*, **2**:1136, 24 September 1864, 374–5.

10 Babington, C C, *Manual of British Botany, containing the Flowering Plants and Ferns Arranged According to the Natural Orders* (London: J Van Voorst, 1851).

11 Gibson, G S, *The Flora of Essex* (London: William Pamplin, 1862).

12 Cited in Picard, L, *Victorian London: the Tale of a City 1840–1870* (New York: St Martin's Griffin, 2005), p.4.

## Chapter 4: Medical student

1 Snow, J, 'Cholera, and the water supply in the south districts of London', *BMJ*, **1**:42, 17 October 1857, 864–5. [See Carpenter, M, *Health, Medicine, and Society in Victorian England* (Santa Barbara, CA: Praeger, 2010).]

2 Carpenter, M, *Health, Medicine, and Society in Victorian England* (2010).

3 Woodham-Smith, C, *Florence Nightingale 1820–1910* (New York: McGraw-Hill, 1951), p.226.

4 Nightingale, F, *Notes on Nursing: What it is and What it is Not* (London: Harrison and Sons, 1860), p.11.

5 Musgrove, F, 'Middle-class education and employment in the nineteenth century', The Economic History Review, **2**:1, 1959, 99–111.

6 Newman, C, *The Evolution of Medical Education in the Nineteenth Century* (1957), p.79.

7 Froggatt, P, '*The Lancet*: Wakley's instrument for medical education reform', *Journal of the Society of Occupational Medicine*, **29**, 1979, 45–53, p.48.

8 Clarke, J F, *Autobiographical Recollections of the Medical Profession* (London: J & A Churchill, 1874), p.70.

9 Newman, p.112.

10 Clarke, J F, (1874), pp.8–9.

11 Peterson, M J, *The Medical Profession in Mid-Victorian London* (1978), p.15.

12 Peterson, p.209.

13 Lane, J, A *Social History of Medicine: Health, Healing* and Disease in England, *1750–1950* (London: Routledge, 2001), pp.29–30.

14 Peterson, p.14.

15 Birken, W, 'The Dissenting tradition in English medicine of the seventeenth and eighteenth centuries', *Medical History*, **39**, 1995, 197–218, p.215.

16 Young, G M, *Victorian England: Portrait of an Age* (London: Oxford University Press, 1953), p.93.

17 Clarke, pp.299–30.

18 Merskey, H, 'Some features of medical education in Great Britain during the first half of the nineteenth century', *British Journal of Medical Education*, **3**:2, 1969, 118–21, p.118.

19 Lawrence, C, 'Lister, Joseph, Baron Lister (1827–1912)', *Oxford Dictionary of National Biography* (Oxford: Oxford University Press, 2004).

20 Bellot, H H, *University College London, 1816–1926* (London: University of London Press, 1929), p.314.

21 Carpenter, M, *Health, Medicine, and Society in Victorian England* (2010), p.25.

22 Brown, H B, 'UCH and Sir William Gowers', BMJ, 1:4400, 5 May 1945, 645.

23 Godlee, R J, *Lord* Lister (Oxford: The Clarendon Press, 1924), p.122.

24 Dobson and Wakely, Edinburgh: Livingstone, p.45.

25 Merrington, W R, *University College Hospital and its Medical School: a History* (London: Heinemann, 1976), p.47.

26 Dobson, J and Wakely, C, *Sir George Buckston Browne* (1957), p.227.

27 Cook, E T, *The Life of Florence Nightingale: Vol 2, 1862–1910* (London: Macmillan, 1913), p.417.

28 Gowers, W R, 'Shorthand and students' [letter], *BMJ*, **1**:1880, 9 January 1897, 113–14, p.113.

29 Critchley, M, *Sir William Gowers 1845–1915: a Biographical Appreciation* (1949), p.18.

30 Seeley, J R, *The London Student*, April 1868, i, 15–16.

31 Reader, W J, *Professional Men: the Rise of the Professional Classes in Nineteenth-Century England* (New York: Basic Books, 1966), p.136.

32 Young, p.16.

33 Dobson and Wakely, p.37.

34 Haley, B, *The Healthy Body and Victorian Culture* (Harvard: Harvard University Press, 1978), p.12.

35 Young, pp.74–5.

36 Arnold, T, *Principles of Church Reform*, 2nd edn (London: Fellowes, 1833), pp.3–4.

37 Temple, F, Williams, R, Baden-Powell, R, Wilson, H B, Goodwin, C W, Pattison, M and Jowett, B, *Essays and Reviews* (London: Parker, 1860).

38 Altholz, J L, *Anatomy of a Controversy: the Debate over Essays and Reviews 1860–1864* (Aldershot: Scholar Press, 1994).

39 Jensen, J V, 'Return to the Wilberforce-Huxley debate', *British Journal for the History of Science*, **21**:2, June 1988, 161–79, p.179.

40 Peterson, p.159.
41 Holmes, G, 'Sir William Gowers at the National Hospital', *BMJ*, **2**:4744, 8 December 1951, 1397–8, p.1397.
42 Leader, 'Sir William Gowers, 1845–1915', *BMJ*, **1**:4395, 31 March 1945, 452, p.282.
43 Bellot, p.275–6.
44 Merrington, p.83.
45 Merrington, p.84.
46 Report, 'Sir William Gowers and the Society of Medical Phonographers', *BMJ*, **2**:1927, 1897, 1657–8.
47 Critchley, p.18.
48 Obituary, 'Sir William Gowers, MD, FRCP, FRS', *BMJ*, **1**:2836, 8 May 1915, 828–30, p.282.
49 Gowers, E A, Notes for Macdonald Critchley, 1948.
50 Gowers, W R, 'An appreciation of Sir William Jenner as a clinical teacher and physician', *BMJ*, **2**:1981, 17 December 1898, 1852.
51 Merrington, p.87.
52 Bellot, p.349.
53 Reynolds, J R, *Lectures on the Clinical Uses of Electricity* (London: J & A Churchill, 1871).
54 Obituary, 'Sir J Russell Reynolds, MD, FRCP, FRS', *BMJ*, **1**:1849, 6 June 1896, 1422–5.
55 In 1863, under a London University Supplementary Charter, the Royal College of Surgeons examination had been incorporated in the MB. The Master of Surgery was created and the whole practical examination in surgery was transferred from the second MB. See Cain, P, *Examination Registers of the University of London 1838–1889* (London: University of London Archives, 1982).
56 Ruskin, J, *The Queen of the Air: being a Study of the Greek Myths of Cloud and Storm* (London: George Allen, 1908).
57 Ruskin, J, *Lectures on Art: delivered before the University of Oxford in Hilary Term, 1870* (London: George Allen & Sons, 1910).
58 Clarke, K, *Ruskin Today* (London: John Murray, 1964), p.xiii.
59 Clarke, p.85.
60 Obituary, 'Sir William Richard Gowers, MD Lond and Dub, FRCP Lond, LL.D Edin. FRS', *Lancet*, **185**:4785, 15 May 1915, 1055–7.
61 Peterson, p.136.
62 Reynolds, H R and Reynolds, J R, *Yes and No; or, Glimpses of the Great Conflict* (London: Macmillan, 1860).
63 Thornton, D, *Mr Mercury: the Life of Edward Baines 1774–1848* (Chesterfield: Merton Priory Press, 2009), p.291.
64 Reid, S J, *Memoirs of Sir Wemyss Reid 1842 to 1885* (Whitefish, MT: Kessinger Publishing) [originally self-published, London, 1905]

## Chapter 5: Choosing neurology

1 Reynolds, J R, *A System of Medicine*, Vol 2, 1st edn (London: Churchill, 1868).
2 Stein, J F and Stoodley, C J, *Neuroscience: an Introduction* (Chichester: Wiley, 2006).
3 Stein and Stoodley, p.4.
4 Neuberger, M, *The Historical Development of Experimental Brain and Spinal Cord Physiology before Flourens* (transl. and ed. Clarke, E) (Baltimore and London: Johns Hopkins Press, 1981 [originally 1897]).

5 Bailey, J B, 'The Medical Societies of London', *BMJ*, **2**:1802, 13 July 1895, 100–4, p.101.
6 Stein, and Stoodley, p.6.
7 Romberg, M H, *A Manual of the Nervous Diseases of Man* (transl. Sieveking, E H) (London: New Sydenham Society, 1853).
8 Hall, M, 'On the reflex function of the medulla oblongata and medulla spinalis', *Philosophical Transactions*, **123**, 1833, 635–65.
9 Hall, M, 'On the theory of convulsive diseases, and especially of epilepsy', *Lancet*, **50**, 1847, 460–7.
10 Reynolds, J R, *The Diagnosis of Diseases of the Brain, Spinal Cord, Nerves and their Appendages* (London: Churchill, 1855).
11 Reynolds, J R, *Epilepsy: its Symptoms, Treatment, and Relation to Other Chronic Convulsive Disease* (London: J & A Churchill, 1861).
12 Rawlings, B B, *A Hospital in the Making: a History of the National Hospital for the Paralysed and Epileptic* (London: Pitman, 1913) p.189.
13 Holmes, G, 'Sir William Gowers at the National Hospital', *BMJ*, **2**:4744, 8 December 1951, 1397–8, p.1397.
14 Perlman Lorch, M, 'The unknown source of John Hughlings Jackson's early interest in aphasia and epilepsy', *Cognitive and Behavioral Neurology*, **17**:3, September 2004, 124–32.
15 Swash, M, 'John Hughlings Jackson: a sesquicentennial tribute', *Journal of Neurology, Neurosurgery, and Psychiatry*, **49**, 1986, 981–5.
16 Anon, *Queen Square and the National Hospital 1860–1960* (London: Edward Arnold, 1960), pp.74–5.
17 Mercier, C, 'The Late Dr Hughlings Jackson: recollections by Dr Mercier', *BMJ*, **1**:2663, 13 January 1912, 85–6, p.85.
18 Buzzard, F E, 'Hughlings Jackson and his influence on neurology', *Lancet*, **224**:5800, 27 October 1934, 909–13, p.910.
19 Gowers, W R, *Epilepsy and other Chronic Convulsive Diseases*, 2nd edn (London: J & A Churchill, 1901), p.261.
20 Worboys, M, 'Bastian, (Henry) Charlton (1837–1915), physician and neurologist', *Oxford Dictionary of National Biography* (Oxford: Oxford University Press, 2004).
21 Buzzard, T, Letter to W R Gowers, 6 December 1905.
22 Critchley, M, *Sir William Gowers 1845–1915: a Biographical Appreciation* (1949), pp.22–3.
23 Hughlings Jackson, J, Buzzard, T, Carter, R B, Bastian, H C, Gowers, W R, Ferrier, D, Ormerod, J.A, Beevor, C E, Tooth, H H, Taylor, J, Risien Russell, J S, Turner, W A, Batten, F E, Semon, F, Horsley, V, Ballance, C A, Gunn, R M, and Cumberbatch, A E, 'The medical staff and the management of the National Hospital for the Paralysed and Epileptic, Queen Square' [letter], *Lancet*, **156**:4014, 4 August 1900, 351–2.
24 Rawlings, B B, *A Hospital in the Making: a History of the National Hospital for the Paralysed and Epileptic* (1913).
25 Hamilton, G H, *Queen Square: its Neighbourhood and its Institutions* (London: Leonard Parsons, 1926), p.125.
26 Hamilton, p.129.
27 Buzzard, T, to W R Gowers, 6 December 1905.
28 Rawlings, p.44–5.
29 Liebreich, R, Letter to QS, 7 November 1872.

30 McHenry, L C, *Garrison's History of Neurology* (Springfield, IL: Charles C Thomas, 1969), p.311.

31 Gowers, W R, *A Manual and Atlas of Medical Ophthalmoscopy*, 1st edn (London: J & A Churchill, 1879).

32 Radcliffe, C B, Letter to QS, 26 October 1872.

33 Radcliffe, C B, Letter to QS, 13 November 1872.

34 Hughlings Jackson, J, Letter to QS, 11 November 1872.

35 Foster, M, Letter to W R Gowers, 9 November 1872.

36 Holmes, p.1198.

37 Critchley, pp.45–6.

38 Gowers, W R and Horsley, V, 'A case of tumour of the spinal cord, with removal and recovery (Royal Medical and Chirurgical Society)', *Lancet*, **131**:3381, 16 June 1888, 1194.

39 Lyons, J B, 'Correspondence between Sir William Gowers and Sir Victor Horsley', *Medical History*, **9**:3, 1965, 260–7, pp.265–6.

40 Gowers W R, to Horsley, 16 November 1891.

41 Gowers W R, to Queen Square Board of Management, 14 March 1874.

### Chapter 6: Gowers and clinical diagnosis

1 Gowers, W R, 'General principles of the diagnosis of diseases of the nervous system (lecture, Queen Square)', *Lancet*, **139**:3573, 20 February 1892, 403–5, p.404.

2 Critchley, M, *Sir William Gowers 1845–1915: a Biographical Appreciation* (1949), p.78.

3 Gowers, W R, 'Mistaken diagnosis' [post-graduate lecture, Queen Square], *BMJ*, **2**:1749, 7 July 1894, 1–3.

4 Brown, H B, 'UCH and Sir William Gowers', *BMJ*, **1**:4400, 5 May 1945, 645.

5 Critchley, M, *Sir William Gowers 1845–1915: a Biographical Appreciation* (1949), pp.77–8.

6 Cited in Critchley, p.79.

7 Critchley, p.81.

8 Holmes, G, 'Sir William Gowers at the National Hospital', *BMJ*, **2**:4744, 8 December 1951, 1397–8.

9 Critchley, p.81.

10 Holmes, G, *The National Hospital Queen Square* (Edinburgh: E & S Livingstone, 1954), pp.47–8.

11 Critchley, pp.82–3.

12 Critchley, pp.81–2.

13 Critchley, p.25.

14 Carswell, and Cruveilhier in 1837, and more fully described later by Friedrichs, Rindfleisch, Vulpian, and Charcot.

15 Critchley, p.23.

16 Clarke, J F, *Autobiographical Recollections of the Medical Profession* (1874), pp.112–30.

17 Gowers, W R, 'A safety hypodermic syringe', *Lancet*, **99**:2526, 27 January 1872, 113.

18 Gowers, W R, 'On the numeration of blood-corpuscles', *Lancet*, **110**:2831, 1 December 1877, 797–8.

19 Critchley, p.25.

20 Gowers, W R, 'A new haemocytometer', *Lancet*, **167**:4307, 17 March 1906, 767.

21 Report, 'Apparatus for the Clinical Estimation of the Haemoglobin in Blood', *BMJ*, **2**:938, 1878, 939.

22 Gowers, W R, 'An apparatus for the clinical estimation of haemoglobin', *Transactions of the Clinical Society of London*, **12**,1879, 64–7.

23 Critchley, p.26.

24 Gowers, W R, 'The estimation of sugar' [letter], *Lancet*, **169**:4372, 15 June 1907, 1673.

25 Gowers, W R, 'A standard dynamometer', *Lancet*, **164**:4223, 6 August 1904, 381.

26 Gowers, W R, 'A triple-wick candle', *Lancet*, **163**:4200, 27 February 1904, 586.

27 Gowers, W R, 'A magnifying otoscope', *Lancet*, **173**:4460, 20 February 1909, 552.

28 Leader, 'Sir William Gowers, 1845–1915', *BMJ*, **1**:4395, 31 March 1945, 452.


### Chapter 7: Gowers the researcher


1 Gowers, W R, 'The art of writing in relation to medical and scientific work', *BMJ*, **2**:1814, 5 October 1895, 817–19.

2 Obituary, 'William Richard Gowers', *Journal of Nervous and Mental Diseases*, **43**:5, May 1916, 485–6, p.486.

3 Critchley, M, 'The beginnings of the National Hospital, Queen Square (1859–1860)', *BMJ*, **1**:5189, 18 June 1960, 1829–37, p.1834.

4 Easton, P G, 'Sir William Gowers', *BMJ*, **2**:5191, 2 July 1960, 72.

5 Critchley, M, *Sir William Gowers 1845–1915: a Biographical Appreciation* (1949), p.30.

6 Jones, E, *Free Associations: Memories of a Psycho-Analyst* (London: The Hogarth Press, 1959), p.120.

7 Critchley (1949), p.24.

8 Critchley (1949), p.29.

9 Wilson, J V K and Reynolds, E H, 'Translation and analysis of a cuneiform text forming part of a Babylonian treatise on epilepsy', *Medical History*, **34**, 1990, 185–98.

10 Adams, F, *The Genuine Works of Hippocrates* (London: Sydenham Society, 1849).

11 Gowers, W R, 'Cases of convulsion from organic brain-disease' [lecture, BMA], *BMJ*, **2**:717, 26 September 1874, 398–400.

12 Gowers, W R, 'Special sense discharges from organic disease' [Hughlings Jackson lecture], *Brain*, **32**:4, 4 March 1910, 303–26.

13 Gowers, W R, *Epilepsy and Other Chronic Convulsive Diseases*, 2nd edn (London: J & A Churchill, 1901).

14 Gowers, W R, *A Manual of Diseases of the Nervous System*, Vol 2, 1st edn (London: J & A Churchill, 1888).

15 Gowers, W R, *The Borderland of Epilepsy: Faints, Vagal Attacks, Vertigo, Migraine, Sleep Symptoms, and Their Treatment* (London: J & A Churchill, 1907).

16 Flourens, M J P, *Recherches Expérimentales sur les Propriétés et les Fonctions du Système Nerveux dans les Animaux Vertébrés* (Paris: Crevot, 1824); Hall, M, *Lectures on the Nervous System and its Diseases* (London: Sherwood, Gilbert & Piper, 1836); Kussmaul, A and Tenner, A, *On the Nature and Origin of Convulsions Caused by Profuse Bleeding, and Also Those of Epilepsy* (transl. Bronner, E) (London: New Sydenham Society, 1859).

17 Hall, M, 'On the reflex function of the medulla oblongata and medulla spinalis', *Philosophical Transactions*, **123**, 1833, 635–65.

18 Hall, M, *Synopsis of Apoplexy and Epilepsy With Observations on Trachelismus, Laryngismus, and Tracheostomy; and a Proposal for a Hospital for Epileptics* (London: Mallett, 1852).

19 Todd, R B, 'On the pathology and treatment of convulsive diseases', *London Medical Gazette*, **8**, 1849, 661–71; 724–9; 66–72; 815–22; 37–46.

20 Reynolds, J R, *The Diagnosis of Diseases of the Brain, Spinal Cord, Nerves and their Appendages* (London: Churchill, 1855).

21 Delasiauve, L J F, *Traité de l'Épilepsie* (Paris: Masson, 1854).

22 Reynolds, J R, *Epilepsy: its Symptoms, Treatment, and Relation to Other Chronic Convulsive Disease* (London: J & A Churchill, 1861).

23 Nothnagel, H, 'Die Entstehung allgemeiner Convulsionen vom Pons und der Medulla oblongata aus', *Virchow's Archives*, **44**, 1868, 1–12.

24 Critchley (1949), p.27.

25 Gowers, W R, *Epilepsy and Other Chronic Convulsive Disorders, their Causes, Symptoms and Treatment* (London: J & A Churchill, 1881); Review, 'Gowers, W R: *Epilepsy and other Chronic Convulsive Diseases* (2nd edn)', BMJ, 1:2140, 4 January 1902, 27.

26 Critchley (1949), p.27. [Gowers' Gulstonian lectures were published as a series in both The *Lancet* and the *BMJ* in 1880.]

27 Gowers, W R, 'The Gulstonian lectures on epilepsy (1)', *Lancet*, **115**:2948, 28 February 1880, 315–18.

28 Gowers, W R, *Epilepsy and Other Chronic Convulsive Disorders, their Causes, Symptoms and Treatment* (1881).

29 Herpin, T, *Des Acces Incomplets d'Epilepsie* (Paris: Ballière, 1867) [published posthumously].

30 Hughlings Jackson, J and Purves Stewart, J, 'Epileptic attacks with a warning of a crude sensation of smell and with the intellectual aura (dreamy state) in a patient who had symptoms pointing to gross organic disease of the right temporo-sphenoidal lobe', *Brain*, **22**:4, 1899, 534–49.

31 Critchley (1949), p.38.

32 Radcliffe, C B, *Epilepsy and Other Convulsive Affections, their Pathology and Treatment* (London: Churchill, 1858).

33 Reynolds, J R, *Epilepsy: its Symptoms, Treatment, and Relation to Other Chronic Convulsive Disease* (1861).

34 Handfield Jones, C, 'Clinical lectures on cases of paralysis agitans', *BMJ*, **1**:635, 1 March 1873, 221–3.

35 Ringer, S, 'A suggestion concerning the condition of the nervous centres in migraine, epilepsy, and other explosive neuroses', *Lancet*, **109**:1877, 228–9.

36 Gowers, W R, 'Minor epilepsy' [clinical lecture, Queen Square], *BMJ*, **1**:2036, 6 January 1900, 1–5.

37 Gowers, W R, *Epilepsy and Other Chronic Convulsive Diseases* (1901).

38 Gowers, W R, 'Insanity and epilepsy in relation to life assurance' [lecture, Association of Life Assurance Medical Officers], *Lancet*, **164**:4233, 15 October 1904, 1061–4.

39 Gowers, W R, 'Heredity in diseases of the nervous system' [Royal Society of Medicine], *Lancet*, **174**:4498, 14 November 1908, 1467–8.

40 Gowers, W R, 'Should epileptics marry?' [letter], *Lancet*, **149**:3834, 20 February 1897, 554.

41 Gowers, W R, *The Dynamics of Life: an Address Delivered Before the Medical Society of Manchester October 3rd, 1894* (London: J & A Churchill, 1894).

42 Gowers, W R, 'Dendrites and disease' [lecture, Queen Square], *Lancet*, **168**:4324, 14 July 1906, 67–9.

43 Critchley (1949), p.71.

44 Gowers, W R, *Epilepsy and Other Chronic Convulsive Diseases* (1901).

45 Herpin, T, *Des Acces Incomplets d'Epilepsie* (1867).

46 Hughlings Jackson, J (ed.), *Selected Writings of John Hughlings Jackson* (London: Hodder & Stoughton, 1932).

47 Gowers, W R, *Epilepsy and Other Chronic Convulsive Disorders, their Causes, Symptoms and Treatment* (1881); Gowers, W R, *Epilepsy and Other Chronic Convulsive Diseases* (1901).

48 Gowers, W R, 'Faints and fainting' [lecture, Queen Square], *Lancet*, **169**:4357, 2 March 1907, 565–8.

49 Gowers, W R, *The Borderland of Epilepsy*, pp.18–19.

50 Gowers, W R, *The Borderland of Epilepsy*, p.65.

51 Airy, H, 'On a distinct form of transient heniopia', *Philosophical Transactions*, **159**, 1870, 247–64.

52 Liveing, E, *On Megrim, Sick-Headache, and some Allied Disorders: a Contribution to the Pathology of Nerve-Storms* (London: Churchill, 1873).

53 Latham, P W, 'Clinical lecture nervous or sick-headaches' (Pt 1), *BMJ*, **1**:586, 23 March 1872, 305–6; (Pt 2), *BMJ*, **1**:587, 30 March 1872, 336–7; Latham, P W, *On Nervous or Sick Headache, its Varieties and Treatment* (Cambridge: Deighton, Bell & Co, 1873).

54 Gowers, W R, *The Borderland of Epilepsy: Faints, Vagal Attacks, Vertigo, Migraine, Sleep Symptoms, and Their Treatment* (1907).

55 Gowers, W R, *A Manual of Diseases of the Nervous System*, 1st edn, Vol.2, (London: J & A Churchill, 1888).

56 Gowers, W R, *A Manual of Diseases of the Nervous System*, 1st edn, Vol 2, (London: J & A Churchill, 1888), p.776.

57 Gowers, W R, *A Manual of Diseases of the Nervous System*, Vol 2, (London: J & A Churchill, 1888), p.778.

58 Gowers, W R, *A Manual of Diseases of the Nervous System*, Vol 2, (London: J & A Churchill, 1888), p.782.

59 Tissot, S A, *Traité des Nerfs et de Leurs Maladies* (Paris: 1840) [originally Paris: Didot, 1780].

60 Liveing, E, *On Megrim, Sick-Headache, and some Allied Disorders: a Contribution to the Pathology of Nerve-Storms* (1873).

61 Gowers, W R, 'The Bradshaw Lecture on Subjective Sensations of Sound', *BMJ*, **2**:1872, 14 November 1896, 1429–36; Gowers, W R, 'Special sense discharges from organic disease' [Hughlings Jackson lecture], *Brain*, **32**:4, 4 March 1910, 303–26; Gowers, W R, *The Borderland of Epilepsy*; Gowers, W R, 'The prodromas of migraine' [address, Westminster Division, BMA], *BMJ*, **1**:2528, 12 June 1909, 1400–3.

62 Du Bois-Reymond, E H, 'De l'hémicrânie ou migraine', *Journal de la Physiologie de l'Homme et des Animaux*, **4**, 1861, 130–7.

63 Möllendorf, 'Ueber Hemikranie', *Virchow's Archives*, **47**, 1867, 385–95.

64 Latham, P W, *On Nervous or Sick Headache, its Varieties and Treatment* (1873).

65 Gowers, W R, 'The prodromas of migraine' [address, Westminster Division, BMA], *BMJ*, **1**:2528, 12 June 1909, 1400–3, p.1400.

66 Gowers, W R, 'The prodromas of migraine'.

67 Report, 'Death of Lord R Churchill', *The Times*, London, 25 January 1895.

68 Wilks, S, 'On syphilitic affections of the internal organs', *Guy's Hospital Reports*, **9**, 1863, 1–16.

69 Wilks, S, *Biographical Reminiscences of Sir Samuel Wilks* (London: Alard & Son, 1911).

70 Gowers, W R, 'The Lettsomian lectures on syphilis and the nervous system (Lecture 1)', *Lancet*, **133**:3411, 12 January 1889, 59–66; Gowers, W R, 'The Lettsomian lectures on syphilis and the nervous system (Lecture 2)', *Lancet*, **133**:3413, 26 January 1889, 159–61.

71 Gowers, W R, 'Visceral syphilis' [Pathological Society], *BMJ*, **1**:838, 20 January 1877, 86–7.

72 Wilks, S, *Lectures on Diseases of the Nervous System* (London: Churchill, 1878).

73 Wilks, S, 'Syphilis and tabes dorsalis', *BMJ*, **1**:1310, 6 February 1886, 273–4.

74 Radcliffe, C B, 'Diseases of the spinal cord', in Reynolds, J R (ed.), *A System of Medicine*, Vol 1, 2nd edn (Philadelphia: Lea's Son & Co, 1879).

75 Maudsley, H, 'Insanity', in Reynolds, J R (ed.), *A System of Medicine*, Vol 1, 2nd edn (Philadelphia: Henry C Lea's Son & Co, 1879).

76 Gowers, W R, 'Syphilitic neuroses' [lecture, BMA], *BMJ*, **1**:948, 1 March 1879, 303–5.

77 Cullen, W, *First Lines of the Practice of Physic* (New York: Duyckinck, Swords, Falconer *et al*, 1805) [originally 1789].

78 Gowers, W R, 'Syphilitic neuroses'.

79 Fournier, J-A, 'De l'ataxie locomotorice d'origine syphilitique', *Annales de Dermatologie et de Syphilologie*, **7**, 1875, 187–97.

80 Wilks, S, 'Syphilis and tabes dorsalis'.

81 Fournier, J-A, 'De l'ataxie locomotorice d'origine syphilitique'.

82 Gowers, W R, 'The Lettsomian lectures on syphilis and the nervous system. The lectures were published in 1892 as a 131-page monograph for which he revised some of the text: Gowers, W R, *Syphilis and the Nervous System (being a revised reprint of Lettsomian Lectures for 1890)* (Philadelphia: Blakiston, 1892).

83 Strümpell, A, *Lehrbuch der speciellen Pathologie und Therapie der innern Krankheiten*, (Leipzig: Vogel, 1883–4). It was present in many later editions of the *Lehrbuch*.

84 Gowers, W R, 'Remarks on the pathology of tabes in relation to general paralysis of the insane' [Pathological Society of London], *BMJ*, **2**:2032, 9 December 1899, 1597–8.

85 Gowers, W R, 'The prognosis and treatment of syphilitic diseases of the nervous system' [lecture, Medical Graduates' College and Polyclinic], *BMJ*, **1**:2205, 4 April 1903, 773–8.

86 Gowers, W R, 'The nature of tabes' [lecture, Queen Square], *BMJ*, **2**:2323, 8 July 1905, 57–61, p.58.

87 Gowers, W R, 'The nature of tabes'.

88 Gowers, W R, 'The dystrophy of tabes and the problem of trophic nerves' [lecture, Queen Square], *BMJ*, **1**:2370, 2 June 1906, 1267–9.

89 Gowers, W R, *A Manual of Diseases of the Nervous System*, Vol 2, 1st edn, p.589.

90 Gowers, W R, *A Manual of Diseases of the Nervous System* 1st edn, Vol 2, p.606.

91 Gowers, W R, 'Paralysis agitans', in Allbutt, C T (ed.), *A System of Medicine*, Vol 8 (London: Macmillan, 1904).

92 Gowers, W R, 'Remarks on two cases of writer's cramp', *Medical Times and Gazette*, **2**, 1877, 536–8.

93 Gowers, W R, 'On some points in the clinical history of chorea: I The irritability of nerve and muscle in chorea; II On the relation of the muscular disturbance in chorea to voluntary movements', *BMJ*, **1**:900, 30 March 1878, 447–9.

94 Gowers, W R, 'On paralytic chorea' [lecture, BMA], *BMJ*, **1**:1060, 23 April 1881, 636–7.

95 Gowers, W R, 'On some points in the clinical history of chorea: I The irritability of nerve and muscle in chorea; II On the relation of the muscular disturbance in chorea to voluntary movements', *BMJ*, **1**:900, 30 March 1878, 447–9; Gowers, W R, 'On some points in the clinical history of chorea: III The distribution of hemichorea', *BMJ*, **1**:901, 6 April 1878, 479–81.

96 Gowers, W R, 'On' athetosis' and post-hemiplegic disorders of movement', *Medico-Chirurgical Transactions*, **59**, 1876, 271–327.

97 Gowers, W R, 'On tetanoid chorea and its association with cirrhosis of the liver', *Review of Neurology and Psychiatry (Edinburgh)*, **4**, 1906, 249–71.

98 Wilson, S A K, 'Progressive lenticular degeneration: a familial nervous disease associated with cirrhosis of the liver', *Brain*, **34**, 1912, 295–509. [At 214 pages this was the longest article ever published in *Brain*.]

99 Lees, A J, Woodward, R M P, Scott, A E M, and Eadie, M J, 'W R Gowers 1895: two unpublished postgraduate lectures', *Brain*, 2012, doi: 10.1093/brain/aws029.

100 Carswell, R, *Pathological Anatomy: Illustrations of the Elementary Forms of Disease* (London: Longman, Rees, Orme, and others, 1835–8); Cruveilhier, J, *Anatomie Pathologique du Corps Humaine*, Vol 2 (Paris: Balliere, 1835–42).

101 Charcot, J M, *Lectures on Diseases of the Nervous System*, Vol 1 (transl. Sigerson, G) (London: New Sydenham Society, 1877).

102 Critchley, (1949), p.17.

103 Lockhart-Clarke, J and Gowers, W R, 'On a case of pseudo-hypertrophic muscular paralysis', *Medico-Chirurgical Transactions*, **57**, 1874, 247–59.

104 Critchley, (1949), p.32.

105 Gowers, W R, *Pseudo-Hypertrophic Muscular Paralysis* (London: J & A Churchill, 1879).

106 Cited in Critchley, (1949), pp.32–3.

107 Duchenne, G B A, 'Recherches sur la paralysie musculaire pseudohypertrophique ou paralysie myosclérotique', *Archives Générales de Médicine*, **11**, 1869, 5–25; 179–209; 305–21; 421–43; 552–88; Meryon, E, 'On granular and fatty degeneration of the voluntary muscles', *Medico-Chirurgical Transactions*, 35, 1851, 73–84.

108 Gowers, W R, 'Myopathy and a distal form' [lecture, Queen Square], *BMJ*, **2**:2167, 12 July 1902, 89–92.

109 Gowers, W R, 'Heredity in diseases of the nervous system' [Royal Society of Medicine], *Lancet*, **174**:4498, 14 November 1908, 1467–8.

110 Gowers, W R, 'Myopathy and syringomyelia' [lecture, Queen Square], *BMJ*, **1**:2523, 8 May 1909, 1101–4.

111 Steinert, H, 'Uber das klinische und anatomische Bild des Muskelschwunds der Myotoniker', *Deutsche Zeitschrift Nervenheilkunde*, **37**, 1909, 38–104.

112 Gowers, W R, 'Polymyositis' [lecture, Queen Square], *BMJ*, **1**:1985, 14 January 1899, 65–7.

113 Gowers, W R, 'The automatic action of the sphincter ani', *Proceedings of the Royal Society of London*, **26**:1 January 1877, 77–84.

114 Gowers, W R, 'The movements of the eyelids' [Royal Medical Chirurgical Society], *Medico-Chirurgical Transactions*, **62**, 1879, 429–40.

115 Gowers, W R, 'Note on a reflex mechanism in the fixation of the eyeballs', *Brain*, **2**:1, 1 April 1879, 39–41.

116 Gowers, W R, 'A study of the so-called tendon-reflex phenomena', *Medico-Chirurgical Transactions*, **62**, 1879, 269–305.

117 Gowers, W R, *The Diagnosis of Diseases of the Spinal Cord*, 2nd edn (Philadelphia: Presley, Blakiston, 1882). We assume that this edition was identical to Gowers, W R, *The Diagnosis of Diseases of the Spinal Cord (revised and partly rewritten, with additions and illustrations)*, 2nd edn (London: J & A Churchill, 1881). However, we have not sighted the 1881 Churchill edition.

118 Gowers, W R, *Clinical Lectures on Diseases of the Nervous System* (Philadelphia: Blakiston, 1895), pp.163–74.

119 Gowers, W R, 'A study of the so-called tendon-reflex phenomena'.

120 Gowers, W R, 'The diagnostic value of the so-called "tendon-reflexes"' [presented to Medical Society of London], *Lancet*, **126**:3245, 7 November 1885, 839–42; Gowers, W R, *Clinical Lectures on Diseases of the Nervous System* (1895).

121 Gowers, W R, 'The rate of nerve impulses', *Nature*, **69**:1038, 3 December 1903, 105.

122 Waller, A D, 'The velocity of a nervous impulse', *Nature*, **69**:1903, 151.

123 Gowers, W R, 'Taste and the fifth nerve', *Journal of Physiology*, **28**:4, 21 July 1902, 300–3.

124 Gowers, W R, 'Lumbago: its lessons and analogues' [lecture, Queen Square], *BMJ*, **1**:2246, 16 January 1904, 117–21.

125 Critchley, (1949), p.64.

### Chapter 8: Gowers the writer and lecturer

1 Note to a house physician, cited in Critchley, M, *Sir William Gowers 1845–1915: a Biographical Appreciation* (1949), p.31.

2 Critchley, M, *Sir William Gowers 1845–1915: a Biographical Appreciation* (1949), p.31.

3 Gowers, E A, *Plain Words: a Guide to the Use of English* (London: HMSO, 1948).

4 Gowers, E A, Notes for Macdonald Critchley, 1948.

5 Gowers, W R, (transl.) *Atlas of Pathological Anatomy of the Eyeball* [translation of Pagenstecher and Genth's *Atlas der pathologischen Anatomie des Gaugapfels*] (Wiesbaden: Kreidel, 1875).

6 Jacyna, L S, A tale of three cities, *Medical History*, Supplement No 9 (London: Wellcome Institute for the History of Medicine, 1989).

7 Gowers, W R, 'The state of the arteries in Bright's disease' [lecture to the BMA], *BMJ*, **2**:832, 9 December 1876, 743–5.

8 Gowers, W R, *A Manual and Atlas of Medical Ophthalmoscopy* (London: J & A Churchill, 1879).

9 Rolleston, H D, *The Right Honourable Sir Thomas Clifford Allbutt* (London: Macmillan, 1929).

10 Bartrip, P W J, 'Churchill, John Spriggs Morss (1801–1875) medical publisher', *Oxford Dictionary of National Biography* (Oxford: Oxford University Press, 2004).

11 Quain, J and Wilson, W J E, *Anatomical Plates of the Human Body* (London: Taylor and Walton, 1836–42).

12 Richardson, R, *The Making of Mr Gray's Anatomy* (Oxford: Oxford University Press, 2008).

13 See 'Calamity' in Richardson, pp.229–55.

14 Obituary, 'Sir William Gowers, MD, FRCP, FRS', *BMJ*, **1**:2836, 8 May 1915, 828–30, p.829.

15 Review, '*A Manual and Atlas of Medical Ophthalmoscopy*', *Lancet*, **114**:2932, 8 November 1879, 694–5.

16 Gowers, W R, *The Diagnosis of Diseases of the Spinal Cord* (London: J & A Churchill, 1880).

17 Critchley, pp.35–7.

18 Gowers, W R, *Lectures on the Diagnosis of Diseases of the Brain*, 1st edn (London: J & A Churchill, 1885).

19 Gowers, W R, *Lectures on the Diagnosis of Diseases of the Brain*, 2nd edn (London: J & A Churchill, 1887).

20 Gowers, W R, *Diagnosis of Diseases of the Brain and of the Spinal Cord*, 1st edn (London: J & A Churchill, 1884).

21 Gowers, W R, *Diagnosis of the Diseases of the Brain and of the Spinal Cord*, 1st edn (New York: William Wood & Co, 1885).

22 Gowers, W R, 'A study of the so-called tendon reflex phenomena' [Royal Medical and Chirurgical Society], *Lancet*, **113**:2892, 1 February 1879, 156–7.

23 Gowers, W R, 'General principles of the diagnosis of diseases of the nervous system' [lecture, Queen Square], *Lancet*, **139**:3573, 20 February 1892, 403–5.

24 Babinski, J, 'Sur le réflexe cutané plantaire dans certains affections organiques du système nerveux centrale', *Comptes-Rendus Hebdomadaires des Séances et Mémoires de la Société de Biologie*, **3**, 1896, 207–8.

25 Holmes, G, *An Introduction to Clinical Neurology*, 2nd edn (Edinburgh: Livingstone, 1952).

26 Illustrations from *A Manual of Diseases of the Nervous System* in this section are taken from the 1st edn: Vol 1 (1886), Vol. 2 (1888) (London: J. & A. Churchill).

27 Gowers, E A, Notes for Macdonald Critchley, 1948.

28 Gowers, W R, *A Manual of Diseases of the Nervous System*, 2nd edn, Vol 1 (London: J & A Churchill, 1892).

29 Romberg, M H, *A Manual of the Nervous Diseases of Man* (1853).

30 Hammond, W A, *A Treatise on Disease of the Nervous System* (New York and London: Appleton & Co, and Turner & Co, 1871).

31 Rosenthal, M and Putzel, L, *A Clinical Treatise in the Diseases of the Nervous System* (New York: Wood & Co, 1879).

32 Wilks, S, *Lectures on Diseases of the Nervous System* (1878).

33 von Ziemssen, G, *A Cyclopaedia of the Practice of Medicine* (New York: Wood & Co, 1878).

34 Reynolds, J R, *A System of Medicine* (London: J & A Churchill, 1868).

35 Ross, J, *A Treatise on the Diseases of the Nervous System*, 1st edn (London: J & A Churchill, 1881); 2nd edn (London: J & A Churchill, 1883).

36 Russell, J S R, Batten, F E and Collier, J, 'Subacute combined degeneration of the spinal cord', *Brain*, **23**, 1900, 39–110.

37 Critchley, p.25. The case of 'Eliza T' (born Joad) was written up in Hughlings Jackson, J, 'Case of large cerebral tumour without optic neuritis and with left hemiplegia and imperception', in Taylor, J (ed.), *Selected Writings of John Hughlings Jackson*, Vol 2, (London: Hodder & Stoughton, 1931).

38 Allbutt, C T (ed.), *A System of Medicine* (London: Macmillan, 1899).

39 Review, '*A Manual of Diseases of the Nervous System*', *BMJ*, **2**:1347, 30 October 1886, 824.

40 M.A.S., '*A Manual of Diseases of the Nervous System*, by W R Gowers', *American Journal of the Medical Sciences*, **95**:6, June 1888, 603–5.

41 J.H.L., 'Recent works on diseases of the nervous system', *American Journal of the Medical Sciences*, **104**:4, October 1892, 450–3.

42 Anon, 'Recent works on nervous diseases', *American Journal of the Medical Sciences*, **93**:185, January 1887, 204–7.

43 Review, '*A Manual of the Diseases of the Nervous System*', *Lancet*, **128**:3294, 16 October 1886, 729. Spillane provided a comprehensive overview of the *Manual* in Spillane, J D, *The Doctrine of the Nerves: Chapters in the History of Neurology* (Oxford: Oxford University Press, 1981).

44 McHenry, L C, *Garrison's History of Neurology* (Springfield: Thomas, 1969), p.15.

45 De Watteville, A, 'Review: *A Manual of the Diseases of the Nervous System*', *Brain*, **2**:1, 1888, 131–3.

46 Critchley, M, *Sir William Gowers 1845–1915: a Biographical Appreciation* (1949), p.50.

47 Gowers, W R, 'Special sense discharges from organic disease' [Hughlings Jackson lecture], *Brain*, **32**:4, 4 March 1910, 303–26.

48 Hunting, P, *The History of the Royal Society of Medicine* (London: Royal Society of Medicine Press, 2001), p.264.

49 Obituary, 'Sir William Gowers, MD, FRCP, FRS', *BMJ*, **1**:2836, 8 May 1915, 828–30.

50 Gowers, W R, 'Introductory lecture' [lecture, UCH], *Lancet*, **124**:3188, 4 October 1884, 582–86, p.582.

51 Gowers, W R, 'A metastatic mystery' [lecture, UCH], *Lancet*, **166**:4792, 2 December 1905, 1593–6, 1593.

52 Gowers, W R, 'A metastatic mystery' p.1593.

53 Brown, H B, 'UCH and Sir William Gowers', *BMJ*, **1**:4400, 5 May 1945, 645.

54 Obituary, 'Sir William Gowers, MD, FRCP, FRS', *BMJ*.

55 Cited in Critchley, p.82.

56 Gowers, W R, 'Birth palsies (1)' [clinical lecture, UCH], *Lancet*, **131**:3372, 14 April 1888, 709–11, p.709.

57 Gowers, W R, 'The Lettsomian lectures on syphilis and the nervous system' [lecture 3:2], *BMJ*, **1**:1468, 16 February 1889, 345–8, p.346.

58 Editorial, 'Continence *versus* syphilis', *Lancet*, **133**:3430, 25 May 1889, 1042–3.

59 Gowers, W R, *Introductory Lecture Delivered on the Opening of the Medical Session at University College, London, October 1st, 1884* (London: H. K. Lewis, 1884).

60 Liddell, E G T, 'Gowers, Sir William Richard (1845–1915)', *Oxford Dictionary of National Biography* (Oxford: Oxford University Press, 2004).

61 Report, 'Dr Gowers', *Lancet*, **133**:3413, 26 January 1889, 186.

62 Gowers, W R, Letter to B Rawlings, undated 1892.

63 Gowers, W R, Letter to B Rawlings, undated 1892.

64 Gowers, W R, 'A case of syringomyelia' [clinical lecture, Queen Square], *Clinical Journal*, **2**, 1893, 65–70.

65 Critchley, M, p.42.

66 Critchley, M, p.51.

67 Obituary, 'Sir William Gowers, MD, FRCP, FRS', *BMJ*.

## Chapter 9: Life outside work


1 Critchley, M, *Sir William Gowers 1845–1915: a Biographical Appreciation* (1949), pp.21–2.

2 Report, 'Typhoid fever in London', *The Times*, London, 13 August 1873.

3 Obituary, 'Sir William R Gowers, FRS', *Nature*, **95**:2376, 1915, 296–7, p.297.

4 1881 census, The family was on holiday at the Isle Wight on census day 1891.

5 Gowers, W R, Letter to T Barlow, 1882. Royal College of Physicians, G92.

6 Gowers, E A, Notes for Macdonald Critchley, 1948.

7 Altholz, J L, *Anatomy of a Controversy: the Debate over Essays and Reviews 1860–1864* (1994), p.12.

8 Gowers, E A.

9 Jessopp, A, *Arcady, for Better for Worse* (London: T Fisher Unwin, 1887).

10 Gowers, W R, 'Chapel of S. Margaret, Mells', *Proceedings of the Suffolk Institute of Archaeology and Natural History*, **8**, 1894, 334–79; Gowers, W R, 'The flintwork inscription in Blythburgh Church', *Proceedings of the Suffolk Institute of Archaeology and Natural History*, **II**, 1903, 51–8.

11 Paget, J, Letter to W R Gowers, 3 September 1889.

12 Gowers, W R, Letter to J J Raven, 9 September 1895. Letter held by Dr Christopher Boes.

13 Hind, A M and Chambers, E, 'Haden, Sir Francis Seymour (1818–1910)', *Oxford Dictionary of National Biography* (Oxford: Oxford University Press, 2004).

14 Haden, F S, Letter to W R Gowers, 9 December 1891.

15 Haden, F S, 'About etching', *Fine Arts Quarterly Review*, new series,1, 1866, 145–60.

16 Haden, F S, Letter to W R Gowers, 9 December 1891.

17 Newbolt, S F, *The History of the Royal Society of Painter-Etchers & Engravers* (London: The Print Collectors' Club, 1930).

18 Haden, F S, Letter to W R Gowers, 10 July 1894.

19 Gowers, W R, *The Dynamics of Life: an Address Delivered Before the Medical Society of Manchester October 3rd, 1894* (1894).

20 Haden, F S, Letter to W R Gowers, 10 July 1894.

21 Prinsep, V, Letter to W R Gowers, 12 November 1888.

22 Gowers, W R, 'Myasthenia and ophthalmoplegia' [an English version of a contribution to the special issue of the *Deutsche Medizinische Wochenschrift*, 28, 278–80, in honour of the 70th birthday of Professor v Leyden], *BMJ*, **1**:1253, 24 May 1902, 1253–6.

23 Report, 'Royal Botanical Society', *The Times*, London, 13 July 1885.

24 Obituary, 'Sir William R Gowers, FRS', *Nature*, **95**:2376, 1915, 296–7.

25 Report, 'The Savile Club', *BMJ*, **2**:3272, 15 September 1923, 472–3.

26 Desmond, A and Moore, J, *Darwin* (London: Michael Joseph, 1991).

27 Cited in Duncan, D, *Life and Letters of Herbert Spencer*, Vol 2 (New York: Appleton, 1908), p.116.

28 Critchley, p.85.

29 Hui-Min, Lo (ed.), *The Correspondence of G E Morrison* (Cambridge: Cambridge University Press, 1976), p.2.

30 Morrison, G E, *An Australian in China: Being the Narrative of a Quiet Journey Across China to Burma* (London: Horace Cox, 1895).

31 Morrison, pp.103–4.

32 Gowers, W R, *A Manual of Diseases of the Nervous System*, 1st edn, Vol 2, (London: J & A Churchill, 1888), p.903.

33 Hui-Min, Lo (ed), *The Correspondence of G E Morrison* (Cambridge: Cambridge University Press, 1976), pp.33–4.

34 Helly, D O and Callaway, H, 'Lugard [nee Shaw], Dame Flora Louise, Lady Lugard (1852–1929)', *Oxford Dictionary of National Biography* (Oxford: Oxford University Press, 2004).

35 Gregory, G S, 'Morrison, George Ernest (Chinese) (1862–1920)', *Australian Dictionary of Biography* (Melbourne: Melbourne University Press, 1986).

36 Gowers, W R, to Morrison, G E, 6 November 1895 (ML MSS 312/42, Morrison, George Ernest—correspondence 1895–1898).

37 Gowers, W R, Letter to G E Morrison, 20 November 1895.

38 Gowers, W R, Letter to G E Morrison, undated 1895.

39 Gowers, W R, Letter to G E Morrison, 16 March 1898.

40 Fitzgerald, C P '*An appreciation*', in Hui-Min Lo (ed.), *The Correspondence of G E Morrison* (Cambridge: Cambridge University Press, 1976), p.vii.

41 Lowry, D, 'Jameson, Sir Leander Starr, baronet (1853–1917)', *Oxford Dictionary of National Biography* (Oxford: Oxford University Press, 2004)

42 Quoted in Zeigler, P, *Legacy: Cecil Rhodes, the Rhodes Trust and Rhodes Scholarships*, (New Haven and London: Yale University Press, 2008), p.11.

43 Gowers, W R, Letter, 'Dr Jameson', *The Times*, London, 3 January 1896.

44 Gowers, W R, 'Dr Jameson's motive', *The Times*, London, 30 July 1896.

45 Gowers, W R, to G E Morrison, 16 March 1898.

46 Gowers, W R, Letter to G E Morrison, 4 November 1895.

47 Vora, S K and Lyons, R W, 'The medical Kipling—syphilis, tabes dorsalis, and Romberg's test', *Emerging Infectious Diseases*, **10**:6, June 2004, 1160–2.

48 Critchley, p.39.

49 Gowers, W R, 'Should epileptics marry?' [letter], *Lancet*, **149**:3834, 20 February 1897, 554.

50 Birkenhead, *Rudyard Kipling* (London: Weidenfeld and Nicolson, 1978), p.178.

51 Kipling, R, Letter to W R Gowers, undated. (c. 1896). Held in Gowers family collection. Kipling never dated these letters. They can be approximately dated by the address on the letterheads.

52 Beckett, I F W, 'Wolseley, Garnet Joseph, first Viscount Wolseley (1833–1913)', *Oxford Dictionary of National Biography* (Oxford: Oxford University Press, 2004).

53 Gregory, J W, Letter to W R Gowers, 3 February 1897.

54 Walford Davies, H, Letter to W R Gowers, 24 February 1913.

55 Jessopp, A, *Arcady, for Better for Worse* (1887).

56 Gowers, W R, *The Dynamics of Life: an Address Delivered Before the Medical Society of Manchester October 3rd, 1894* (1894).

57 Kipling, R, Letter to Gowers, undated.

58 Flood, A, *The Guardian*, 9 April 2010.

59 Critchley, p.93.

60 Gilmour, D, *The Long Recessional: the Imperial Life of Rudyard Kipling* (London: Pimlico, 2002), p.135.

61 Kipling, R, Letter to W R Gowers, undated 1898.

62 Birkenhead, *Rudyard Kipling* (1978), p.184.
63 Critchley, p.93.
64 Kipling, R, to W R Gowers, undated 1898.
65 Gowers, W R, Letter to G E Morrison, 13 September 1899.
66 Gowers, W R, Letter to G E Morrison, 30 August 1898.
67 Gowers, W R letter to C Fleming, 15 November 1899. SxMs53/3/2/1, AlRefNo 1/9.
68 Birkenhead, *Rudyard Kipling* (1978), p.240.
69 Critchley, p.93.
70 Critchley, p.61.
71 Obituary, 'Sir William Gowers, MD, FRCP, FRS', *BMJ*, pp.829–30.
72 Report, 'Phonographic jubilee of Mr T A Reed', *The Times*, London, 24 November 1892.
73 Gowers, W R, 'President's annual address, Society of Medical Phonographers', *Phonographic Record*, **2**:6, July 1896, 81.
74 Dr Ken Tyler began a project a century later to have Gowers' articles transcribed. Tyler, K L, 'Pioneers in neurology: William Richard Gowers (1845–1915)', *Journal of Neurology*, **250**, 2003, 1012–13; Tyler, K L, Roberts, D and Tyler, H R, 'The shorthand publications of Sir William Richard Gowers', *Neurology*, **55**, 2000, 289–93. An incomplete set of the journals is held in the British Library.
75 Gowers, W R, 'Valedictory address by the late President', *Phonographic Record*, **5**:1, January 1899, 1–6.
76 Kennedy, F, 'William Gowers (1845–1915)', in Haymaker, W and Schiller, F (ed.), *The Founders of Neurology* (Springfield, IL: Charles C Thomas, 1953), p.444.
77 Gowers, W R, 'A post-graduate lecture on acute myelitis' [Queen Square], manuscript, 27 November 1895, Queen Square Library, Archive and Museum. See Lees, A J, Woodward, R M P, Scott, A E M, and Eadie, M J, 'W R Gowers 1895: two unpublished postgraduate lectures', *Brain*, 2012, doi: 10.1093/brain/aws029.

### Chapter 10: 'Grand old man' of neurology

1 Taylor, J, *Paralysis and other Diseases of the Nervous System in Children and Early Life* (London: J & A Churchill, 1905).
2 Hughlings Jackson, J (ed.), *Selected Writings of John Hughlings Jackson* (London: Hodder & Stoughton, 1932).
3 Lyons, J B, 'Correspondence between Sir William Gowers and Sir Victor Horsley', *Medical History*, **9**:3, 1965, 260–7, p.266.
4 Purdon Martin, J, 'Reminiscences of Queen Square', *BMJ*, **283**, 6307, 19–26 December 1981, pp.1640–2.
5 Critchley, M, *Sir William Gowers 1845–1915: a Biographical Appreciation* (1949), p.59.
6 Gowers, W R, *The Dynamics of Life: an Address* (Philadelphia: Blakiston, 1894), pp.1–8.
7 Gowers, W R, *The Dynamics of Life*, pp.65–6.
8 Gowers, W R, 'The new neurology' [lecture, Queen Square], *Lancet*, **153**:3933, 14 January 1899, 71–3.
9 Gowers, W R, 'Abiotrophy' [lecture, Queen Square], *Lancet*, **159**:4102, 12 April 1902, 1003–7.
10 Gowers, W R, 'Heredity in diseases of the nervous system' [Royal Society of Medicine], *Lancet*, **174**:4498, 14 November 1908, 1467–8.

11 Gowers, W R and Taylor, J, *A Manual of Diseases of the Nervous System*, Vol 1, 3rd edn (London: J & A Churchill, 1899).

12 Gowers, W R, 'The diagnosis of diseases of the spinal cord' [an address to the Medical Society of Wolverhampton], *Medical Times and Gazette*, **2**:Nov–Dec 1879, 524–6, 575–7, 657–9, 683–5.

13 Gowers, W R, *A Manual of Diseases of the Nervous System*, Vol 1, 1st edn (London: J & A Churchill, 1886) p.32.

14 Gowers, W R, 'Local panatrophy', *Review of Neurology and Psychiatry (Edinburgh)*, *1*:1903, 3–4.

15 Brain, W R and Walton, J N, *Diseases of the Nervous System*, 7th edn (Oxford: Oxford University Press, 1969).

16 Gowers, W R, 'A case of unilateral optic neuritis from intracranial tumour' [lecture, UCH], *Lancet*, **174**:4480, 10 July 1909, 67–8.

17 Kennedy, F, 'Retrobulbar neuritis as an exact diagnostic sign of certain tumors and abscesses in the frontal lobes', *American Journal of Medical Science*, **142**, 1911, 355–68.

18 Henson, R A, 'Commentary on de Watteville review', *Brain*, **110**:4, August 1987, 1082–3.

19 Gowers, W R, Letter to S Weir Mitchell, 14 July 1884. Yale University archives.

20 Osler, W, *On Chorea and Choreiform Affections* (Philadelphia: Blakiston, 1894).

21 Gowers, W R, Letter to W Osler, 18 July 1912. Osler Library of the History of Medicine: G723d 1890 BO2786.

22 Weir Mitchell, S, Letter to W R Gowers, 13 March 1897.

23 Purves Stewart, J and Collier, J, Letter to W R Gowers, 22 June 1897.

24 Barlow, T, Letter to W R Gowers, 29 June 1897.

25 Beevor, C E, Letter to W R Gowers, 27 June 1897.

26 Poore, G V, Letter to W R Gowers, 23 June 1897.

27 Hughlings Jackson, J, Letter to W R Gowers, 22 June 1897.

28 Lister, Letter to W R Gowers, 26 June 1897.

29 Mackenzie, S, Letter to W R Gowers, 22 June 1897.

30 Wakley, T, Letter to W R Gowers, 26 June 1897.

31 Kipling, R, Letter to W R Gowers, 25 June, 1897.

32 Beaumont, F G, Letter to W R Gowers, 22 June 1897.

33 Mercier, C, Letter to W R Gowers, 27 June 1897.

34 The practice of buying honours became a scandal when Lloyd-George was prime minister a few years later.

35 Report, 'Sir William Gowers and the Society of Medical Phonographers', *BMJ*, **2**:1927, 1897, 1657–8.

36 Kipling, R, Letter to Dr James M Conland, 17–18 December 1897, cited in Pinney, T, *The Letters of Rudyard Kipling, Vol 2 1890–99* (London: Macmillan, 1990), p.329.

37 Broderick, S, Letter to W R Gowers, 19 August 1904.

38 Letter, 'Factory girls' country holiday fund (Mrs Temple, Mrs Creighton, Sir William Gowers, Lord Haversham et al.) letter about the appeal', *The Times*, London, 26 August 1911.

39 Letter, 'National Hospital for the Paralysed and Epileptic (strife between doctors and board)', *The Times*, London, 14 March 1901.

40 Report, 'The crisis in the Church', *The Times*, London, 29 April 1899.

41 Report, 'The conference of churchmen', *The Times*, London, 1899.

42 Report, 'Sir W Gowers on the lunacy laws', *The Times*, London, 21 November 1902.

43 Gowers, W R, 'The metric system in pharmacy' [letter], *Lancet*, **160**:4127, 4 October 1902, 956.

44 A.P.C., 'Sir William Gowers', *Postgraduate Medical Journal*, **25**:288, October 1949, 507.

45 See http://www.lond-amb.nhs.uk/about_us/who_we_are/our_story/a_brief_history.aspx.

46 Letter, 'Metropolitan Street Ambulance Association', *The Times*, London, 29 February 1904.

47 'Street noises in Marylebone', *The Times*, 28 October 1904, p.4.

48 Gowers, W R, 'Lumbago: its lessons and analogues' [lecture, Queen Square], *BMJ*, **1**:2246, 16 January 1904, 117–21, p.121.

49 Critchley, M, *Sir William Gowers 1845–1915: a Biographical Appreciation* (1949), p.29.

50 Compston, A, 'Editorial', *Brain*, **130**:7, 2007, 1709–11.

51 Gowers, W R, 'Special sense discharges from organic disease' [Hughlings Jackson lecture, Neurological Section of the Royal Society of Medicine], *Lancet*, **174**:4503, 18 December 1909, 1803–8.

52 Critchley, p.94.

53 Butterfield, E K, *The Making of a Neurologist: the Letters of Foster Kennedy 1884–1952 to His Wife* (Cambridge: private, 1981), pp.32–3.

54 Report, 'The King and Queen', *The Times*, London, 30 October 1909.

55 Report, 'High Court of Justice, King's Bench Division: claim for an electric shock on a tramcar', *The Times*, London, 3 March 1909.

56 Critchley, p.75.

57 Tedder, H R, Letter to W R Gowers, 6 December 1912.

58 Gowers, W R to W Osler, 18 July 1912. Osler Library of the History of Medicine: G723d 1890 BO2786.

59 Mercier, C to W R Gowers, 27 June 1897.

60 See also Sacks, O, 'Gowers' memory', *Neurology*, **46**, 1996, 1467–9.

61 Cited in Critchley, p.94.

62 Gowers, E A, Letter to W Osler, 5 May 1915. Osler Library of the History of Medicine: G723d 1881 BO2783.

63 Cameron Blair, M, Letter to W F Gowers, 14 June 1915.

64 Scott, R D, 'Gowers of Uganda: The Public and Private Life of a Forgotten Colonial Governor', *Australasian Review of African Studies*, 30:2, 2009, 12–31.

65 Annotation, 'A fruitful century', *Lancet*, **275**:7138, 18 June 1960, 1336–7.


### Chapter 11: Gowers the man, his work, and his legacy


1 Jones, E, *Free Associations: Memories of a Psycho-Analyst* (1959), p.119.

2 De Lehoczky, T, 'On recent biographies of two great physicians: Gowers and Cushing', *Journal of Nervous and Mental Diseases*, **166**:6, December 1952, 506–10, p.509.

3 Brown, H B, 'UCH and Sir William Gowers', *BMJ*, **1**:4400, 5 May 1945, 645.

4 Critchley, M, *Sir William Gowers 1845–1915: a Biographical Appreciation* (1949), p.37.

5 Martin, J P, 'Medicine and books: personal account of a career in neurology', *BMJ*, **284**:6329, 1982, 1624.

6 Kennedy, F, in Haymaker, W and Schiller, F (ed.), *The Founders of Neurology* (Springfield, IL: Charles C Thomas, 1953), p.444.

7 Howard, R and Willison, H, 'The nature of catalepsy and the model for Percy Trevelyan', *The Sherlock Holmes Journal*, **20**:4, 1992, 128–30.

8 Reynolds, J R, 'Paralysis and other disorders of motion and sensation dependent on idea', *BMJ*, **2**:462, 1869, 483–5.

9 Gowers, W R, *Epilepsy and Other Chronic Convulsive Disorders, their Causes, Symptoms and Treatment* (London: J & A Churchill, 1881).

10 Symonds, C, 'Disease of the mind and disorder of brain' [Gowers Memorial Lecture given 23 June 1960], *BMJ*, **2**:5191, 1960, 1–5, p.1.

11 Walshe, F, 'The nature and dimension of nosography in modern medicine' [first Gowers Memorial Lecture given on 15 November 1956], *Lancet*, **268**:6952, 24 November 1956, 1059–63, p.1059.

12 Taylor, J (ed.), *Neurological Fragments (John Hughlings Jackson)* (London: Oxford University Press Medical, 1925), p.11.

13 Critchley, p.90.

14 Obituary, 'Death of Sir W Gowers: a famous nerve specialist', *The Times*, London, 5 May 1915.

15 Obituary, 'Sir William Richard Gowers, MD Lond and Dub, FRCP Lond, LL.D Edin. FRS', *Lancet*, **185**:4785, 15 May 1915, 1055–7, p.1056.

16 Obituary, 'William Richard Gowers', *Journal of Nervous and Mental Diseases*, **43**:5, May 1916, 485–6.

17 Leader, 'Sir William Gowers, 1845–1915', *BMJ*, **1**:4395, 31 March 1945, 452.

18 Critchley, p.96.

19 Critchley, M, 'The Beginnings of the National Hospital, Queen Square (1859–1860)', *BMJ*, **1**:5189, 18 June 1960, 1829–37.

20 Kinnier Wilson, S A, *Neurology* (London: Edward Arnold, 1940).

21 Critchley citation: recorded by his house physician Stanley Barnes, in *Transactions of the Clinical Society of London*, 36.

22 Critchley citation: recorded by his house physician, Walter Spencer, in a letter to *The Lancet*, 1886.

23 Critchley citation: recorded by Stanley Barnes.

24 Critchley, pp.95–6.

25 Holmes, G, 'Sir William Gowers at the National Hospital', BMJ, **2**:4744, 8 December 1951, 1397–8, p.1399.

26 McHenry, L C, *Garrison's History of Neurology* (Springfield, IL: Charles C Thomas, 1969), p.12.

27 Obituary, 'Sir William Gowers, MD, FRCP, FRS', *BMJ*, **1**:2836, 8 May 1915, 828–30.

28 Walshe, p.1063.

# Index

The manufacturer's authorised representative in the EU for product
safety is Oxford University Press España S.A. of El Parque Empresarial
San Fernando de Henares, Avenida de Castilla, 2 - 28830 Madrid
(www.oup.es/en or product.safety@oup.com). OUP España S.A. also acts
as importer into Spain of products made by the manufacturer.
Printed and bound by CPI Group (UK) Ltd, Croydon, CR0 4YY
14/09/2026
02216309-0003